Foreword

From the Australian bush, to the md the need for
and celebrate the pleasures of the c   id well being.
The outdoors is where we can go to   fe, or relax.
Freedom to access outdoor spaces i.

So in an ideal world, this book would r   when services are
developed for people with dementia the   are often ignored. In construction
projects we often see access to the outdoors being restricted or denied as a cost
cutting issue, or because of lack of foresight and planning. This results in long term
problems for people living with dementia, that could be preventable. Outdoor
access can reduce agitation, restlessness, and other behavioural symptoms that
cost staff time and may lead to overuse of medication, both of which can have
expensive and unpleasant consequences.

This book addresses the big question of how we design and deliver the right types
of outdoor spaces for people with dementia. It demonstrates many positive
examples of good practice from across the globe in the design and use of outdoor
spaces. It challenges decision makers and designers to think about the care of
people with dementia and those who care for them.

Books are sometimes described as "groundbreaking"... and this one is certainly
revolutionary in that sense. But it also carries a plea on behalf of all people with dementia to everyone who commissions, designs, or builds for them – keep dementia
and its needs uppermost in your mind. Before you even break the ground, remember the outdoor spaces. And give us space to enjoy the open air.

Colm Cunningham	Prof June Andrews
Director, The Dementia Centre	Director, DSDC
HammondCare	University of Stirling
Australia	United Kingdom

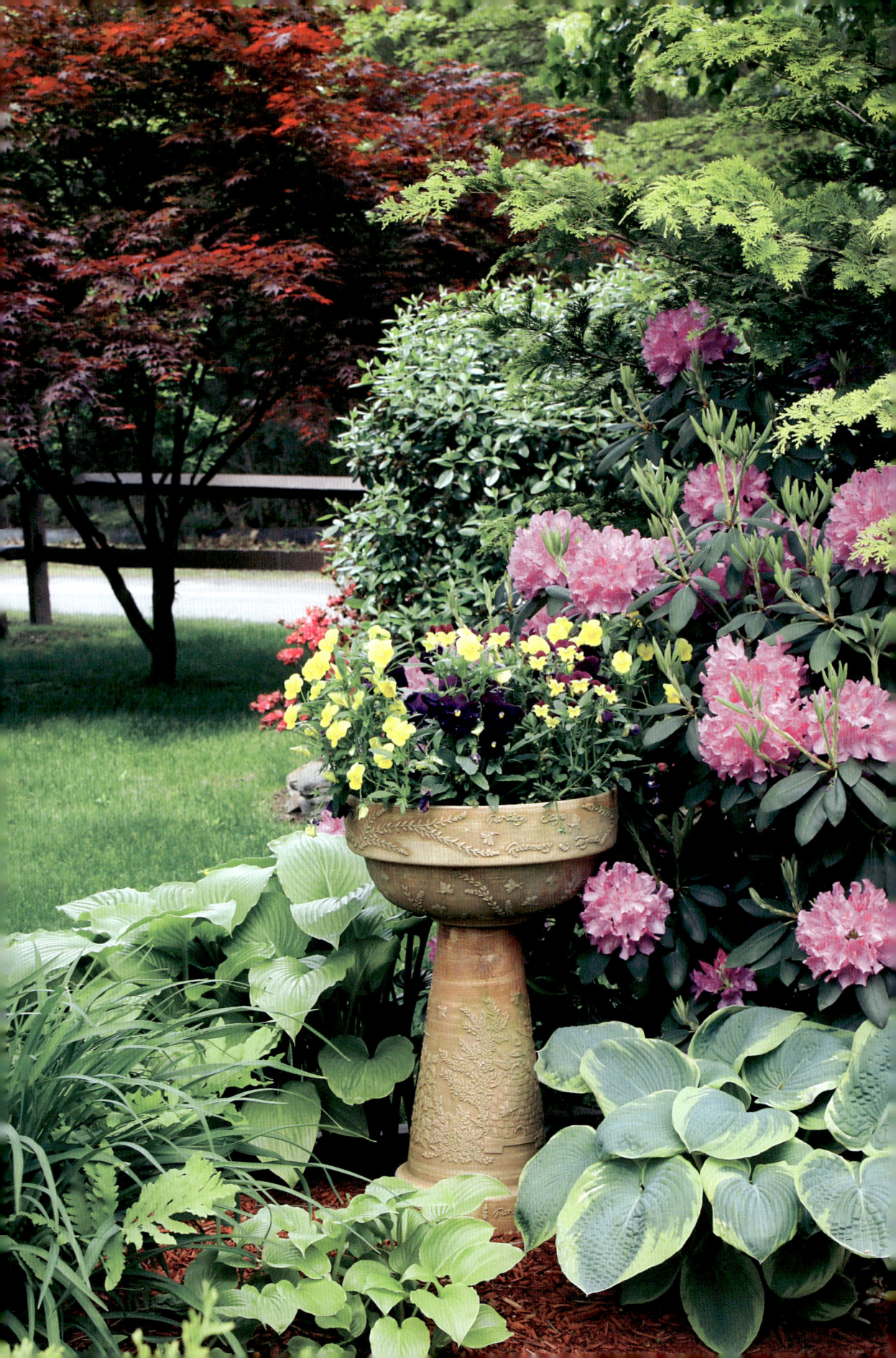

Contents

Designing outdoor spaces for people with dementia
Annie Pollock and Mary Marshall (Editors)

Dedication: Annie Pollock
Contributors: Authors, Consultants and Editors
Introduction: Annie Pollock and Mary Marshall

PART 1: WHY THE OUTDOORS IS IMPORTANT

Chapter 1	Perspectives from people with dementia and relatives	17
	Alec Lindsay, John Killick, Fay Godfrey & two carers	
Chapter 2	Going outside is essential for health and wellbeing	23
	Annie Pollock & David McNair	
Case study 1	The Living Garden at the Family Life Centre	49
	Clare Cooper Marcus	

PART 2: CIVIL LIBERTY AND CULTURAL CONSIDERATIONS

Chapter 3	Going out - rights and responsibilities	53
	Donald Lyons	
Case study 2	The gardens at Plaisir Villa Ichikawa	59
	Yuji Okubo	
Chapter 4	Being outside 'down under'	67
	Stephen Judd	
Case study 3	Werruna: Creating an appropriate environment for rural Australians living with dementia	75
	Peter Birkett	
Chapter 5	Culturally appropriate design of outdoor spaces	79
	Kirsty Bennett	
Case study 4	Haugmotun Sensory Garden: a therapeutic garden for people with dementia	89
	Ellen-Elisabeth Grefsrød & Nancy Gerlach-Spriggs	

PART 3: DESIGN GUIDANCE

Chapter 6	Site and climate consideration	93
	Annie Pollock, Richard Pollock, Clifford McClenaghan; Consultant: Fan Wang	
Chapter 7	Dementia-friendly neighbourhoods – a step in the right direction	119
	Lynne Mitchell & Elizabeth Burton	
Case study 5	Back Porch Garden	135
	Jack Carman	
Chapter 8	Design principles that apply to all outside spaces	139
	Clare Cooper Marcus, Mary Marshall, Annie Pollock, Richard Pollock	
Case study 6	Sydenham Court	161
	Clifford McClenaghan & Sally Visick	

PART 4: USING THE OUTDOORS

Chapter 9	Activities and outside space	167
	Teresia Hazen & Maria McManus	
Case study 7	Charnley Fold	179
	Garuth Chalfont	
Chapter 10	Using outside space at night	185
	Colm Cunningham	
Chapter 11	How relatives, friends and staff can facilitate being outside	191
	Edith Macintosh	
Case study 8	Blairgowrie Community Hospital	201
	Annie Pollock	

CONCLUDING REFLECTIONS	205
Annie Pollock & Mary Marshall	
APPENDIX	210
Image credits	224

Dedication

This book is dedicated to all those people who have or had a close relative or friend with dementia.

And to my father, who served in the Royal Navy from the age of 14 until he retired at 52.

He survived two submarine disasters before the Second World War, served in minesweepers during the war, and was the last captain of the battleship HMS Vanguard.

I didn't realise that, at the time of his retirement, he already had the beginnings of vascular dementia, almost certainly as a result of wartime and services lifestyle.

We suffered continuous re-telling of naval stories, irascible and often unpredictable behaviour and we found life with him increasingly difficult – but of course, no-one really understood or knew much about dementia in those days.

The last time I saw him, he was in hospital and he asked me to take him home – to the house we had lived in when I was seven years of age…

Now I understand!

Hence my wish to dedicate this book to my father who passed away at the age of 72, some 30 years ago!

How far we have come since then in our understanding!

I hope that this book will help in achieving a better quality of life for people with dementia.

Annie Pollock, April 2012

Contributors: authors

Kirsty Bennett (Australia)

Kirsty Bennett is an architect who has specialised in designing for older people and people with dementia for many years. Kirsty has been responsible for the briefing, design, documentation and contract administration of residential aged-care facilities in many parts of Australia. A number of these projects have been for indigenous people. Kirsty has undertaken research and written a number of articles on designing for people with dementia, and has been invited to speak at international conferences on this topic.

Peter Birkett (Australia)

Peter Birkett is the Chief Executive Officer of Hesse Rural Health in Winchelsea, Australia. Peter has successfully merged a career in nursing, midwifery and commerce working in both metropolitan and rural sectors. Over the past 15 years he has developed Hesse into a rural, integrated care facility. He holds degree and Masters qualifications in business and is a sitting Board member on Maryville Aged Care, a denominational aged care service in Geelong, Australia.

Elizabeth Burton (Engand)

Elizabeth Burton is Professor of Sustainable Building Design and Wellbeing and founder/director of the WISE (Wellbeing in Sustainable Environments) research unit at the University of Warwick, UK. Having qualified as an architect and urban designer, Elizabeth took up a research career, with the aim of developing an evidence base for architectural practice. Her research investigates the social aspects of sustainability and how the built environment (architecture and urban design) influences people's wellbeing, quality of life and mental health. She has particular expertise in ageing research, including dementia-friendly design. Elizabeth is now seeking to promote design for wellbeing in the built environment through the development of new cross-disciplinary courses.

Jack Carman (USA)

Jack Carman is President of Design for Generations LLC, a landscape architect with 20 years of experience in the analysis, planning, design and management of outdoor spaces with a particular specialisation in the creation of therapeutic exterior environments for senior communities and healthcare facilities. He has designed over 30 memory care gardens for individuals with dementia and is the founder and Co-Chair of the Healthcare and Therapeutic Garden Professional Practice Network of the American Society of Landscape Architects (ASLA).

Garuth Chalfont (England)

Garuth Chalfont is published and acknowledged internationally for his expertise on design and his efforts to evolve care practice and management. By integrating the design of landscape and architecture, his designs enable optimal use of both indoors and outdoors for connection to nature. His book Design for Nature in Dementia Care (2008) was recently translated as Naturgestutzte Therapie (Huber, 2010) for therapeutic horticulture practice in Germany.

Clare Cooper Marcus (USA)

Clare Cooper Marcus is a professor emerita in the Departments of Architecture and Landscape Architecture at the University of California, Berkeley, and principal of Healing Landscapes in Berkeley, California, a consulting firm that specialises in researching the effectiveness of restorative landscapes in healthcare settings. She has written several books and is the co-author/editor (with Marni Barnes) of *Healing Garden: Therapeutic Benefits and Design Recommendations.* She is a regular contributor to Chicago Botanic Garden's certificate course on Healthcare Garden Design.

Colm Cunningham (Australia)

Colm Cunningham is Director of the Dementia Centre, HammondCare in Sydney, Australia. The Centre is an international leader in education, consultancy, research and developing publications in dementia care. Colm is an international expert with over 20 years experience in older age care. A general and intellectual disability nurse and social worker, Colm has been the deputy director at the UK Dementia Centre, University of Stirling and has written extensively and undertaken research in a wide range of issues about dementia including design, pain care, hospital care, night time care and intellectual disability.

Nancy Gerlach-Spriggs (USA)

Nancy Gerlach-Spriggs is author of the book Restorative Gardens: the Healing Landscape. She received a BSLA from City College in New York and an MLA from Harvard University. She teaches in the landscape design and horticultural therapy programs at the New York Botanical Garden and has collaborated with Ellen-Elisabeth Grefsrød on several projects.

Fay Godfrey (Scotland)

Fay Godfrey, Registered Mental Nurse, has worked with Alzheimer Scotland, managing the Falkirk Services since 1998.

Ellen-Elisabeth Grefsrød (Norway)

Ellen-Elisabeth Grefsrød is author of several books and a DVD, among them the book *Gardens for People with Dementia*: *Design and Use* (2008). She received a MLA from the Norwegian University of Life Sciences. She has been teaching as well as working as a project landscape architect and now she works for the firm COWI.

Teresia Hazen (USA)

Teresia Hazen has been with Legacy Health System (LHS) in Portland, Oregon since 1991 as the coordinator of Therapeutic Gardens and Horticultural Therapy (HT). This is a not-for-profit integrated healthcare network including five hospitals and related services. LHS promotes gardens in healthcare to create supportive environments of care for patients, families, visitors, staff and neighbours. This is the only healthcare system in the USA to offer a horticultural therapy certificate program authorised by the American Horticultural Therapy Association (AHTA).

Dr Stephen Judd (Australia)

Dr Stephen Judd is Chief Executive of HammondCare, an independent Australian charity. During his tenure as Chief Executive, HammondCare has grown at 20% p.a. compound, with revenues of $120 million, making it one of the top 50 Australian charities serving more than 2500 patients, residents and clients. It is acknowledged as Australia's leading dementia-specific service provider and is unique in its development of a continuum of care encompassing residential, at home and sub-acute health and hospital services.

He is passionate about creating environments for people with dementia, the rights of older citizens and the excellent use of technology.

Dr Judd co-edited Design for Dementia (1998) with Mary Marshall and Peter Phippen.

John Killick (Scotland)

John Killick has worked as a poet with people with dementia for 17 years. His most recent publication is The Elephant in the Room (2009). Forthcoming from Jessica Kingsley is Creativity and Communication in Persons with Dementia, co-authored with Claire Craig.

Alec Lindsay (Scotland)

Alec Lindsay was raised in a small house not far from Oxford Street, London and when old enough left home to become a nurse. All old hospitals were in the countryside, which he preferred. His breaks were spent backpacking alone by the sea, hence his preference of Mother Nature over gods. He is now a member of the Scottish Dementia Working Group, an effective educational and campaigning body for people with dementia.

Donny Lyons (Scotland)

Donny Lyons has been Director (now Chief Executive) of the Mental Welfare Commission for Scotland since 2003. He was previously a Consultant Old Age Psychiatrist in Glasgow. He was heavily involved in Commission reports on dementia care.

Edith Macintosh (Scotland)

Edith works as the Rehabilitation Consultant for the Care Inspectorate, supporting the care sector to improve the quality of care in care homes and day services for older people in relation to rehabilitation. She trained as an Occupational Therapist (OT) and has worked previously in health and social care as a clinician, and latterly as OT service manager in Perth and Kinross.

Maria McManus (Northern Ireland)

Maria McManus is a registered Occupational Therapist. She undertook this work while she was the Director of the Northern Ireland office of the Dementia Services Development Centre of the University of Stirling.

Clifford McClenaghan (Northern Ireland)

Clifford McClenaghan has been a qualified architect since 1985 when he started his own practice. As principal of The Bridge Studio, he has designed sheltered accommodation and homes for people with dementia. One scheme received an award for innovation in social housing. His special interest is the study of acoustics in relation to the design of care homes.

David McNair (Scotland)

David McNair has been a lighting engineer since 1975 and is a Fellow of the Institution of Lighting Professionals. He was President of the Institution in 2003 and has presented papers at many lighting conferences. Presently he is an independent lighting specialist, working with the Dementia Services Development Centre at the University of Stirling to acquire and disseminate knowledge on the benefits of good lighting for people with dementia.

Lynne Mitchell (England)

Lynne Mitchell is a Senior Research Fellow and co-founder of the WISE (Wellbeing in Sustainable Environments) research unit in the School of Health and Social Studies at the University of Warwick. She is also a Chartered Member of the Royal Town Planning

Institute. Lynne's research interests lie in the social aspects of sustainability and how the indoor and outdoor built environment (architecture, planning and inclusive urban design) influences people's health and wellbeing. She has particular expertise in researching the design needs of older people and people with dementia. Lynne is a partner in the EPSRC Research Consortium, Inclusive Design for Getting Outdoors (I'DGO), considered to be an international 'centre of excellence'.

Yuji Okubo (Japan)

Yuji Okubo received his BSc in Social Science at Waseda University in 1981. He worked as a marketing consultant for 15 years. Yuji then established the Social Welfare Corporation. He obtained an MSc in Social Work at Kanagawa University of Human Services in 2009. He is now chairman of the Social Welfare Corporation Sosaykai in Kanagawa prefecture, Japan.

Richard Pollock (Scotland)

Richard Pollock has worked as a consultant architect at the Dementia Services Development Centre (DSDC) at the University of Stirling since 1999 and became Director of Architecture in 2009. Richard has lectured widely and authored several research papers including writing and editing the *DSDC publications Designing Interiors for People with Dementia* and *Light and Lighting Design for People with Dementia.* Richard also founded the architectural and planning consultancy Burnett Pollock Associates in 1974. Since then, the Edinburgh-based practice has established both design and research expertise in sustainable development, disabilities and dementia-friendly design.

Sally Visick (Northern Ireland)

Sally Visick is a chartered landscape architect with more than 30 years experience in a broad range of landscape practice for public and private sector clients throughout Northern Ireland and beyond. She has been in private practice since 1984 and is a partner in Designs Matter in Belfast. Sally has been responsible for award-winning landscape projects, including the £1.15 million Cookstown Town Centre EI Scheme, the largest of its kind when completed in 1998. More recently, she designed the landscape works around the Ulster Museum (winner of the 2010 Art Fund Prize) when it underwent a major three-year renovation.

Our two carer contributors wished to remain anonymous. One is a daughter-in-law and the other a wife.

Contributors: consultants

Liz Fuggle (Scotland)

Liz Fuggle has been a chartered architect since 2006 and has always had a particular interest in designing for mental health. Working at Burnett Pollock Associates has enabled a focused approach in good architecture for the elderly, implementing best practice for designing for dementia as documented by Stirling University's research. She often undertakes freelance graphic design and illustration, as well as this being part of her day-to-day work.

Fan Wang (Scotland)

Fan Wang studied first Physics and then Architectural Technology in Zhejiang University. He won two major scholarships to continue his research in University of Sheffield in the UK. Subsequently, he joined the School of Built Environment at Heriot Watt University where he now teaches subjects in architectural engineering and carries out research in airflow and thermal modelling. His special interests are in building ventilation systems in hot climates, wind safety and comfort in built environments, and building/system thermal performance modelling.

Editors:

Annie Pollock (Scotland)

Annie Pollock is a qualified architect and landscape architect. Having undertaken consultancy work for the Dementia Services Development Centre (DSDC) at the University of Stirling for several years, she became Director of Landscape Design and Architecture in 2009. She has lectured widely and authored the DSDC publication *Designing Gardens for People with Dementia* (2001). Annie is principal of the Edinburgh-based landscape practice Arterre, specialising in design for frail elderly people and people with dementia. In 1999, she designed a show garden for Alzheimer Scotland at the Royal Horticultural Show in Scotland and in 2002 the courtyard garden for the Iris Murdoch Building at Stirling University, both of which won awards.

Mary Marshall (Scotland)

Mary Marshall is a professor emeritus at the University of Stirling where she was the director of the Dementia Services Development Centre for 16 years until 2005. She now writes and lectures about dementia care and dementia design.

Introduction *Mary Marshall and Annie Pollock*

The need for this book has become apparent as the design team at the University of Stirling's Dementia Services Development Centre has undertaken increasing numbers of design audits and design training.

It is clear that many people in the field of dementia care are not aware of the importance of being outdoors for people with dementia as many buildings for people with dementia either lack suitable outside space or the design makes it difficult for this space to be reached. Often the door leading to this space is locked.

This book seeks to help anyone involved in procuring, designing or advising on facilities for people with dementia. It aims to draw together a wide range of information and expertise about optimal design and use of outside spaces, as well as providing the ammunition should expenditure and effort require justifying. It comprises four parts:

1. Why the outdoors is important
2. Civil liberty and cultural considerations
3. Design Guidance
4. Using the outdoors

There is also a set of case studies showing examples of successful outdoor space; some of these specifically relate to the sections that they are set within. Designers, for example, need to know about activities in order to provide a sufficiently flexible space. It is probably important to say at the outset that there is always a balance of factors to be achieved, which is optimal in the particular set of circumstances. This is not an area for hard and fast rules; a good understanding of dementia and of the latest thinking provides a clear steer for the direction of travel. The aim is to provide input on the factors that need to be taken into account in all circumstances.

Whilst there is little research, per se, on the efficacy of outside space on the quality of life and behaviour of people with dementia, examples of relevant research have been provided to illustrate our points. This relevant research is problematic for many reasons:

- outside spaces are very different one from another
- there are a whole set of issues around access, staff attitudes and behaviour
- people with dementia have very different attitudes and experience.

It is known that access to outside space at will is beneficial to people with dementia. Namazi and Johnson (1992) in their small study found less challenging behaviour in people with dementia who had open access to the outdoors.

There is a lot of research on the importance of being outside for older people generally, which is covered in this book. Where there is no dementia-specific research, we have turned to people with dementia and their carers for their views; we have also added our own experience and that of others gleaned through many years of work in this field.

However, this is not an academic guide to research; it is a book for people in practice. Rodiek and Schwarz (2006 and 2007) have edited two excellent books, which provide plenty of guidance on research in this area.

This book develops and expands existing garden design guides, such as Pollock (2001), Berentsen, Grefsrød and Eek (2008) and Cochrane (2010).

The statistics for the UK (2010) as noted on the Alzheimer's Society website are as follows, and it is assumed that these will be proportionally similar in most developed countries:

- there are currently 750,000 people with dementia in the UK (population in 2010 was 62,262,000)
- there are over 16,000 younger people with dementia in the UK
- there are over 11,500 people with dementia from black and minority ethnic groups in the UK
- there will be over a million people with dementia by 2021
- two thirds of people with dementia are women
- the proportion of people with dementia doubles for every five-year age group
- one third of people over 95 have dementia
- 60,000 deaths a year are directly attributable to dementia
- delaying the onset of dementia by five years would reduce deaths directly attributable to dementia by 30,000 a year
- the financial cost of dementia to the UK is over £20 billion a year
- family carers of people with dementia save the UK over £6 billion a year
- 64% of people living in care homes have a form of dementia
- two thirds of people with dementia live in the community while one third live in a care home
- only 40% of people with dementia receive a diagnosis.

This book is inevitably mainly about care homes, except for the specific chapter on town and city neighbourhoods. Care homes present particular challenges, but nevertheless the design advice is appropriate for all people with dementia whether or not they are in a care home. 'Dementia-friendly' design works for everyone.

Almost everything in this book is equally applicable to any building for older people, and in particular assisted living (USA), sheltered housing (UK), hostels and nursing homes (Australia), hospital wards, day centres and day hospitals.

Dementia

The term dementia is an umbrella term for a set of diseases of the brain, all of which are progressive. Currently, the internationally accepted definition is from the ICD-10 Classification of Mental and Behavioural Disorders, World Health Organization, Geneva, 1992:

"Dementia is a syndrome due to disease of the brain, usually of a chronic or progressive nature, in which there is disturbance of multiple higher cortical functions, including memory, thinking, orientation, comprehension, calculation, learning capacity, language, and judgment. Consciousness is not clouded. Impairments of cognitive function are commonly accompanied, and occasionally preceded, by deterioration in emotional control, social behaviour, or motivation. This syndrome occurs in Alzheimer's disease, in cerebrovascular disease, and in other conditions primarily or secondarily affecting the brain."

The set of diseases includes Alzheimer's disease, vascular dementia and Lewy body dementia. Alzheimer's disease is the most common and often occurs together with vascular dementia. This medical definition needs to be seen alongside a social or disability approach, suggesting that it is the interaction between the brain damage, the person and the social and built environment, which results in the actual experience of dementia. Thus, personal factors such as life experience, mental and physical health, diet, sleep and exercise are crucially important as are the relationships with people and the physical environment itself. The last of these includes outside space and buildings.

Most people with dementia are older people and experience the same sort of impairments as other older people such as impaired sight, hearing and mobility. These are exacerbated for people with dementia because they may forget they have these impairments and may be unable to understand and deal with them. This means that the environment has to help them.

Many people with dementia, especially those living in places like care homes and hospitals, have behaviour that challenges those around them. This can result from the brain damage itself but is often the only way they are able to communicate their feelings. It is important that the environment assists staff in efforts to reduce challenging behaviour. There is increasing interest in non-pharmacological approaches to help the behaviour of people with dementia and the environment is part of these approaches. By enabling people to do what they want to do, reducing their frustration, and helping them remain calm, the experience of dementia should be less stressful for all parties.

Kinds of outside space

Most of the world is outside buildings so it is necessary to put some limits of what can be covered in this book. The main types of outside space included in this book are:

- town and city neighbourhoods
- gardens
- courtyards
- outside spaces above the ground floor.

Some technical information is provided which applies to all outside spaces, such as climatic considerations. A very specific research study has been drawn upon which looks at how the urban environment can be improved to assist people with dementia. Following this, design features of domestic outside spaces are discussed. Case studies provided are used as illustrations.

Editors' notes

Audience

This book is written for a wide readership, which is why it avoids jargon and technical language as far as possible. It will be useful for:

- people who own and commission buildings for people with dementia
- architects and landscape architects
- managers of facilities for people with dementia
- medical, nursing and care staff as well as professions allied to medicine such as occupational therapists and physiotherapists
- relatives of people with dementia and people with dementia themselves.

Structure

This book comprises four sections as mentioned earlier. The chapters within each section clearly need to overlap and they do. This means that most chapters have a lead author or two, but many of the authors have also contributed and commented on other chapters.

We are very grateful to our contributors. They include authors and consultant colleagues who have assisted us in advising, assisting and checking. Their brief biographies can be found on pages 6-10. They are all experts in their field, several of international standing. Our authors live in the USA, Japan, Australia and Norway as well as the UK. We are very much alert to cultural differences in attitudes to outdoor spaces. Although most of the chapters reflect the experience of industrialised societies, we have included a very different perspective in Kirsty Bennett's chapter, about Australian aboriginal people to make the point that cultural diversity has to be taken very seriously, and also Case study 3 which looks at a facility for rural Australians, many of whom were farmers.

Language

We realise that some terms are culturally specific, such as *elders* and *seniors*, which would be terms used in the USA but not generally in the UK, where *older people* is the more usual term. These have been left, but we have replaced all references to people with dementia with this term, as we wish to emphasise very strongly that we are talking about people first and the condition second.

We have had some difficulty with words used to describe people who live in various kinds of establishments, so have opted for *residents* for nursing homes and residential homes and *service users* for day care centres. We have also used the term *care home* to refer to nursing homes and residential homes; this is normal in Scotland where the distinction no longer exists.

Focus

This book is about older people with dementia. About 3% of people with dementia are younger than 65 and we had to make a decision about whether to include them given space constraints. We agreed on our focus because we believe that almost everything in this book applies equally to younger people with the possible exception of some of the activities. In constantly mentioning age and cultural appropriateness, we hope readers will include cohorts younger than 65 in their consideration.

Other materials

There is an increasing number of books about domestic outside spaces; we refer to these and provide references throughout. The balance between providing a comprehensive text and directing readers to more substantial, detailed and technical sources is not easy. This book should provide enough material for readers to understand the basics, and give information about further sources for those who want to look at a topic in depth. We hope the book provides enough information to enable the reader to make a strong case for outside space for people with dementia, as well as material help to design it optimally.

Acknowledgments

We are most indebted to all those that have contributed to this book, in writing, advice and providing illustrations.

We also thank those who have painstakingly undertaken proofreading and in particular Eileen Richardson, library and information services manager at the Dementia Services Development Centre, University of Stirling, for her dedication in resourcing research articles, correcting references and text.

References

Alzheimer's Society. (2011). *About dementia: Statistics.* Retrieved from http://www.alzheimers.org.uk/site/scripts/documents_info.php?documentID=341

Berentsen, V.D., Grefsrød, E.-E. & Eek, A. (2008). *Gardens for people with dementia: Design and use.* Tønsberg, Norway: Aldring og helse.

Cochrane, T.G. (2010). *Gardens that care: Planning outdoor environments for people with dementia.* Adelaide: Alzheimer's Australia SA Inc.

Namazi, K.H. & Johnson, B.D. (1992). Pertinent autonomy for residents with dementias: Modification of the physical environment to enhance independence. *American Journal of Alzheimer's disease and other dementias,* 7(1), 6-12.

Pollock, A. (2001). *Designing gardens for people with dementia.* Stirling, UK: Dementia Services Development Centre.

Rodiek, S. & Schwarz, B. (Eds.) (2006). *The role of the outdoors in residential environments for aging.* New York, NY: Haworth Press.

Rodiek, S. & Schwarz, B. (Eds.) (2007). *Outdoor environments for people with dementia.* New York, NY: Haworth Press.

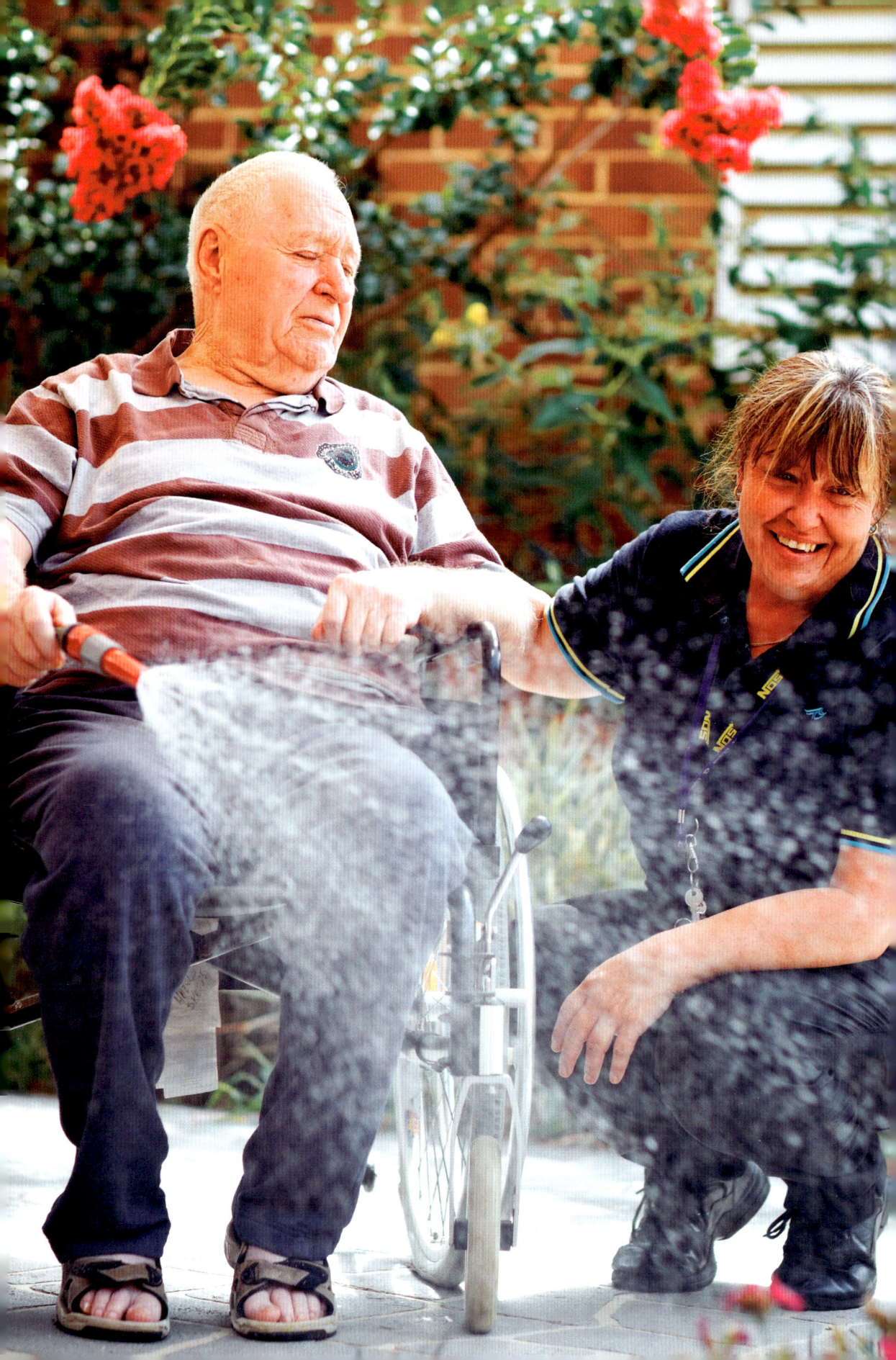

PART 1 WHY BEING OUTSIDE IS IMPORTANT

Chapter 1
Perspectives from people with dementia and relatives

Alec Lindsay, John Killick, Fay Godfrey and two carers

Anyone with dementia or a relative will tell you how important a garden or other outside space is to someone with dementia. The reasons will differ from person to person, but the strength of feeling is unanimous. Alec Lindsay, from the Scottish Dementia Working Group, kindly wrote a contribution about his garden. John Killick provides the other voice of a person with dementia, by recording the words of people with dementia and presenting them as poems. The poem included in this chapter is from work he undertook for Cambridgeshire County Council and published in 2009 in a collection called **The Elephant in the Room.** *The members of Alzheimer Scotland gardening group in Falkirk were asked for quotes for this book and we have simply listed these to show a range of views. Our two relative's contributions are from friends of ours who prefer to remain anonymous.*

Alec Lindsay

Based on my own experience I find that it is essential to have space outside. Sitting indoors makes me vegetate and offers no stimulus. TV and the media make people housebound and we need that time-out from four walls. I am fortunate to have a back and front garden. I spend a lot of time buying ornaments for them. The front has Grecian statues and a sundial and to lighten things up I have a few funny and quirky ornaments. These make people laugh and encourage conversation. My back garden is mostly to my wife's taste. We have an agreement of sorts:

1. She decides on the plants etc
2. I go out with a carer and buy them
3. We get family members to do the planting.

Space is necessary to stop people like me with dementia from becoming too introverted. Although Martin, the coordinator of the Scottish Dementia Working Group, and others who meet me, see me as a bit extrovert, I feel the need for space to think without interruption. These moments out in the garden give me strength to keep going and also lift my spirits. As an agnostic, I don't talk to any gods or clerics, but I have great faith in Mother Nature who can be both predictable and unpredictable. This stimulates me. I go out in all weather for a few minutes to clear my mind. It also takes me away from the mind-numbing and boring TV soaps and a certain Fountain of useless knowledge who appears each weekday morning with his usual gallery of social misfits. I remarked to my good wife that I was quite partial to "Loose Women", and I dare not print her reply. That was cleared up when she discovered it was a

TV show. I have just spent about 40 minutes in my garden and now I feel able to discuss gardens and space. Having had my space and fresh air I am now composing a letter to the media. There are so many things to complain about that I am spoiled for choice. Space outside four walls stops me developing mental space or vacuum. I am off to the garden now with a ciggie and to consult my muses: Victor Meldrew, Alf Garnet etc.

John Killick
FASCINATED BY FOLIAGE

Look at it out there ---

have you ever seen anything like it?

It's this all the way in ---

you go in and you come out.

The first time I went into it

I thought 'I could die here!'

You've got to admit it's lovely.

I wake up every morning

and I look out and I think

this whole place is fantastic!

Have you seen that foliage there?

Just turn around and look.

As far as the eye can see

I love every bit of it.

It wasn't always like that.

When I first came I thought

they look so weird, those things,

you know, those things dangling down.

I used to get really fanky.

My husband said "Those are trees!"

I said "Well I'll have to go

somewhere else!"

But it's a long time ago,

and now I think they're outstanding.

They're not just trees, are they?

They're different. I know it's odd ---

look how high it is, and

the way they come down from the top

instead of up from the ground.

When I first came I'd say

"Come and look at these things!"

And he'd say "Have a look down here."

And I'd say "I'm not interested in down there, it's all sticks and dead things. It's them ---

I don't want them in my garden!"

But I got used to it. They're wonderful.

I think they're just fascinating.

I've been mesmerised with them

ever since we moved here.

Members of the gardening group at the Alzheimer Scotland service in Falkirk

Fay Godfrey is the service manager for the Alzheimer Scotland service in Falkirk where Julie Shankland is the gardener/group leader for the gardening group.

Fay says:

"The group has been a great way to gently introduce people to services in an informal way as three of the men who attended refused all support prior to this, all three went on to accept support in terms of day care or outreach. One of the gentlemen

still refuses traditional support, however, he loves coming along to the garden and we have managed to get funding on an individual basis to continue this. They've done lots of jobs in the garden ranging from weeding, planting seeds, tending the veg patch, cutting the hedge and painting the fence as well as building a bug house and sorting out the compost heap. It has saved me a lot of time as I used to come over at the weekends and potter but am less able to do so now."

Fay collected some quotes from members of the group:

I really enjoy being outside in the fresh air and sunshine.

I have always enjoyed gardening.

Canny be bothered with sitting about inside.

I really love the smell of that flower – it reminds me when I was a wee girl.

My granny used to make soup with this.

Doing gardening keeps you fit.

I didn't know I could do this anymore.

The colours are just really beautiful.

Oh! Look at the butterflies - aren't they gorgeous!

I like getting my hands dirty.

I just love gardening, always have done.

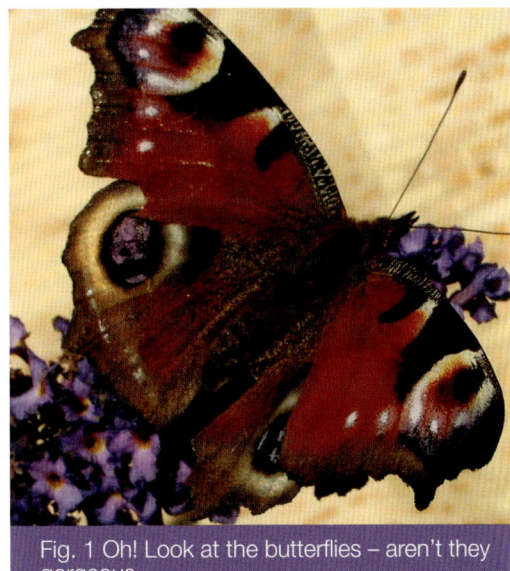

Fig. 1 Oh! Look at the butterflies – aren't they gorgeous

A daughter-in-law

My father-in-law is 62 years old and approximately three years ago he was diagnosed with Alzheimer's disease. Following diagnosis, his condition quickly deteriorated and he is now resident in a specialist facility in a hospital.

My father-in-law loved being outdoors and spent vast amounts of time gardening, which was one of his hobbies. In fact, following his retirement from a senior position in the police force, he took up a small part-time role as a gardener at a local stately home, which he loved. Unfortunately, as his condition worsened he was unable to continue with this job.

Caring for an individual with Alzheimer's disease is very difficult. Unfortunately, after several months of looking after my father-in-law, his condition rapidly worsening, my mother-in-law placed him in a care home on the outskirts of the town. This was an extremely difficult time for all the family, but even more difficult (as you can imagine) for my father-in-law. He missed his home, his family and his freedom. He was no longer able to come and go as he pleased. The facility, whilst having a small grass area, was not secure and therefore my father-in-law had to be accompanied at all times whilst outdoors. It was not, therefore, possible for my father-in-law to spend the time in the outside that he wanted, and often complained about being 'trapped' in what he called 'the jail'.

After a few months of his arrival, it was apparent that my father-in-law was extremely unhappy with the facility within which he'd been placed. Whilst his symptoms were such that he would forget what he ate for lunch and struggled to engage in verbal conversation, he still knew his own mind and was extremely frustrated both by his condition and his surroundings.

Eventually my father-in-law was placed in hospital, which, whilst it was a secure ward, had a garden that he could access without being accompanied and he could 'potter', sit in the fresh air, and help the staff with some gardening etc. He was much happier in this facility, but unfortunately this was a short-term placement and an alternative long-term facility was required to be found.

After a few weeks my father-in-law was placed again in a short-term facility, but this time it was at another hospital. This placement was principally aimed at assessment and trying to treat his condition as well as possible under the circumstances. The facility in this hospital again had a large secure garden and my father-in-law could access it at will. He spent hours in the garden and when we went to visit, this was our first port of call. Nine times out of ten we would find him there. When he was in the garden it brought back memories of his past life and for the hours that he was out there, he seemed happier.

After a month or so my father-in-law was placed in a longer-term ward in the same hospital. Whilst the staff are terrific and extremely caring, the ward is two floors up with no access to a garden. The only fresh air that my father-in-law gets is when the staff take him for an occasional walk around the grounds of the hospital. His condition has significantly worsened since being placed in this ward. Whilst I am sure, from a medical diagnosis point of view, this is consequent to his illness with which he has been diagnosed, I believe that if this facility allowed him access to a garden, his quality of life would be improved. At least for the short time he was in the garden he might be allowed a small amount of happiness and to engage in the hobby he enjoyed for so many years, escaping the feeling of being 'trapped' and imprisoned.

Watching a relative disappear before your eyes as a result of a condition such as Alzheimer's disease is absolutely heart-breaking. I believe that anything we can do to make this awful condition more bearable and provide the best quality of life possible should be pursued.

A daughter

My mother is aged 92 and lives in a sheltered flat that is attached to a care home for older people, and part of the same building. She has quite a lot of physical problems and is sometimes unsteady on her feet. She has fallen a few times but often doesn't remember what happened or even that she fell. The most distressing part of her growing older is the loss of her short-term memory. She expresses anxiety and distress about this. She has no fear of death – she says with real conviction that she is past her 'sell by' date and ready to go. She says she hopes to die before she completely loses her mental abilities.

It is upsetting for us as well, as she often doesn't remember what happened in the last few minutes/hours/days. Her long-term memory is quite good, although she sometimes forgets about things like the death of a family member years before, and she feels the distress of the bereavement all over again.

Increasingly, I have noticed that my mother sits out in the garden much more than she used to. She used to be happy for us to take her out of the complex but she no longer likes to do that, and this may be why she spends more time in the garden. She also likes to go for a little walk with us when we visit her, just around the garden to the car park.

I asked her how important she felt it was to be able to go out to the garden when you want? This is what she said:

"Oh, very important. I like to go out and sit down and get the fresh air. I would really miss it if I wasn't able to do this... It's nice to be able to go out and sit down when the sun is out but I like to sit in the shade and enjoy the sunshine. I would say it is very important for old people to have a garden to sit in and it is very good for our health... There are usually two or three other people sitting in the same part of the garden but I don't really chat to them because I mainly like to enjoy the peace and quiet."

My own opinion is that having access to a nice, spacious and well-tended garden has really improved my mother's quality of life as her physical health and memory have deteriorated, and I am thankful she lives in such a caring environment.

Key points

- these are simply a set of perspectives from a small number of people with dementia and their relatives – they are not meant to be typical
- people with dementia and their relatives are as different from one another as any other people in the population – everyone's pathway through dementia is different
- everyone wants different things from their outside spaces
- we have to design for diversity.

References

Killick, J. (2009). *The elephant in the room: Poems by people with memory loss in Cambridgeshire.* Cambridge: Cambridgeshire County Council.

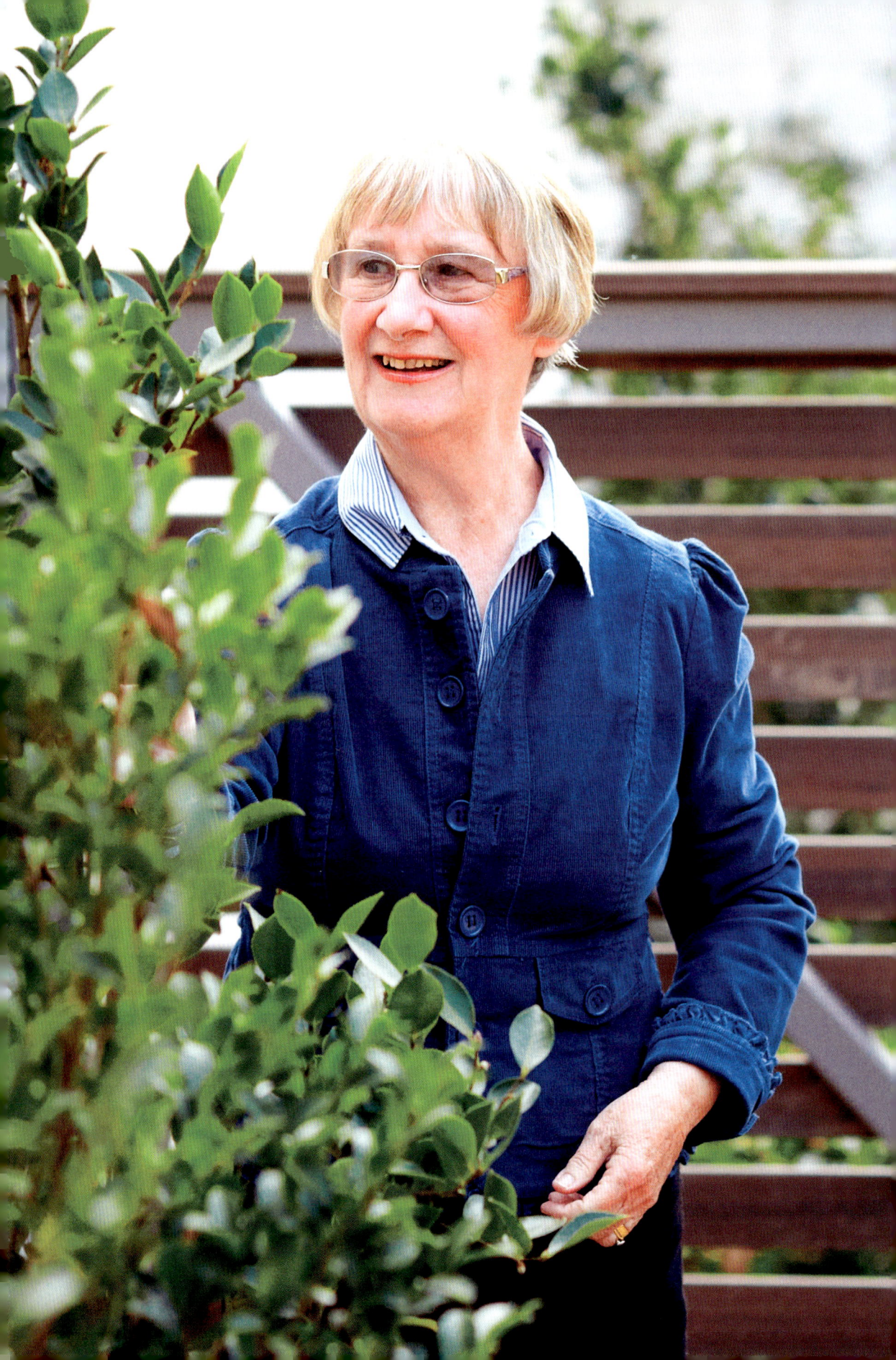

Chapter 2
Going outside is essential for health and wellbeing

Annie Pollock and David McMair

Whilst there is little research on the benefits of being outside, specifically in respect to people with dementia, there is a lot of research that shows the benefits for the population at large, both of spending time outdoors and of having a good view out from a building.

When we consider older people, most will have health problems of some sort, usually associated simply with ageing. However, for those with the added disability of dementia, which affects mainly older people (5% of over 65s and 30% of over 90s), it is vital that their general health is as good as possible to allow them to deal positively with this incurable illness.

This chapter looks at the advantages of having suitable outdoor areas that promote good health for people with dementia, who can use at will, and for the staff that care for them.

Background

The concept of having gardens within healthcare settings dates back at least to Greek and Roman times and was seen as part of a patient's therapy. In Roman military hospitals, a courtyard was the main feature and fresh air and exercise were central to recovery. Hospices in the Middle Ages had gardens and/or vineyards. In the Renaissance, public hospitals with central courtyards were standard.

In the late 19th century, hospitals experienced a loss of garden and open space even though Florence Nightingale said:

"Second only to fresh air… I should be inclined to rank light in the importance for the sick. Direct sunlight, not only daylight, is necessary for speedy recovery… I mention from experience… in promoting recovery, the being able to see out of a window, instead of looking at a dead wall; the bright colours of flowers; the being able to read in bed by the light of the window close to the bed-head.

It is generally said the effect is on the mind. Perhaps so, but it is not less so upon the body on that account."

Today, landscape in the modern health-care setting is all too often relegated to small courtyards at the entrance or within the building to provide light to surrounding rooms and corridors but to which there may be no public access.

Today's generation of people with dementia grew up in an era when there was a general belief that fresh air was health-giving and, indeed, it is true that sunlight kills some types of bacteria and colds and flu-like viruses. These are also spread less easily outdoors than in internal spaces because of the superior airflow.

In that immediate postwar era:

- central heating was rare, yet people often slept with their bedroom windows open the year round
- babies were frequently put outside

in their prams in cold weather, well wrapped, to benefit from the fresh air

- people did their shopping for food every day, usually on foot or bicycle to local shops, as few people owned a refrigerator or a car
- gardens or allotments were often used to grow vegetables or even to keep chickens
- hospitals often had balconies or outdoor areas where patients were encouraged to sit to access the 'health-giving' fresh air and sunshine. Sadly, few modern hospitals now have such a facility.

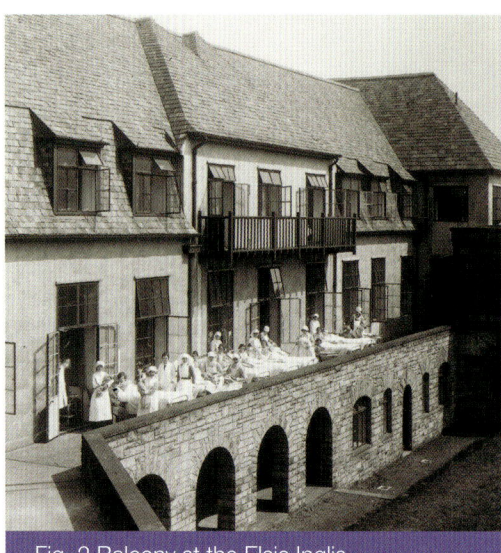

Fig. 2 Balcony at the Elsie Inglis Memorial Pavilion, Edinburgh, c. 1935

Yet in many facilities for people with dementia, these same people, who are usually in their late 70s, 80s or 90s, often have little or no access to the outdoors and to fresh air. They lack physical activity, are frequently lethargic, are physically frail, have poor sleeping patterns and sometimes show challenging behaviour.

A report by the Mental Welfare Commission for Scotland (2009) noted that over half of all people in the care homes they looked at never went out of the care home and a further 25% rarely went out. They also found that whilst 52% of care homes did have gardens that were accessible and safe, they were not necessarily suitable for people with dementia. In addition, the majority of people did not get the chance to use the gardens and outside areas regularly.

England's Department of Health in its publication *'Care Homes for Older People: National Minimum Standards'* (2003) notes as a minimum standard:

"There is outdoor space for service users, accessible to those in wheelchairs or with other mobility problems, with seating and designed to meet the needs of all service users including those with physical, sensory and cognitive impairments" and that *"Opportunities are given for appropriate exercise and physical activity; appropriate interventions are carried out for service users identified as at risk of falling."* It also notes *"You will be able to move around easily in the house and its grounds."*

A study (Hoe, Hancock, Livingston & Orrel, 2006) on the quality of life of people with dementia in residential care homes concluded that:

"Despite most having severe dementia, residents' views of their own quality of life were strongly linked to their mood, suggesting that improving mood would increase quality of life."

"Care staff and health professionals should be aware that the quality of life of people with dementia in

residential homes might primarily relate to their mood in terms of both anxiety and depression. Maximising their enjoyment and enhancing well-being along with the identification and treatment of mood disorders should therefore be prioritised in care plans."

In recent years there has been a lot of research related to the way a green and natural environment impacts on people's general mood and wellbeing. Maller, Townsend, Pryor, Brown and St. Leger (2005) noted that 'natural areas can be seen as one of our most vital health resources'.

In this chapter, we aim to provide a snapshot of some of the research that demonstrates positive health benefits and cost saving results of having access to appropriate outdoor space, although there is clearly a great need for further research, specifically on the benefits for people with dementia of access to an outdoor space and activity.

We propose to look at benefits of being outdoors under the following headings:

1. Health benefits of being outdoors
2. The benefits of vitamin D
3. Psychological benefits of being outdoors
4. Reduction in use of drugs.

1. Health benefits of being outdoors

Being outside is an intrinsic part of being human – mankind started out as 'hunter gatherers', learning how to cultivate crops, farm animals, and support themselves by working the countryside, and thereby spent the majority of waking hours outside. For many in Europe this changed with the industrial revolution in the late 18th century. People worked long hours in factories or down mines; smoke and pollution reduced the amount of daylight and sunlight reaching ground level in towns and cities and there was an epidemic of rickets in industrial cities Europe-wide.

It is worth noting that complete cloud cover reduces UV energy by 50% and shade, including that produced by severe pollution, can reduce UV energy by 60% (Wharton et al., 2003). So people in countries that have frequent cloud cover and in cities where there are large amounts of pollution may not get sufficient vitamin D from sunlight if they do not access the outdoors frequently or seek an unpolluted environment.

Rickets is a disease that affects the bone development of children, causing the softening and weakening of bones; this can lead to deformities, such as bowed legs and curvature of the spine. The most common causes are lack of vitamin D or calcium. Although in the 1940s the incidence of rickets vastly reduced, there has been a reported increase in the UK in recent years. Children from Asian, African, Caribbean or Middle Eastern origin are at higher risk because their skin is darker and they need more sunlight to get enough vitamin D. However, any child that does not go outside very often, that is frequently covered up or has a diet low in vitamin D or calcium, can also be at risk (www.nhs.uk/choices).

A study (Galbraith and Westphal, 2003) of the Martin Luther Alzheimer Garden at a Third State Alzheimer's Dementia Unit in Holt, Michigan, USA found that, in respect of eight variables (aggressive and non-aggressive behaviour; physician ordered and as-needed medication; pulse rate; diastolic and systolic blood pressure; and weight change) residents who spent as little as 10 to 15 minutes each day of unprogrammed activity in the garden during the summer months showed significant improvements on virtually every parameter (none deteriorated and one stayed the same).

So we can see the importance for everyone, including people with dementia, of getting enough sunshine, fresh air and exercise to aid good health and strong bones.

Exercise for mental and physical health

We all benefit from being outdoors and having contact with nature; we recall childhood games and memories, the joy of eating outdoors in good weather, walks, holidays, working in the garden and so on.

It is well known that exercise has very positive health benefits in the following ways:

- it reduces the risk of heart disease, stroke, and high blood-pressure and lowers cholesterol levels
- it helps with lower back pain (in particular, pain due to osteoarthritis) and slows bone degeneration
- it reduces the likelihood of developing diabetes and certain cancers
- it can prevent and help with the treatment of mental illness and stress
- it can help manage weight problems.

This is not new. England's Department of Health produced their Strategy Statement on Physical Activity in 1996. This recommended levels of physical activity, which are now widely used.

These are:

- adults should accumulate at least 30 minutes of moderate intensity physical activity on five or more days a week
- young people should accumulate at least 60 minutes of moderate intensity physical activity each day, and that at least twice a week this should include activity that can improve bone health, strength and flexibility.

In 2008 The National Institute for Clinical Excellence (NICE) noted that:

"The maintenance of physical activity in later life is central to improving physical health. Regular exercise has beneficial effects on general health, mobility and independence, and is associated with a reduced risk of depression and related benefits for mental wellbeing, such as reduced anxiety and enhanced mood and self-esteem."

A further study (Jacobs et al., 2008) has shown that people in their 70s who go out daily reported much less musculoskeletal pain, sleep problems, urinary incontinence and decline in activities of daily living. The conclusion is that this is beneficial for independent older people and correlates with reduced functional decline and improved health.

It should also be noted that falls in people over 65 years of age cost the National Health Service (NHS) in England and Wales over £4.6 million a day and that evidence has shown if elderly people take part in exercise programmes specifically designed to improve strength and balance, the risk of falls can be cut by up to 55% (Age UK, 2010). See also sections on vitamin D and reduction in the use of drugs.

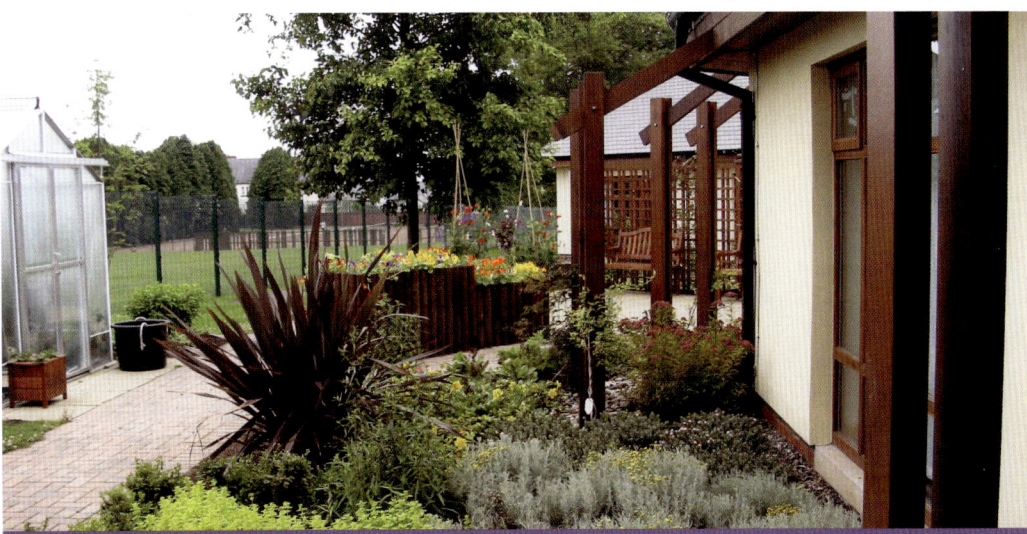
Fig. 3 Outdoor activities at a hospital specialist palliative unit

So, by providing good outdoor space with associated activities for all in care homes, day centres, hospital wards and so on, the general health of those using them (staff and residents) is likely to be improved and/or maintained for longer and there will unquestionably be substantial savings in healthcare costs.

Reduction in cognitive decline

Cognitive decline is generally associated with ageing and is a particular symptom of the various dementias. However, keeping the brain active and exercised is an essential contribution towards preventing or lessening this decline and helps to maintain an active and fulfilling lifestyle.

The outdoors provides a substantial range of opportunities for participating in activities that help people to retain their cognitive abilities and enable them to continue taking an active part in society for as long as possible; these are discussed in greater detail in Part 4 of this book.

The New Scientist, (17 December, 2005), in an article called 'Use it don't lose it' by Lisa Melton (science writer-in-residence at the Novartis Foundation in London) noted that, whilst mental activity really can cushion people against age-related decline, results from a study in Dublin, Ireland, suggest that physical activity can also be beneficial and that exercise has a remarkable impact on mental performance.

This is borne out by a study undertaken in the USA at the Group Health Cooperative in Seattle (Larson et al., 2006) of a group of 1740 people aged 65 or over, all of whom had good cognitive function at the outset. After six years, 158 of these had developed dementia (of whom 107 had Alzheimer's). But those who had exercised at least three times a week were, on average, 38% less likely to have developed dementia. Other studies, such as one undertaken in the Gironde (Fabrigoule et al., 1995) in France, concur with this.

Verghese et al., (2003) noted that the general conclusion from this and other research projects is that "Participation in leisure activities is associated with a reduced risk of development of dementia, both Alzheimer's disease and vascular dementia".

However, the reduction in risk is related to the frequency of participation, for example, elderly people who did crossword puzzles four days a week (four activity-days) had a risk of dementia that was 47% lower than that among subjects who did puzzles once a week (one activity-day).

For people who have dementia, does activity (physical and mental) slow down their cognitive decline? There is some evidence that it does.

A planned walking programme of half-an-hour three times a week for people with Alzheimer's resulted in significant benefits in their ability to communicate (Friedman & Tappen, 1991).

Several studies have linked exercise with improved cognitive function. Heyn, Abreu and Ottenbacher (2004) concluded that exercise training increases fitness, physical function, positive behaviour and cognitive function (measured with MMSE[1]) in people with dementia and related cognitive impairments. Lautenschlager et al. (2008) demonstrated that exercise improves cognitive function in older adults with subjective and objective mild cognitive impairment and this benefit lasted for at least 12 months after the intervention had been discontinued.

A study by Erickson et al. (2009) noted that the deterioration of the hippocampus[2] leads to memory impairment and dementia. The results of this study clearly demonstrate that higher aerobic fitness levels are associated with greater hippocampal volumes in elderly humans. Larger hippocampal volumes translate to better spatial memory function.

In addition, bright light has a modest benefit in improving some cognitive and non-cognitive symptoms of dementia (Riemersma-van der Lek et al., 2008). Further information on the benefits of bright light is presented overleaf.

However, perhaps whether being outside reduces cognitive decline or not is really a side issue. The main issue is that being outside gives most older people, and in particular those in a care-home environment, a great deal of pleasure, sense of freedom and a resource for exercise, activity, conversation, reflection and so on, at a time when their lives are changing irrevocably.

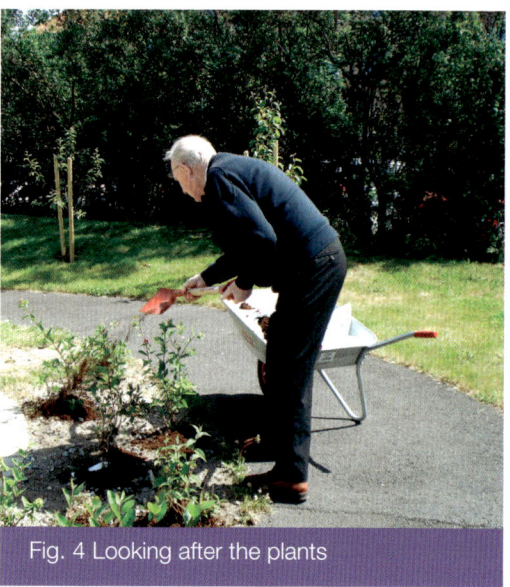
Fig. 4 Looking after the plants

For older people living in nursing homes, visiting an outdoor green space is associated with better concentration and improved mood (Rappe & Kivelä, 2005) and being able to go outside enables people to perceive their health as better (Rappe & Kivelä, 2006).

---

1 The mini-mental state examination (MMSE) is the most commonly used instrument for screening cognitive function.
2 Hippocampus: a major component of the human brain. It plays important roles in the consolidation of information from short-term memory to long-term memory and spatial navigation.

Improved sleep patterns and circadian rhythm[3]

Exposure to bright morning light, in particular, triggers a burst of energy that makes people active. At the same time, it contributes to good quality sleep by training the circadian rhythms and reducing the incidence of any symptoms of seasonal depression. Daylight is as effective as sunlight and if this exposure to light is achieved by taking exercise outdoors, even if only pottering about in the garden, this further aids the quality of sleep.

However, whilst many older people, given half a chance, would take a nap in the afternoon after a good lunch, all too often in the care-home environment they sleep at abnormal times during the day (for example in the morning) and this can be correlated with disturbed sleep patterns at night. This may well be exacerbated by the lack of anything to do and general boredom. There is often little opportunity for participation in activity other than at mealtimes, and generally there is no allowance for early or late eating preferences.

Sleep disturbance is a symptom shared by all neurodegenerative illnesses and can be a significant factor in seeking institutional care. Van Someren, Mirmiran, and Swaab (1993) noted that:

"Restlessness and awakenings during the evening and night are serious problems and were even found to be a primary factor in the decision of a caregiver to have an elderly relative institutionalised."

Sleep disturbances result in great demands on carers in domestic settings and staff in residential settings. However, long-term care facilities in particular may cause their residents to suffer disturbed sleep because of noise, light and disturbance by staff on the night shift; this is a management issue that should always be given attention.

Researchers have found that interruption of the circadian rhythm is also an important factor in sleep disturbance and that this tended to become greater with progression of dementing disease (Harper et al., 2004). In addition, people in institutional environments have been found to have lower daytime and higher night-time exposure to light than the community-dwelling elderly. This is also linked to increased sleep disturbance (Shochat, Martin, Marler & Ancoli-Israel, 2000).

Therefore if the circadian rhythm can be positively influenced, people with dementia might be able to live more independent lives for longer. In care homes, improved sleep patterns can help to reduce challenging behaviour and this in turn can improve staff morale.

So how can the circadian rhythm be improved? It is accepted that scheduled exposure to bright light and to darkness are effective tools for regulating the human circadian clock. Specifically of interest here is the capacity of bright light during the day combined with darkness at night to maintain a 'normal' rhythm. Van Someren concluded in his randomised control trial (Riemersma-van der Lek et al., 2008) that:

"the simple measure of increasing the illumination level in group care facilities ameliorated symptoms of disturbed cognition, mood, behaviour, functional abilities, and sleep."

A number of studies have found that the output from standard light boxes can produce the desired stabilisation of circadian rhythm when used for the time

---

3 Circadian rhythm: a 'built-in', roughly 24-hour cycle in biochemical, physiological or behavioral processes. It is adjusted to the environment by external cues, the primary one being daylight.

and at the distance recommended by the manufacturer. For example, a Norwegian study (Fetveit, Skerjve, & Bjorvatn, 2003) used 6000 to 8000 lux[4] at a distance of 60 to 70 cm to expose people to bright light for about two hours during the period 8am to 11am and found 'substantial improvement in sleep among demented nursing home patients'.

However, using light boxes can cause visual discomfort (as has been observed by experimenters, Smith, Revell and Eastman, 2009), whereas being outside gives one exposure to the necessary light levels without stress or discomfort and at no cost.

In a typical UK city, external daylight exceeds 6,000 lux for about 80% of a 9am to 5pm working day. The necessary illumination will be received even if people are outside in the shade.

In addition, external exposure to daylight may well involve activity that is beneficial to health and has a significant therapeutic benefit.

Improved appetite

Many older people are dehydrated and malnourished (Scottish Government, 2011). There are many possible reasons for this, including depression, constipation, medication and difficulties in chewing and swallowing (Dementia Services Development Centre 2009).

The Alzheimer's Society has a series of useful factsheets, one of which is on eating and drinking. This includes lack of exercise as a further reason for lack of appetite. (http://www.alzheimers.org.uk/site/scripts/documents.php).

There are plenty of materials that promote ways of tackling the problems such as the DSDC DVD *Oh good, lunch is coming.*

However, being outdoors can help promote appetite in the following ways:

- by providing an attractive and social setting for a snack, picnic or barbeque which, by the smell of food cooking, can trigger appetite
- by providing opportunities for exercise and activity, which may help with depression, lessen physical discomfort and ease constipation.

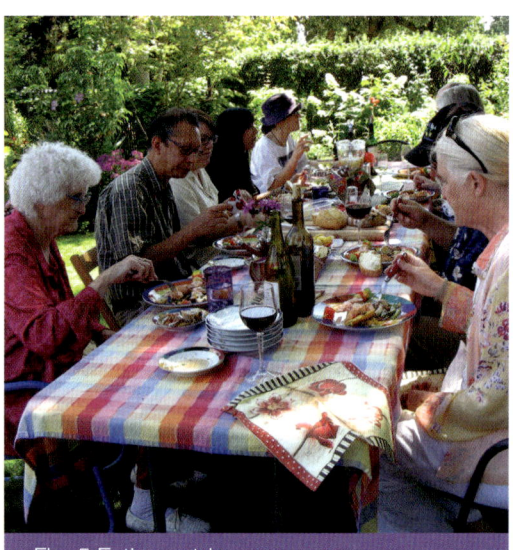

Fig. 5 Eating outdoors

Healthy eating will increase energy levels and promote a better night's sleep. If it is possible to eat outside sometimes, the benefits of bright light may also help with problems of poor vision.

Less incontinence

All types of incontinence are common among older men and women and the prevalence increases with age. Women are more likely to suffer urinary

---

4 Lux is the standard international unit of illumination

incontinence, while the prevalence of faecal incontinence and double incontinence is similar in both men and women.

Stenzelius (2005) noted that the ability to be continent is largely dependent on whether a person can find the way to and reach the toilet in time. A person with walking and mobility problems could be incontinent just because it takes him or her too long to get to the bathroom, to remove the necessary clothes and to sit down on the toilet. Other contributing factors could be the ability to use hands, to remember and, in particular, to see clearly where the toilet is located.

He also noted that 'intervention studies' to prove earlier studies have shown positive results, such as walking exercise to reduce urinary and faecal incontinence.

Faecal incontinence can also be a result of constipation, which may be caused by many different things, for example, lack of fibre, change of eating habits, drinking insufficient liquids, anxiety/stress/depression, or as a side effect of medication. However, it may also be caused by immobility or lack of exercise.

The UK's NHS Choices (2010) notes that:

"Keeping active is a very important part of leading a healthy lifestyle, and it can help to prevent a number of serious health conditions, including urinary incontinence. Make sure that you do a minimum of 30 minutes of exercise at least five times a week."

The exercise too will help strengthen muscles and in turn may help some people with pelvic floor control, thereby aiding continence. Being as physically healthy as possible means that the person with dementia is more likely to get to a toilet in time as long as it is clearly signed and getting there is not stressful. Consequently, there are many benefits in having a toilet that can be easily seen and reached from the outdoor areas that are used for exercise and activity.

Key points

- easily accessible outdoor space will encourage exercise, which in turn can increase body fitness and enhance appetite
- eating outside in a social atmosphere can also enhance appetite
- bright light can stabilise the circadian rhythm, thereby improving sleep patterns
- cognitive decline in older people is slowed down by exercise and activity
- the more frequent the outdoor visits, the better people rated their heath
- better mobility and more exercise may help incontinence problems but clear signage and easy access to toilets is essential.

All these benefits have a double impact on carers – directly by improving their own sleep and health, and indirectly by improving the sleep and health of the people they are looking after.

2. The benefits of vitamin D

Vitamin D is perhaps best known for its role in preventing rickets. It is crucial to the maintenance of bone and muscle strength. In addition to this, deficiency of vitamin D is associated with an increased risk of malignancies, particularly of colon, breast and prostate gland and of chronic inflammatory and autoimmune diseases e.g. type 1 diabetes, inflammatory bowel disease, multiple sclerosis, rheumatoid arthritis, as well as of metabolic disorders (metabolic syndrome[5], hypertension) (Peterlik & Cross, 2009).

People with Alzheimer's disease have an increased prevalence of vitamin D deficiency but it is not known whether this is a cause or consequence of Alzheimer's disease. Venning (2005) noted that:

"Vitamin D deficiency among elderly people is much more common than previously recognised. It constitutes a serious public health problem for residents of old people's homes, nursing homes, and long-stay wards and housebound people in the community."

How vitamin D is obtained

As glass and plastics absorb the critical ultraviolet (UV) wavelengths of light, it is necessary to be directly exposed outdoors to sunlight, rather than just to daylight, before the body can start to produce vitamin D.

Generally older people or those who have darker skin need a longer exposure to sunlight to make vitamin D. Non-smokers, younger people and those with lighter skin all need less exposure than their opposites.

A minimum daily dose of vitamin D of around 800 IUs[6] for older people (70+) is generally recommended (http://ods.od.nih.gov/factsheets/vitamind/). Holick (2004) notes that:

"Sensible sun exposure (usually 5–10 min of exposure of the arms and legs or the hands, arms, and face, 2 or 3 times per week) and increased dietary and supplemental vitamin D intakes are reasonable approaches to guarantee vitamin D sufficiency."

However, it has been found that in elderly people living in the community in Europe, 36% of men and 47% of women had vitamin D concentrations at levels often taken as the lower limit of sufficiency (van der Wielen et al., 1995). Curiously, the lowest values were found in Southern Europe and this was attributed to attitudes towards sunlight, daily living activities and wearing clothing with long sleeves.

Low fish consumption has also been associated with a reduced vitamin D status.

At latitudes above 37°N and below 37°S, sunlight is insufficient to induce cutaneous vitamin D3 synthesis during the winter months. Researchers recommend that exposure to direct sunlight of no more than five to ten minutes between 10am and 3pm in spring, summer and autumn in the northern hemisphere will prevent vitamin D inadequacy (Holick, 2006).

However, in Australia, where the UV radiation levels are higher (compared to Europe and North America) with an increased risk of developing skin cancers, researchers recommend exposure before 10am and after 2pm standard time in the summer months (11am to 3pm daylight saving time) (Osteoporosis Australia, 2011).

---

5 Metabolic syndrome is a name for a group of risk factors that occur together and increase the risk for coronary artery disease, stroke, and type 2 diabetes. Symptoms: Extra weight around the waist (central or abdominal obesity).
6 IU: International Unit: unit of measurement for the amount of a substance, based on biological activity or effect. It is used to quantify vitamins, hormones, some medications, vaccines, blood products, and similar biologically active substances.

It is a fortunate coincidence that such exposure in the morning would additionally provide the bright light necessary to entrain the circadian rhythm towards aiding or encouraging or establishing maximum sleep efficiency and minimising the risk of seasonal affective disorder (see sections overleaf).

As vitamin D cannot be synthesised by the body in northern latitudes between October and March inclusive (Macdonald et al., 2008), winter requirements have to be met from a combination of stores accumulated in fat during the summer and dietary intake.

As a guide, each of the following would provide the daily requirements of 800 IUs:

- 170 grams of salmon
- 440 grams of tuna fish, canned in water and drained
- 1615 grams of liver or beef
- 39 sardines (from a drained can)
- 19 egg yolks
- just less than a tablespoon of cod liver oil (but be aware that more could lead to vitamin A toxicity).

Quantities such as these with the foods that are the most rich in vitamin D would be somewhat challenging to manage. Therefore, at times when the skin cannot produce enough vitamin D, supplements should be considered. However, there is no doubt of the importance of access to outdoor space to get direct sunshine during the summer months.

The time of exposure to sunlight will obviously vary with latitude and, of course, this must be balanced against the dangers of sunburn, which can lead to melanoma (a type of cancer). Care therefore needs to be taken by applying sunblock to avoid sunburn.

Vitamin D and falls

Analysts from the Health Economics Consortium at the University of York (Scuffham, Chaplin & Legood, 2003) examined national databases to evaluate how many people over 60 had experienced a severe fall in 1999. The study looked at the number of Accident and Emergency (A&E) visits and hospital admissions in patients aged 60 to 64, 65 to 69, 70 to 74 and 75 and over and found that there were almost three times the number of A&E attendances among the over-75s compared to those in the other age groups. Furthermore, the over-75s were also found to be 11 times more likely to be hospitalised after a fall compared to those aged 60 to 64. Most falls in all age groups occurred when a person was walking on a level surface.

Gordon Lisham, Director General of Age Concern England, noted that the findings of this survey were "extremely worrying", observing that:

"Even minor falls can cause older people to lose their confidence to get on with everyday life."
(BBC News, 2003)

Adequate levels of vitamin D are very good at reducing falls in older people. They work by maximising calcium and phosphorous absorption, which improves bone production, and lowering levels of parathyroid hormone that would otherwise decrease bone density and weaken muscles.

In a French study of 3270 women living in nursing homes or apartment houses for elderly people, it was found that giving supplements of vitamin D (800 IU daily) and calcium (1.2 gm daily) reduced the risk of hip fractures by 43% and that of other fractures by 32% (Chapuy et al., 2002).

The researchers stated that "vitamin D insufficiency, especially in institutionalised subjects, is due mainly to a lack of exposure to sunshine that is not compensated for by increased dietary vitamin D intake".

A two-year follow-up study of a further 583 institutionalised women produced almost identical results.

A meta-analysis (Bischoff-Ferrari et al., 2009) of eight randomised control trials revealed that levels of vitamin D above a daily intake of 700 IU reduced falls by between 19% and 26% and concluded that a daily intake is warranted in all people over 65. It was also found that below this threshold of 700 IU daily the vitamin produced no effect. (Note: International Units for vitamin D: 1 IU equals 0.025 micrograms in food.) Some other studies have found that doses of 400 IU daily are ineffective in reducing falls and fractures (Lips, Graafmans, Ooms, Bezemer & Bouter, 1996; Meyer et al., 2002).

Vitamin D and general health

Researchers have consistently identified that people with higher vitamin D levels in their blood are less likely to have a range of medical conditions.
For example:

- an analysis of five epidemiological studies (Gorham et al., 2007) found a 50% decrease in the risk of colorectal cancer in those with high vitamin D levels
- a six-year study (Wang et al., 2008) reported that, after adjustment for conventional risk factors, the risk for a first cardiovascular event was 62% higher in people with low vitamin D.

After an earlier study suggested that the central nervous system might be influenced by vitamin D levels (Bischoff-Ferrari et al., 2009), researchers found that in elderly people generally and in people with mild Alzheimer's disease vitamin D deficiency was associated with low mood and impaired cognitive function (Wilkins, Sheline, Roe, Birge & Morris,. 2006; Oudshoorn, Mattace-Raso, van der Velde, Colin & van der Cammen, 2008). However, it is important to note that the researchers could not rule out deficiency as a marker rather than a contributor of disease, and called for more research.

Some stated that their results supported a recommendation for preventative vitamin D supplementation in older people at risk (Oudshoorn et al., 2008).

Key points

- lack of vitamin D is due mainly to lack of exposure to sunshine and is associated with many diseases
- people with Alzheimer's disease have an increased prevalence of vitamin D deficiency and it is essential for their health to address this shortfall
- vitamin D deficiency can be addressed by a suitable diet and safe exposure to direct sunlight with appropriate vitamin D supplements in the winter months
- managed well, there should be little downside in relation to risk
- even if the only benefit of vitamin D were a reduction in falls, this would be very important in care environments and would achieve great savings to health services. If other benefits are eventually proven, the importance of vitamin D can only increase.

3. Psychological benefits of being outdoors

People relax, worry less and smile more when the climate is amenable and comfortable. Particularly in countries with variable weather, they all cheer up and spirits rise when the clouds clear away and the sun comes out.

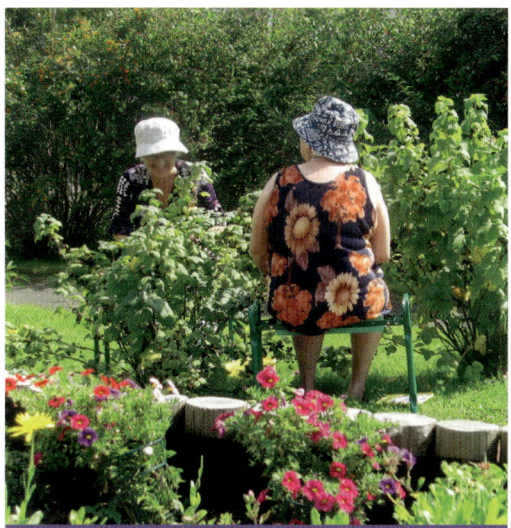
Fig. 6 Enjoying the sunshine, picking berries

This is probably much more an issue in the far northern and southern hemispheres, where seasonal change also means, in the winter, short days compared with the summer, and correspondingly a huge reduction in daylight and sunlight hours. According to the World Health Organisation, half of the suffering due to ill-health in Western Europe is due to mental illness and the bulk of this to depression and anxiety.

A good overview of research into the positive impact of light is provided by Joseph (2006), who noted that exposure to daylight leads to the following:

- reduced depression among patients with seasonal affective disorder and bipolar depression
- decreased length of stay in hospitals
- improved sleep and circadian rhythms
- lessened agitation among people with dementia and less pain
- improved adjustment to night-shift work among staff.

Interaction with green spaces can provide significant benefits for older people. It provides a means to maintain physical activity, concentration, reduce stress and overall improved quality of life. In Case study 2, Mrs Endo, Director of Plaisir Villa Ichikawa, clearly states that the rooftop garden calms the confusion of her residents with dementia.

The opportunities for social interaction that green spaces can provide are important for alleviating stress (Milligan, Gatrell & Bingley, 2004). The aesthetics of the outside and a wtranquil environment have been found to be beneficial for mental wellbeing (Kweon, Sullivan & Wiley, 1998).

Interaction with green spaces has also been found to contribute to feelings of personal worth (Newton, 2007).

Seasonal Affective Disorder and bright light exposure

Seasonal Affective Disorder (SAD) is a type of depression that leaves people tired, lethargic, stressed and unhappy (www.nhs.uk/Conditions/Seasonal-affective-disorder/). It tends to appear when the days are shorter and usually symptoms disappear in the spring.

When it is dark and gloomy, many people without SAD feel more lethargic and less sociable, with mood, appetite and energy levels affected. Up to one in eight people in the UK experience these milder symptoms (known as sub-syndromal SAD or sub-SAD).

People tend to associate the prevalence of SAD and sub-SAD with increased latitude.

However, the research does not entirely support this association and has found that the following are important factors:

- climate
- genetic vulnerability
- social-cultural context.

Studies comparing the incidence in different continents found it to be twice as high in the USA as in Europe, whereas the opposite would be expected since the latitudes used in the European studies were higher (Mersch et al., 1999).

On the other hand, a highly positive correlation with cloudiness (Potkin, Zetin, Stamenkovic, Kripke & Bunney, 1986) has been found together with significant correlations between mood and minutes of sunshine, length of daylight and temperature (Molin, Mellerup, Bollwig, Scheike & Dam, 1996). A study of Icelandic descendants in Canada found the rate of winter SAD was nearer the lower rate of Iceland, compared to the higher rate in Canada. This led to speculation, but no proof, about genetic adaptation (Magnusson & Axelsson, 1993) playing a role, or the influence of omega-3 essential fatty acids from fish in the diet (and therefore vitamin D). Cott and Hibbeln (2001) noted a similar and unexpected previous finding of a low prevalence of SAD in Japan (which also has a high per capita intake of fish).

Exposure to light has been found to be an effective agent for relieving the symptoms of SAD and sub-SAD. Typical exposures quoted are about 2500 lux for two to four hours or 10,000 lux for about 30 minutes, at a distance of one metre from a light device (Tonello, 2008).

Clearly, sitting for 30 minutes in front of a light only a metre away would be difficult to achieve for residents in a care home setting, and hard for them to understand. However, McNair, Cunningham, Pollock and McGuire, (2010) further note that exposure outdoors to morning daylight for about 30 minutes daily, failing which, internal exposure to bright light of about 5000 lux on the face for about one hour daily, is recommended to minimise the effects of SAD/sub-SAD and this should be achievable.

An experimental study that compared the effect of morning and evening light on patients with winter depression found that morning light was twice as effective as evening light in treating SAD (Lewy et al., 1998). This may be because the bright light suppresses the production of the (sleep) hormone melatonin and promotes the production of the (activity) hormone serotonin.

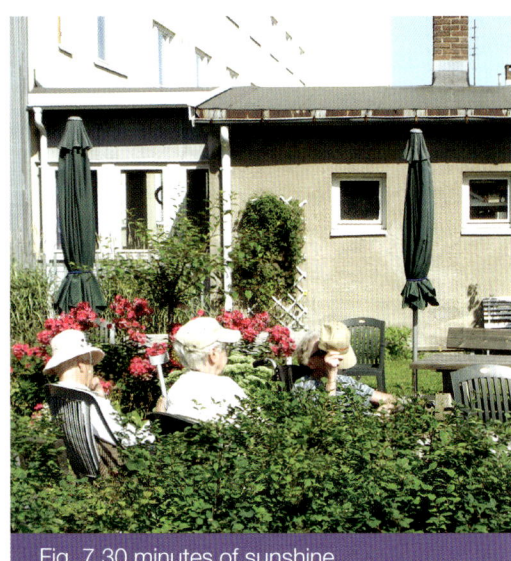
Fig. 7 30 minutes of sunshine

Reduction in aggressive behaviour and increase in positive mood

Of all the things that staff find most difficult about caring for people with dementia, not being able to communicate with the resident (18%) and dealing with aggressive/violent/abusive behaviour (17%) top the list (Alzheimer's Society 2007).

The National Association for Providers of Activities for Older People (NAPA) notes that boredom, frustration and isolation increase the risk of behaviour that care staff may find challenging:

"People with dementia who are bored and do not have 'people to see, places to go and things to do' are more likely to resort to behaviour which others find challenging in an attempt to get their needs met."

Surely this is common sense? Boredom and frustration at being trapped indoors can lead to perfectly understandable aggressive and challenging behaviour. This is borne out by research undertaken as long ago as the early 1990s:

- a study by Mooney and Nicell (1992) showed that violent behaviour by residents with dementia decreased when the residents had access to secure outdoor environments; in facilities where this was removed, violent behaviour increased

- a study by Namazi and Johnson (1992) found that the number of agitated behaviours in five categories decreased with unlocked doors to outdoor space.

The chart below (adapted from one in Namazi and Johnson's paper) shows that repeated requests, talking to one's self and verbal abuse, all significantly declined with an unlocked door to the outside. Screaming and being uncooperative (a small number in any case) disappeared.

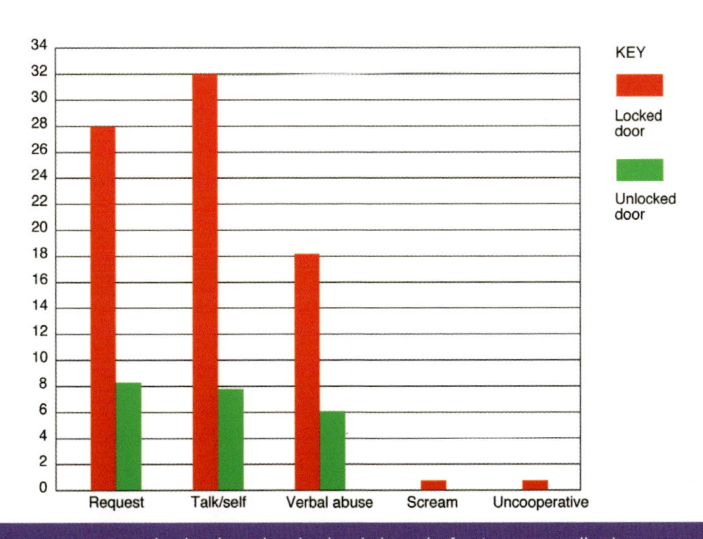

Fig. 8 Verbal responses to a locked and unlocked door (refer to appendix 1 on page 210 for enlarged version)

Residents in care homes and hospital patients with dementia can often be seen to congregate at brightly lit fire-doors at corridor ends and they become irritated by not being able to go outside. This should be recognised in the design process and 'designed out'.

Other ways of minimising aggression and agitation are indicated by the research noted below:

- **exercise:** in a study undertaken in a dementia unit on structured walking (Holmberg, 1997), the central finding was that resident-to-resident and resident-to-staff aggression was significantly less on those days when physically able people with severe dementia participated in a group walking session

- **exercise not immobilisation:** another report (Scherder, Bogen, Eggermont, Hamers & Swaab, 2010) concluded by noting that "institutionalisation and the use of physical restraints reduces and minimises the level of physical activity, respectively, and together aggravate behavioural disturbances such as agitation". They also noted that "agitation should not be treated by immobilisation but by an increase in physical activity, i.e. by participation in an exercise programme"

- **exposure to bright morning light:** this has been shown to reduce agitation among elderly patients with dementia. When they were exposed to 2500 lux for two hours in the morning for two ten-day periods, their agitation reduced. Patients were significantly more agitated on non-treatment days (Lovell, Ancoli-Israel & Gevirtz, 1995).

The possibility that nature can improve outcomes even in patients with late-stage dementia has received some support from a quasi-experimental study that found reduced levels of agitated aggressive behaviour were associated with a shower bath when recorded nature sounds (birds, babbling brook) and colour pictures were present (Whall et al., 1997).

Mood is influenced by activity. How many of us have come back after a long walk feeling much better, mentally as well as physically, than when we started out? Fresh air, rosy cheeks, good circulation resulting in better oxygen levels and red blood cell levels, warm even in cold weather.

A study (Matsouka, Kabitsis, Harahousou & Trigonis, 2005) looked at elderly and sedentary women, aged between 60 and 75. Exercise was performed between one and three times a week. Those who exercised three times a week had significantly more positive mood profiles than those who only exercised once a week or not at all.

Interestingly, however, where we exercise is important. A study conducted by Mind (2007), a leading mental health charity in the UK, benchmarked the effects of green therapy on 20 members of their local groups. The results demonstrated that 71% of participants reported decreased levels of depression following a country walk, whereas 22% had an increase of depressive symptoms after walking through an indoor shopping centre. The 'green' walks reduced stress levels and had a surprising knock-on effect of increasing self-esteem: 90% of participants stated that they felt better about themselves after a country walk.

One of the report's recommendations was that "access to green space should be considered as a key issue for all care planning and care assessment processes".

A Canadian study (Beauchemin & Hays, 1996) compared the lengths of stay in hospital of depressed patients in sunny rooms with those of patients in dull rooms. Those in sunny rooms had an average stay of 16.9 days compared to 19.5 days for those in dull rooms, a difference of 2.6 days (15%).

Stress reduction and self-rated health

We are all probably happier living without undue stress. When we are in control of our lives, we can usually keep stress to a manageable level.

However, people with dementia may be extremely stressed. Not only are they aware that their memory is failing, that they are finding their environment difficult to understand and everyday tasks difficult to undertake, but in many cases they have been 'removed' from their home to a care setting where their environment is unfamiliar and the freedoms they were accustomed to have been taken away.

It is well understood that people's mental health is strongly influenced by having the freedom to do what they want when they want – and, in particular, the freedom to go outdoors without unreasonable restriction. The Joseph Rowntree Foundation's report of the *Older People's Inquiry* (2006) noted that older people considered the ability to get out and about and keep active an important part of their lives. Why should people with dementia feel any different?

Nature has a strong attention-holding capacity and this may be associated with improved pain tolerance when looking at plants and natural landscapes (Kaplan & Kaplan, 1989). Coping better with pain and other troubles when going outside may decrease stress and result in people actually rating their health better.

Staff as well can feel stressed. This will in turn influence the people that they are caring for. A recent Turkish study (Alimoglu & Donmez, 2005), investigating 'burnout' in nurses, found that a lack of windows in the workplace contributes to stress and that a lack of daylight in the work setting can be a predictor of job burnout. A minimum of three hours of exposure to daylight seemed to reduce stress and burnout (however, the study did not specify the extent of the reduction). In addition, with fewer staff suffering from stress, staff turnover is reduced.

Research also suggests that access to nature in the workplace is related to lower levels of perceived job stress and higher levels of job satisfaction (Kaplan & Kaplan, 1989).

Benefits of a view from a building to the outside

The next best thing to being able to go outside, or to staying in when the weather is inclement, is at least to be able to see out and remain aware of what is going on in the world outside. Some people are much happier watching things outside than being there or participating. Many people with dementia become so impaired that all they can do is sit and watch.

Fig. 9 A place to watch outside activity

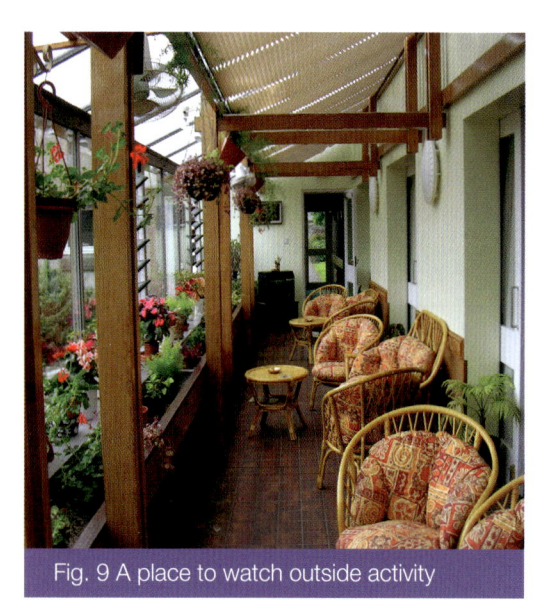

Research is providing mounting and convincing evidence that visual exposure to nature improves outcomes, such as stress and pain. For example, a study in a Swedish hospital found that heart-surgery patients in Intensive Care Units, who were assigned a picture with a landscape scene with trees and water, reported less anxiety/stress and needed fewer strong doses of pain relieving drugs than a control group assigned no pictures (Ulrich, 1991; Ulrich, 2001). Interestingly, another group of patients assigned an abstract picture had worsened outcomes compared to the control group, so it does matter what is being looked at.

A questionnaire study undertaken on windowless environments found that patients (generally wheelchair dependent and elderly) and staff have a strong preference for having views of nature, with artificial views (photos etc) preferred less than real views (Verderber, 1986).

A study (Ulrich, 1984) based on records between 1972 and 1981 indicated that 23 surgical patients assigned randomly to rooms with windows looking out on a natural scene, had shorter post-operative hospital stays, received fewer negative comments in nurses' evaluations, and took fewer potent analgesics than 23 similar patients randomly assigned to rooms with windows facing a brick wall.

The powerful effect of windows is also seen amongst the prison population where windows take on a meaning of 'life and freedom'. Prisoners with windows facing meadow or mountains had significantly lower rates of stress-related sick calls than inmates with a view of the prison courtyard and buildings (Moore, 1981).

A Canadian literature review in 2001 confirmed the outcome of many studies: that people prefer natural rather than urban views (Farley & Veitch, 2001). Recovery times have been found to be shorter and analgesic intake reduced for surgical patients with a view of nature (Ulrich, 1984), and stress found in office workers was less with those who had a natural view (Leather, Pyrgas, Beale & Lawrence, 1998).

Velarde, Fry, and Tveit (2007) provide a good summary of the many research papers on the health effects of viewing landscapes.

However, not only do people with dementia enjoy a view where something is happening – a village square, a bus stop, a footpath, any situation where they can take an interest in events and perhaps even interact with passers-by – but most actually like to be outdoors in the fresh air. So a garden with scope for activities seems an obvious way to provide a therapeutic view, fresh air and activities.

Key points

- to minimise the effects of SAD/sub-SAD, external exposure to morning daylight for about 30 minutes daily, failing which internal exposure to bright light of about 5000 lux hours on the face for about one hour daily, is recommended
- structured walking, bright morning light and the freedom to go outside to a garden area through an unlocked door minimises aggression and agitation in people with dementia
- exposure to daylight and access to nature can reduce stress
- exercise and activity significantly improves mood
- views out to a natural landscape or a place of activity, for residents and staff alike, are therapeutic.

4. Reduction in need for drugs

Why are drugs given to people with dementia? There may be many reasons including the following:

- providing pain relief
- help in sleeping at night
- relieving depression
- minimising challenging behaviour.

Pain, poor sleeping patterns and depression can all contribute to challenging behaviour.

Having shown how being outside, getting bright light and vitamin D, exercising and taking part in activities can all contribute to better health, improved mood, better cognition and reduction in challenging behaviour, it is sad to note the prevalence of antipsychotic drugs for people with dementia.

It was reported in the New Scientist magazine (17 October, 2009) that up to 60% of people with Alzheimer's disease in Europe and North America were prescribed antipsychotic drugs. In the UK alone, this was estimated to cost £80 million a year, despite the fact that studies have shown that compared with a taking a placebo, the benefits seem modest at best (Cochrane Database of Systematic Reviews, DOI: 10.1002/14651858.CD003012.pub2). Furthermore, the risks of these drugs are large, according to the UK Medicines and Healthcare Regulatory Agency website. This medication produces a threefold increase in the risk of a stroke and a 1–2% increased risk of mortality compared with no treatment. A study (Hartikainen, Lönnroos & Louhivuori, 2007) concluded that CNS[7] medicines, especially psychotropic drugs, seemed to be associated with increased risk of falling.

In December 2008, the UK All-Party Parliamentary Group (APPG, 2009) on Dementia announced that it would be undertaking an inquiry into the dementia-care skills of care home staff and staff supporting people with dementia living in their own homes. A key stimulus for this inquiry was the previous APPG report into the prescription of antipsychotic drugs to people with dementia living in care homes. Subsequently, England's Department of Health commissioned a report from Professor Sube Banerjee (2009).

---

[7] CNS drugs, those that act on the Central Nervous System

In this report, Banerjee noted that:

"Antipsychotic drugs are used for the management of behavioural and psychological symptoms in dementia" but that *"They can cause major problems for people with dementia and their carers and are a legitimate focus for intervention to decrease distress and harm, and increase quality of life."*

He also noted that of those being treated with antipsychotic drugs, approximately 20% only derived some benefit. Banerjee noted the need for further research to be completed, including work assessing the clinical and cost effectiveness of non-pharmacological methods of treating behavioural problems in dementia.

The Alzheimer's Society *Home from Home* report (2007) noted that:

- 54% of carers reported that their relative did not have enough to do in a care home
- the typical person in a care home spent just two minutes interacting with staff or other residents over a six-hour period of observation (excluding time spent on care tasks)
- the availability of activities and opportunities for occupation is a major determinant of quality of life, affecting mortality, depression, physical function and behavioural symptoms, but these activities are seldom available.

If the use of drugs can be reduced, there would be an enormous saving in the cost of care of older people. If these savings could be used in the creation of therapeutic outdoor spaces, there would be a great more happy residents and carers.

Enabling people to get outdoors and be active, and in poor weather to be involved in activities that relate to the outside, could make a major contribution to their wellbeing and the cost-effectiveness of their care (see Chapter 9, Activities outside).

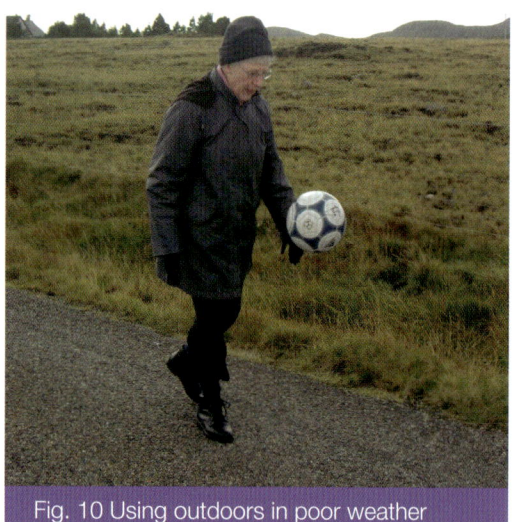

Fig. 10 Using outdoors in poor weather

Key points

- boredom and lack of free access to the outside contribute to challenging behaviour, all too frequently treated with antipsychotic drugs which have been shown to cause severe health problems and yet achieve remarkably few positive results
- the cost of these drugs is enormous and the side effects can lead to dditional medical costs
- how many therapeutic outdoor spaces and increased numbers of staff could this same amount of money provide?

References

Age UK. (2010). *Falls in the over 65s cost NHS £4.6 million a day*. Retrieved from www.ageuk.org.uk/latest-news/archive/cost-of-falls

All-Party Parliamentary Group on Dementia. (2009). *Prepared to care: Challenging the dementia skills gap*. London: All-Party Parliamentary Group on Dementia.

Alimoglu, M.K., & Donmez, L. (2005). Daylight exposure and the other predictors of burnout among nurses in a University Hospital. *International Journal of Nursing Studies, 42*(5), 549-555.

Alzheimer's Society. (2010). *Eating and drinking: Fact sheet*. Retrieved from http://www.alzheimers.org.uk/site/scripts/documents_info.php?documentID=149

Alzheimer's Society. (2007). *Home from home: Quality of care for people with dementia living in care homes*. Retrieved from http://www.alzheimers.org.uk/site/scripts/download_info.php?downloadID=70

Banerjee, S. (2009). *The use of antipsychotic medication for people with dementia: Time for action*. London: Department of Health.

BBC News. (2003). *£1 billion cost of elderly falls*. Retrieved from http://news.bbc.co.uk/1/hi/health/3167005.stm

Beauchemin, K.M., & Hays, P. (1996). Sunny hospital rooms expedite recovery from severe and refractory depressions. *Journal of Affective Disorders, 9*(40), 49–51.

Bischoff-Ferrari, H.A., Dawson-Hughes, B., Staehelin, H.B., Orav, J.E., Stuck, A.E., Theiler, R., & Henschkowski, J. (2009). Fall prevention with supplemental and active forms of vitamin D: A meta-analysis of randomised control trials. *British Medical Journal, 339*: b3692.

Bischoff, H.A., Stähelin, H.B., Dick, W., Akos, R., Knecht, M., Salis, C., & Conzelmann, M. (2003). Effects of vitamin D and calcium supplementation on falls: A randomized controlled trial. *Journal of Bone and Mineral Research, 18*(2), 343-351.

Chapuy, M.C., Pamphile, R., Paris, E., Kempf, C., Schlichting, M., Arnaud, S., & Meunier, P.J. (2002). Combined calcium and vitamin D_3 supplementation in elderly women: Confirmation of reversal of secondary hyperparathyroidism and hip fracture risk: The Decalyos II study. *Osteoporosis International, 13*(3), 257-264.

Cott, J., & Hibbeln, J.R. (2001). Lack of seasonal mood change in Icelanders (letter to the editor). *American Journal of Psychiatry, 158*(2), 328.

Department of Health (England). (2003). *Care homes for older people: National minimum standards*. London: The Stationery Office.

Department of Health (England). (1996). *Strategy statement on physical activity*. London: Department of Health.

Dementia Services Development Centre. (2009). *Food and nutrition for people with dementia*. Stirling: DSDC.

Erickson, K.I., Prakash, R.S., Voss, M.W., Chaddock, L., Hu, L., Morris, K.S., & Kramer, A.F. (2009). Aerobic fitness is associated with hippocampal volume in elderly humans. *Hippocampus, 19*(10), 1030–1039.

Fabrigoule, C., Letenneur, L., Dartigues, J.F., Zarrouk, M., Commenges, D., & Barberger-Gateau, P. (1995). Social and leisure activities and risk of dementia: A prospective longitudinal study. *Journal of the American Geriatrics Society, 43*(5), 485-90.

Farley, K.M.J. & Veitch, J.A. (2001). *A room with a view: A review of the effects of windows on work and well-being: IRC Research Report RR-136*. Ottawa: Institute for Research in Construction.

Fetveit, A., Skerjve, A., & Bjorvatn, B. (2003). Bright light treatment improves sleep in institutionalised elderly: an open trial. *International Journal of Geriatric Psychiatry, 18*(6), 520-526.

Friedman, R., & Tappen, R.M. (1991). The effect of planned walking on communication in Alzheimer's disease. *Journal of the American Geriatrics Society, 39*(7), 650–654.

Galbraith, J., & Westphal, J. (2003). *Therapeutic garden design: Martin Luther Alzheimer Garden* [Juried abstract and presentation]. Charleston, SC: Proceedings of the Council of Educators in Landscape Architecture.

Gorham, E.D., Garland, C.F., Garland, F.C., Grant, W.B., Mohr, S.B., Lipkin, M., & Holick, M.F. (2007). Optimal vitamin D status for colorectal cancer prevention: A quantitative meta-analysis. *American Journal of Preventive Medicine, 32*(3), 210-216.

Jacobs, J., Cohen, A., Rozenburg-Hammerman, R., Azoulay, D., Maaravi, Y., & Stessman, J. (2008). Going outdoors daily predicts long-term functional and health benefits among ambulatory older people. *Journal of Aging and Health, 20*(3), 259-272.

Hartikainen, S., Lönnroos, E. & Louhivuori, K. (2007). Medication as a risk factor for falls: Critical systematic review. *Journal of Gerontology: Medical Sciences, 62A*(10), 1172–1181.

Harper, D.G., Stopa, E.G., McKee, A.C., Satlin, A., Fish, A., & Volicer, L. (2004). Dementia severity and Lewy bodies affect circadian rhythms in Alzheimer disease. *Neurobiology of Aging, 25*(6), 771–781.

Heyn, P., Abreu, B.C., & Ottenbacher, K.J. (2004). The effects of exercise training on elderly persons with cognitive impairment and dementia: A meta-analysis. *Archives of Physical Medicine and Rehabilitation, 85*(10),1694–1704.

Hoe, J., Hancock, G., Livingston, G., & Orrel, M. (2006). Quality of life of people with dementia in residential care homes. *British Journal of Psychiatry, 188*(5), 460-464.

Holick, M.F. (2004). Sunlight and vitamin D for bone health and prevention of autoimmune diseases, cancers, and cardiovascular disease. *American Journal of Clinical Nutrition, 80*(6 suppl), 1678S–1688S.

Holick, M.F. (2006). High prevalence of vitamin D inadequacy and implications for health. *Mayo Clinic Proceedings, 81*(3), 297-29.

Holmberg, S. K. (1997). Evaluation of a clinical intervention for wanderers on a geriatric nursing unit. *Archives of Psychiatric Nursing, 11*(1), 21-28

Joseph, A. (2006). *The impact of light on outcomes in healthcare settings*. Concord, CA: Center for Health Design.

Kaplan, R., & Kaplan, S. (1989). *The experience of nature: A psychological perspective*. Cambridge: Cambridge University Press.

Kirsch, I. (2009). Dump the drugs; as we live longer we face the horrors of Alzheimer's disease – and the very worst kind of treatment for its symptoms. *New Scientist*, October 17, 26.

Kweon, B.S., Sullivan, W.C., & Wiley, A.R. (1998). Green common spaces and the social integration of inner-city adults. *Environment and Behavior, 30*(6), 832-858.

Larson, E.B., Wang, L., Bowen, J.D., McCormick, W.C., Teri, L., Crane, P., & Kukull, W. (2006) Exercise is associated with reduced risk for incident dementia among persons 65 years of age and older. *Annals of Internal Medicine, 144*, 73-81.

Lautenschlager, N.T., Cox, K.L., Flicker, L., Foster, J.K., van Bockxmeer, F.M., Xiao, J., & Almeida, O.P. (2008). Effect of physical activity on cognitive function in older adults at risk for Alzheimer disease: A randomized trial. *Journal of the American Medical Association, 300,* 1027-37.

Leather, P., Pyrgas, M., Beale, D., & Lawrence, C. (1998). Windows in the workplace: Sunlight, view and occupational stress. *Environment and Behaviour, 30*(6),739–762.

Lewy, A.J., Bauer, V.K., Cutler, N.L., Sack, R.L., Ahmed, S., Thomas, K.H., & Jackson, J.M.L. (1998). Morning vs. evening light treatment of patients with winter depression. *Archives of General Psychiatry, 55*(10), 890–896.

Lips, P., Graafmans, W.C., Ooms, M.E., Bezemer, P.D., & Bouter, L.M. (1996). Vitamin D supplementation and fracture incidence in elderly persons: A randomized placebo-controlled trial. *Annals of Internal Medicine, 124*(4), 400-406.

Lovell, B.B., Ancoli-Israel, S., & Gevirtz, R. (1995). Effect of bright light treatment on agitated behavior in institutionalized elderly subjects. *Psychiatry Research, 57*(1), 7–12.

Macdonald, H.M., Mavroeidi, A., Barr, R.J., Black, A.J., Fraser, W.D., & Reid, D.M. (2008). Vitamin D status in postmenopausal women living at higher latitudes in the UK in relation to bone health, overweight, sunlight exposure and dietary vitamin D. *Bone, 42*(5), 996–1003.

McNair, D., Cunningham, C., Pollock, R., & McGuire, B. (2010). *Light and lighting design for people with dementia.* Stirling: DSDC.

Magnússon, A., & Axelsson, J. (1993). The prevalence of seasonal affective disorder is low among descendants of Icelandic emigrants in Canada. *Archives of General Psychiatry, 50*(12), 947-51.

Maller, C., Townsend, M., Pryor, A., Brown, P., & St. Leger, L. (2005). Healthy nature healthy people: 'Contact with nature' as an upstream health promotion intervention for populations. *Health Promotion International, 21*(1), 45-54.

Matsouka, O., Kabitsis, C., Harahousou, Y., & Trigonis, G. (2005). Mood alterations following an indoor and outdoor exercise program in healthy elderly women. *Perceptual and Motor Skills, 100*(3 Pt 1), 707-15.

Medicines and Healthcare Products Regulatory Agency. (2011). *Antipsychotic drugs.* Retrieved from http://www.mhra.gov.uk/Safetyinformation/Generalsafetyinformationandadvice/Product-specificinformationandadvice/Product-specificinformationandadvice-A-F/Antipsychoticdrugs/index.htm

Melton, S. (2005). *Use it don't lose it. New Scientist,* 17 December, 32.

Mental Welfare Commission. (2009). *Remember, I'm still me.* Retrieved from http://reports.mwcscot.org.uk/Visiting_monitoring/RememberImStillMe/Remember_Still_me.aspx [Accessed 19 January 2012]

Mersch, P.P., Middenthorp, H.M., Bouhuys, A.L., Beersma, D.G., & van den Hoofdakker, R.H. (1999). Seasonal affective disorder and latitude: a review of the literature. *Journal of Affective Disorders, 53*(1), 35-48.

Meyer, H.E., Smedshaug, G.B., Kvaavik, E., Falch, J.A., Tverdal, A., & Pedersen J.I. (2002). Can vitamin D supplementation reduce the risk of fracture in the elderly?: A randomized controlled trial. *Journal of Bone and Mineral Research, 17*(4), 709-15.

Milligan, C., Gatrell, A., & Bingley, A. (2004). Cultivating health: Therapeutic landscapes and older people in northern England. *Social Science and Medicine, 58*(9), 1781-1793.

Mind. (2007). *Ecotherapy: the green agenda for mental health.* London: Mind.

Molin, J., Mellerup, E., Bollwig, T., Scheike, T., & Dam, H. (1996). The influence of climate on development of winter depression. *Journal of Affective Disorders, 37*(2-3), 151-155.

Mooney, P., & Nicell, P.L. (1992). The importance of external environments for Alzheimer's residents: Effective care and risk management. *Healthcare Management Forum, 5*(2), 23-9.

Moore, E.O. (1981). A prison environment's effect on health care service demands. *Journal of Environmental Systems, 11*(1), 17-34.

Namazi, K.H., & Johnson, B.D. (1992). Pertinent autonomy for residents with dementias: Modification of the physical environment to enhance independence. *American Journal of Alzheimer's Disease and Other Dementias, 7*(1), 16-21.

NHS Choices. (2010). *Seasonal affective disorder.* Retrieved from http://www.nhs.uk/conditions/seasonal-affective-disorder/Pages/Introduction.aspx

NHS Choices. (2010). *Preventing urinary incontinence*. Retrieved from http://www.nhs.uk/conditions/incontinence-urinary/pages/prevention.aspx

Newton, J. (2007). *Wellbeing and the natural environment: A brief overview of the evidence.* Bath: University of Bath, Wellbeing in Developing Countries (WeD) Research Group.

National Institute for Health and Clinical Excellence. (2008). *Occupational therapy interventions and physical activity interventions to promote the mental wellbeing of older people in primary care and residential care.* London: NICE.

Osteoporosis Australia. (2011). *Preventing osteoporosis.* Retrieved from http://www.osteoporosis.org.au/about/about-osteoporosis/preventing-osteoporosis-vitamin-d/

Oudshoorn, C., Mattace-Raso, F.U.S., van der Velde, N., Colin, E.M., & van der Cammen, T.J.M. (2008). Higher serum vitamin D_3 levels are associated with better cognitive test performance in patients with Alzheimer's disease. *Dementia and Geriatric Cognitive Disorders, 25*(6), 539-543.

Peterlik, M., & Cross, H.S. (2009). Vitamin D and calcium insufficiency-related chronic diseases: Molecular and cellular pathophysiology. *European Journal of Clinical Nutrition, 63*(12),1377-86.

Potkin, S.G., Zetin, M., Stamenkovic, V., Kripke, V., & Bunney, W.E. (1986). Seasonal affective disorder: Prevalence varies with latitude and climate. *Clinical Neuropharmacology, 9* (Supp.4). 181-183.

Rappe, E., & Kivelä, S.L. (2005). Effects of garden visits on long-term care residents as related to depression. *HortTechnology, 15*(2), 298-303.

Rappe, E., Kivelä, S.L. & Rita, H. (2006). Visiting outdoor green environments positively impacts self rated health among older people in long-term care. *HortTechnology, 16*(1), 55.

Raynes, N., Clark, H., & Beecham, J. (Eds.) (2006). The report of the Older People's Inquiry into 'That Bit of Help'. Retrieved from http://www.jrf.org.uk/sites/files/jrf/9781859354612.pdf

Riemersma-van der Lek, R.F., Swaab, D.F.,Twisk, J., Hol, E.M., Hoogendijk, W.J.G., & Van Someren, E.J.W. (2008). Effect of bright light and melatonin on cognitive and noncognitive functioning elderly residents of group care facilities: A randomized controlled trial. *Journal of the American Medical Association, 299*(22), 2642-2655.

Shochat, T., Martin, J., Marler, M., & Ancoli-Israel, S. (2000). Illumination levels in nursing home patients: Effects on sleep and activity rhythms. *Journal of Sleep Research, 9*(4), 373-379.

Scottish Government. (2011). Older people living in the community: Nutritional needs, barriers and interventions: A literature review. Retrieved from http://www.scotland.gov.uk/Publications/2009/12/07102032/0

Scuffham, P., Chaplin, S., & Legood, R. (2003). Incidence and costs of unintentional falls in older people in the United Kingdom. *Journal of Epidemiology and Community Health, 57*(9), 740–744.

Scherder, E.J.A., Bogen, T, Eggermont, L.H., Hamers J.P., & Swaab, D.F. (2010). The more physical inactivity, the more agitation in dementia. *International Psychogeriatrics, 22*(8), 1203.

Smith, M.R., Revell, V.L., & Eastman, C.I. (2009). Phase advancing the human circadian clock with blue-enriched polychromatic light. *Sleep Medicine, 10*(3), 287-294.

Stenzelius, K. (2005). *Urinary and faecal incontinence among older women and men in relation to other health complaints, quality of life and dependency.* Lund: Department of Health Sciences, Faculty of Medicine, Lund University, Sweden. Bulletin No. 20 from the Unit of Caring Sciences.

Tonello, G. (2008). Seasonal affective disorder: Lighting research and environmental psychology. *Lighting Research and Technology, 41*(3), 103-110.

Ulrich, R.S. (1984). View through a window may influence recovery from surgery. *Science, 224*(4647), 420-421.

Ulrich, R.S. (1991). Wellness by design: Psychologically supportive patient surroundings. *Group Practice Journal, 40*(4), 10-19.

Ulrich, R.S. (2001). Effects of healthcare environmental design on medical outcomes. In A. Dilani, (Ed.) *Design and health: Proceedings of the Second International Conference on Health and Design.* Stockholm: SvenskByggtjanst, 49-59.

Van der Wielen, R.P., Lowik, M.R., van den Berg, H., de Groot, L.C., Haller, J., Moreiras, O., & van Staveren, W.A. (1995). Serum vitamin D concentrations among elderly people in Europe. *Lancet, 346*(8969), 207-10.

Van Someren, E., Mirmiran, M., & Swaab, D.F. (1993). Non-pharmacological treatment of sleep and wake disturbances in aging and Alzheimer's disease: Chronobiological perspectives. *Behavioural Brain Research, 57*(2), 235-253.

Velarde, M.D., Fry, G., & Tveit, M. (2007). Health effects of viewing landscapes: Landscape types in environmental psychology. *Urban Forestry and Urban Greening, 6*(4), 199–212.

Venning, G. (2005). Recent developments in vitamin D deficiency and muscle weakness among elderly people. *British Medical Journal, 330*(7490), 524-6.

Verderber, S. (1986). Dimensions of person-window transactions in the hospital environment. *Environment and Behaviour, 18*(4), 450.

Verghese, J., Lipton, R.B., Katz, M.J., Hall, C.B., Derby, C.A., Kuslansky, G., & Buschke, H. (2003). Leisure activities and the risk of dementia in the elderly. *New England Journal of Medicine, 348*(25), 2508-2516.

Wang, T.J., Pencina, M.J., Booth, S.L., Jacques, P.F., Ingelsson, E., Lanier, K., & Vasan, R.S. (2008). Vitamin D deficiency and risk of cardiovascular disease. *Circulation, 117*(4), 503-11.

Walch, J.M., Rabin, B.S., Day, R., Williams, J.N., Choi, K., & Kang, J.D. (2005). The effect of sunlight on postoperative analgesic medication usage: A prospective study of spinal surgery patients. *Psychosomatic Medicine, 67*(1), 156–163.

Whall, A.L., Black, M.E., Groh, C.J., Yankou, D.J., Kupferschmid, B.J., & Foster, N.L. (1997). The effect of natural environments upon agitation and aggression in late stage dementia patients. *American Journal of Alzheimer's Disease and Other Dementias, 12*(5), 216-220.

Wharton, B., & Bishop, N. (2003). Rickets. *Lancet, 362*(9393), 1389–4000.

Wilkins, C.H., Sheline, Y.I., Roe, C.M., Birge, S.J., & Morris, J.C. (2006). Vitamin D deficiency is associated with low mood and worse cognitive performance in older adults. *American Journal of Geriatric Psychiatry, 14*(12), 1032–40.

Case Study 1
The living garden at the family life center

Clare Cooper Marcus

The Living Garden is at the Family Life Center in Grand Rapids, Michigan, USA. This is a day centre for people with Alzheimer's disease, other forms of dementia, schizophrenia, multiple sclerosis, Parkinson's, or Huntington's Disease, and who live at home with their families. The oldest patient is 90; the youngest is 36.

The garden was designed by Martha Tyson of Douglas Hills Associates in Evanston, Illinois.

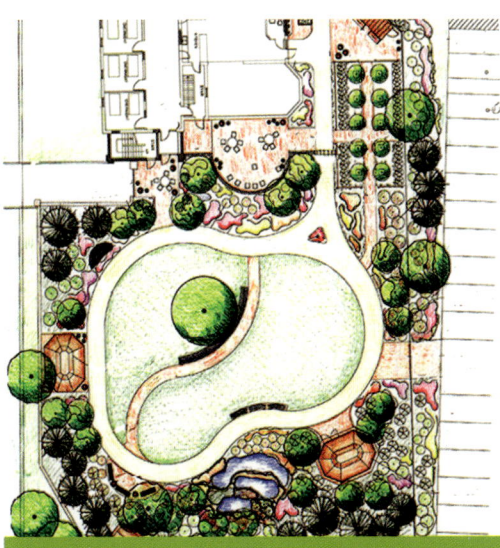

Fig. 11 The garden layout (north is to the top) (refer to appendix 1 on page 211 for enlarged version)

There are two main components to the half-acre site: the main strolling and viewing garden and the working garden.

The working garden is a rectangular area, east of the building with raised beds and trellises for horticultural therapy, a potting area with shade and a sink, a garden shed, a small orchard, a butterfly garden, and an umbrella-shaded area for seating near the atrium entry door.

The larger component, the main garden, is entered via an arbour from the working garden and consists of lawns, paths, perennial beds, gazebos, a waterfall and pond, and various places to sit.

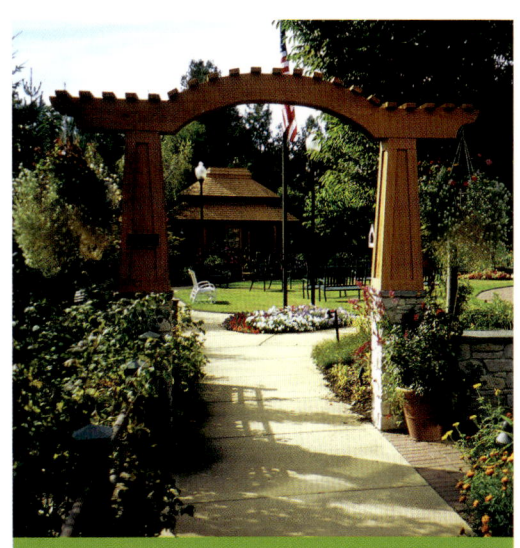

Fig. 12 An arch marks the transition from the working garden to the strolling garden. A view to a gazebo provides a destination point

Founded in 1991, the Family Life Center is a healthcare facility housed in what was once a convent. A dining/activity room and a large, glass-roofed atrium have views and access to the garden. Also overlooking the garden is a large conservatory, heavily used in colder weather for indoor horticultural activities.

The Family Life Center has spacious views to the garden and entries to it from the atrium and the dining room. The doors remain unlocked during the day.

This ensures that people with dementia can see it and have easy access to it. Some patients at the Family Life Center, who do not need to be watched, constantly and freely go back and forth from the building to the garden. But many do need constant care and they are accompanied on garden visits twice a day.

The design of this garden works extraordinarily well for scheduled activities organised by the staff. There are chairs in a semicircle on the lawn for conversation; a large gazebo (The Garden House) which is wired for lighting, fans, and music and which has comfortable peripheral seating; a flat lawn for croquet; a concrete path for wheelchair 'races'; access to water, raised beds, tables, and a potting shed for gardening. "The garden also works very, very well for physical therapy staff working with people who have had a stroke or need help walking," says Sherry Gaines, the program and activity manager. "It has a wonderfully calming effect on people who are agitated. The facility has a ratio of staff to customers of one to five, and when volunteers and interns are factored in, it is two to one."

The design of the garden allows users to see the layout at a glance and offers a simple circular or figure-of-eight circulation system. The main garden has a clear perimeter path of tinted concrete bisected by a curving brick pathway, thus allowing patients (who tend to be restless) a number of alternatives for moving around the garden. One trip around the six-foot-wide loop path provides a 300-foot route with changing details but no anxiety-provoking choices in way finding, as too many choices can lead to confusion, agitation, and even aggression. The entry arbour, a flagpole, a grotto with a statue of the Virgin Mary (50% of the centre's users are Roman Catholic), and bird feeders hanging from trees provide landmarks to aid in orientation. Places such as the working garden and the lawn provide gathering places encouraging physical and social activity. Two wooden gazebos (the Garden House and the Tea House) provide destination points and comfortable settings for scheduled activities. The building, walls, fence, and peripheral plantings provide edges defining the space.

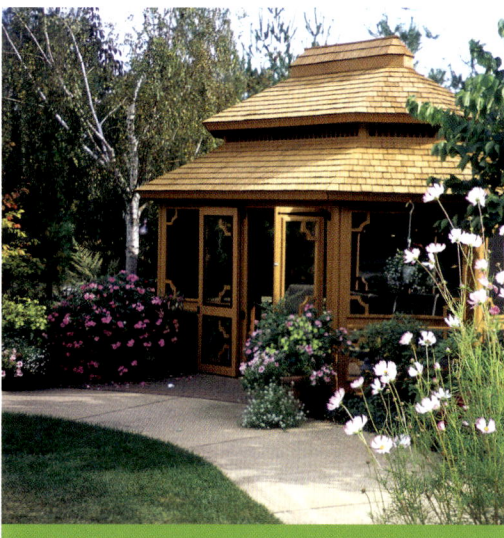

Fig. 13 A gazebo provides a popular setting for events programmed by the staff such as singing and music. It is wired for sound, and has bug screens and fans so that it is comfortable on summer evenings

The garden has plenty of seating where people, alone or in a group, can find a place to sit for a while. There is seating inside the two gazebos; three comfortable gliders (swinging seats) alongside the perimeter path; patio seating with tables and umbrellas outside the conservatory; a curved stone seating wall; and numerous movable chairs scattered throughout the garden. The only unattractive seating consists of three marble slabs inscribed 'In Loving Memory'. In the gardens of nursing homes, hospices, and Alzheimer's facilities, family members often want to dedicate a tree, a flower border, an arbour, or a bench in memory of someone who has died. But one has to wonder how this feels for the living, reminded of death each time they walk in the garden?

The garden is visually enclosed so that people who might want to 'find their way home' are not exposed to tempting or frustrating views of 'the outside world'. It is bounded on the north side by the building and conservatory; on the west and south sides by high walls of mellow, buff-coloured brick; and on the east side (facing the parking area) by a steel fence. The walls and fences are virtually invisible, screened by a variety of trees – mostly evergreen – so that even in winter, the boundaries of the garden are blurred. One exception is a steel gate that allows entry from the parking lot for service personnel and people arriving for an event in the garden.

While the boundaries of the garden are marked by moderately tall trees stepping down in height to shrubs (lilac, roses, rhododendrons, and dogwood) and perennial borders, the centre of the garden is open lawn that is in turn bounded by the circular concrete path. The slightly mounded western lawn is partially bounded by a stone seating-wall (permitting transfer from a wheelchair onto the grass) and punctuated by a beech tree and a playhouse with steps and a slide for visiting grandchildren.

On a visit in early October, over 25 varieties of flowers were in bloom.

Staff use these flowers to stimulate conversation about the seasons, next year's garden, and memories of flowers from childhood; in dried form, for arts and crafts in the winter. Star jasmine and tobacco flowers smell good and the feathery blooms of amaranthus and the seedheads of coneflower tempt visitors to reach out and touch them. Colour and smell stimulate parts of the brain not reached by 'intellectual' activities, and even those with little cognitive ability seem able to sense the tranquility and beauty of a garden on a precognitive, affective basis. It also facilitates talking about growth, blossoming, maturity, decay, and renewal.

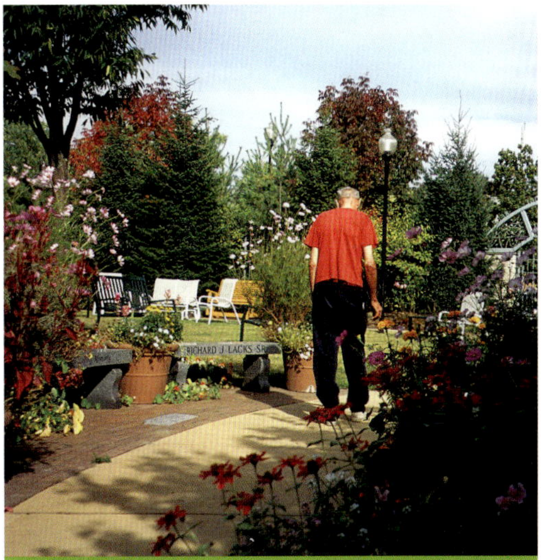

Fig. 14 A meandering figure-of-eight path offers a pleasant, 90-metre route for those who are prone to frequent 'wandering'

In one corner of the garden, there is a semi-private staff patio, providing an essential respite from the stress of work and the demands of patients. Though few of the staff leave this patio, they still have an expansive view of the garden, its colours and innumerable shades of green, the sounds of birdsong and breezes moving through the trees. All of these have a remarkable effect on reducing stress, as researchers such as Roger Ulrich have discovered, even in as short a time as five to ten minutes.

Perhaps the only element in this garden that doesn't work so well is the waterfall at southern end of the garden.

The sound of falling water adds a soothing touch, but to keep some residents from getting into the water, the pond and waterfall had to be screened from view by shrubs.

To understand the use of gardens for individuals with Alzheimer's, we need more post-occupancy evaluation studies such as that conducted by Charlotte Grant at the Living Garden as part of her PhD dissertation. She mapped activities in this garden for 10-minute periods at 20-minute intervals from 9am to 4pm during five days of observation in mid-September 2001. Of those using the garden, 45% were day clients, 38% were staff (paid and volunteer) working with clients, and 17% were maintenance staff. Of the day clients in the garden, 41% were walking, sitting, or talking on the loop path; 27% were in the Garden House (gazebo) participating in organised activities; 20% were in the working garden; and 11% sitting in the Tea House (a gazebo on the west side of the garden). A large number of staff was observed on the patio reserved for their use.

PART 2 CIVIL LIBERTY AND CULTURAL CONSIDERATIONS

Chapter 3
Going out – rights and responsibilities

Donald Lyons

In 2006, the National Association for the Provision of Activities for Older People (NAPA) raised an important issue that was widely reported in the media. Prisoners in the UK must have at least one hour of fresh air each day. People with dementia in care establishments often get much less access to fresh air than this. Do they not have a right to at least as much fresh air as a prisoner?

The Mental Welfare Commission for Scotland exists to safeguard the rights and welfare of people with mental disorders, including dementia. We visit individuals in a variety of care settings, can investigate deficiencies in care and give advice on applying best legal and ethical principles to people's care and treatment. We decided to look into whether people with dementia had access to fresh air when we visited hospitals and care homes. All too often, we found that they did not.

We looked into the care of people with dementia in NHS continuing care wards in Scotland in 2007 in *Older and Wiser,* (Mental Welfare Commission for Scotland, 2007). Of 16 wards we visited, only nine had access to enclosed garden areas. Seven of these were designed to be suitable for people with dementia. We looked in detail at care plans for 29 people across these 16 wards. We found that only 12 of those 29 people had been outside during the previous three months. Nine people had not been out at all since they were admitted.

When we looked at care homes for people with dementia, we found a similar picture. In our joint report with the Scottish Commission for the Regulation of Care, *Remember, I'm Still Me* (2009), we found that just over half of a sample of 30 care homes had safe and accessible gardens.

They were not necessarily 'dementia-friendly' and not necessarily used. Over half of the people whose personal plans we studied never went out. The few people who went out regularly were relying on family and friends to take them out.

We found that care staff did not think creatively enough about the use of people's own money. There are many legal ways to use people's money for their benefit, even after they lose capacity to manage their own money. Care staff were often unaware of the options available. While they have the duty to provide much of the person's care from within their resources, they should look at ways to use people's own money to improve their quality of life. This could include arranging trips to places of interest for individuals or groups of people with a common interest.

We found some good practice. Some care homes helped people to use their own money to pay for taxis to places of interest and used money from fundraising to organise outings. Recently, we found a care home where there were several male residents with dementia who used to enjoy car maintenance. The staff put an old car in a secure garden area where the men could enjoy tinkering with it. Unfortunately, we found that good practice was the exception. Far too many people with dementia in care establishments were denied access to outside facilities and to the community.

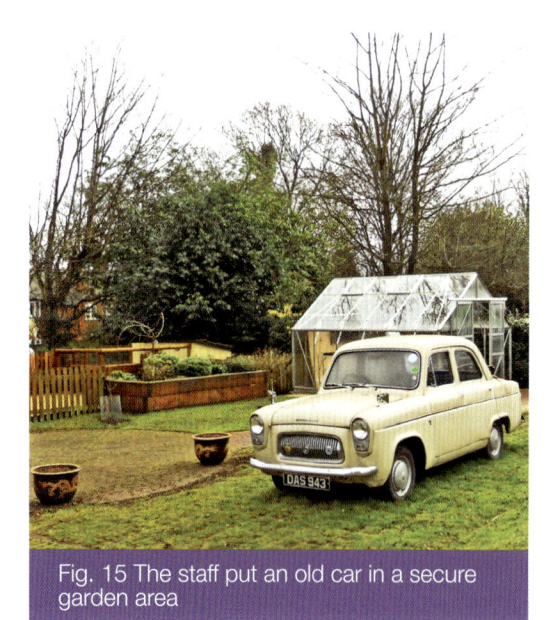

Fig. 15 The staff put an old car in a secure garden area

Why is this important? Do people with dementia have the right to fresh air and activity? Do service providers have the duty to provide this? Our reading of human rights law says yes. Also, the principles of legislation on mental health and incapacity in Scotland impose duties on care providers. While I use Scots law as an example of rights-based legislation, the approach we advocate is consistent with human rights legislation and is, we argue, no more than people with dementia deserve and should expect.

Human rights law confers rights on individuals and duties on public authorities. Everybody has the right to liberty under Article 5 of the European Convention on Human Rights (ECHR). While "persons of unsound mind" may be deprived of their liberty, this must be achieved using a procedure prescribed by law and the person must have the right of appeal to a competent court. Surely a person who is deprived of fresh air is being deprived of liberty to some degree? The same argument applies to people who used to enjoy activities within their community and are now prevented from doing so. If people have the capability to enjoy being outside and active, and are prevented from doing so, this would not be compatible with Article 5.

Article 8 of ECHR asserts the right to privacy, dignity and family life. Is it dignified to be confined to indoor life? Are people being prevented from enjoying activities they might still be capable of enjoying with family and friends? Our findings suggest that care providers may not be providing care that affords people this right.

The Nuffield Council on Bioethics (2009) published a report on a wide variety of ethical issues in the care of people with dementia. Among other issues, the report considered the issue of restraint. Care establishments for people with dementia need to consider restraint in its broadest sense. It is more than direct physical or mechanical restraint; it also involves locks, passive alarms, sensors and surveillance. The report identifies general issues that must be considered within the legal frameworks in place. It recommends that all UK regulators should provide guidance similar to the Mental Welfare Commission for Scotland's *Rights, Risks and Limits to Freedom* (2006).

In Scotland, human rights are enshrined in incapacity legislation, not least in its principles. Where a person lacks capacity to decide on aspects of their own welfare, any intervention must comply with the principles of the Adults with Incapacity (Scotland) Act 2000. These principles provide an excellent guide as to how to care for the person with dementia.

The first principle is one of benefit. Any intervention must benefit the person. Fresh air, activity and exercise benefit all of us. When physical or mental ill-health restricts the ability of the person to get access to fresh air and exercise, there are duty of care services to intervene for the person's benefit. This means helping the person to get the benefit of fresh air.

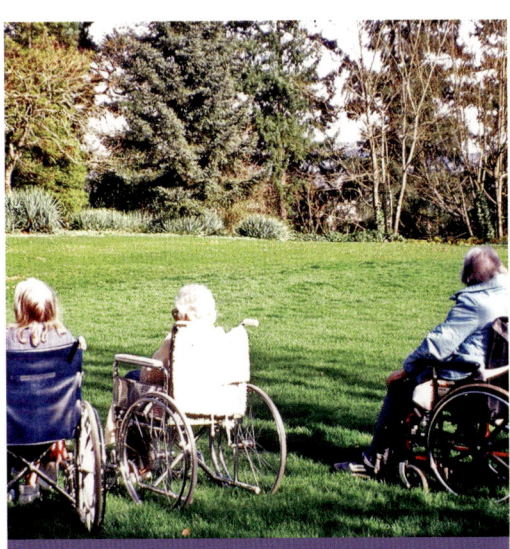

Fig. 16 This means helping the person to get the benefit of fresh air

Secondly, any intervention must be the least restrictive of the person's freedom. Where the person with dementia loses judgement, it may be less safe for him/her to go out. There is then a danger that care becomes over-restrictive, either by confining the person to his/her own home or by admission to a care facility.

Where this happens, care services have a duty to restrict freedom as little as possible. They must make sure that the person is able to enjoy the freedom of being outside in a way that is safe.

The person's past and present wishes and feelings must be taken into account. This is critical to helping the person achieve the benefit of being outside. Care staff must be familiar with the person's interests, likes and dislikes and tailor the care they provide accordingly. In both reports, *Older and Wiser* and *Remember and I'm Still Me*, we found too little use of life stories. Care was 'one size fits all' and not geared towards the person as an individual. Outings and activities are of greatest value when they comply with this principle.

There is a duty, where reasonable and practical, to take account of the views of those who know the person well. Again, information from reliable informants will help decide the best outings and activity as it is based on their knowledge of what is likely to be of most benefit.

Finally, there is a duty imposed on some people under the Act (but good for all to bear in mind) to help the person use existing skills and develop new skills. For people with dementia, retaining existing skills, abilities and interests is crucial to good care. Where this involves outdoor activities that the person used to enjoy, care staff should do all they can to help the person maintain that interest.

Although following these principles is mandatory in Scotland, I recommend them as a framework for the care of people with dementia wherever they are and whatever the local legislative framework says. By applying these principles to the issue of fresh air and exercise, it is clear that people with dementia have a right to expect this.

Those who provide care have a duty to meet this expectation.

It can be difficult to provide this level of care. Poor design of care environments, lack of access to garden space and constraints on staff time mean that care providers cannot give people with dementia the time out of the unit that they would like to. Our findings demonstrate this and we think that everyone needs to work to improve people with dementia getting access to outside space and stimulation.

Action needed

It is wrong that people with dementia get little access to outside space and activity. They have the right to get this access. We all have a responsibility to make sure they get that right. The key points that follow show that people with dementia, carers, independent advocates, care providers, care regulators and governments all have a part to play.

Key points

- people with dementia should make advance statements about their wishes; these could include records of the sort of activities that they enjoy and a desire to continue these wherever practicable

- friends and relatives can help by providing support for outings where possible and by expecting more of care establishments

- care providers must remember that activity and getting out are central to the person's care and not an optional extra; care plans must reflect this and must record the way that outside activity benefits the person

- external inspection is necessary; people with dementia, especially if there are no close friends or family, may not be able to assert their own rights and need someone to check they are having their needs met and their rights respected

- independent advocacy is a right in Scotland for anyone with a mental disorder; even if the person cannot instruct an advocate, non-instructed advocacy, individual or group, can be very helpful in raising issues like this with care providers

- governments must make sure that they prescribe standards of care that include access to fresh air and outside activities

- we all have a role to play as a society; we are living longer and more likely to develop dementia ourselves. Would we like to spend all our time inside a care establishment? We should do all we can to welcome, encourage and assist people with dementia to remain involved in our communities.

References

Mental Welfare Commission for Scotland. (2007). *Older and wiser*. Retrieved from http://www.mwcscot.org.uk/nmsruntime/saveasdialog.asp?IID=936&sID=720

Nuffield Council on Bioethics. (2009). *Dementia: Ethical issues.* Retrieved from http://www.nuffieldbioethics.org/dementia

Scottish Commission for the Regulation of Care. (2009). *Remember, I'm still me*. Retrieved from http://www.mwcscot.org.uk/web/FILES/Publications/CC__MWC_joint_report.pdf

Scottish Executive. (2000). *Adults with Incapacity (Scotland) Act*. Retrieved from http://www.hmso.gov.uk/legislation/scotland/acts2000/20000004.htm

Further reading

Great Britain. Parliament (1998). *Human Rights Act.1998*. Retrieved from http://www.opsi.gov.uk/ACTS/acts1998/ukpga_19980042_en_1

Mental Welfare Commission for Scotland. (2006). *Rights, risks and limits to freedom.* Retrieved from http://reports.mwcscot.org.uk/web/FILES/Frredom_restriction_restraint/Rights_Risks.pdf

National Association for the Provision of Activities for Older People. (NAPA). Retrieved from http://www.napa-activities.co.uk/

To find out more about the work of the Mental Welfare Commission for Scotland, visit http://www.mwcscot.org.uk

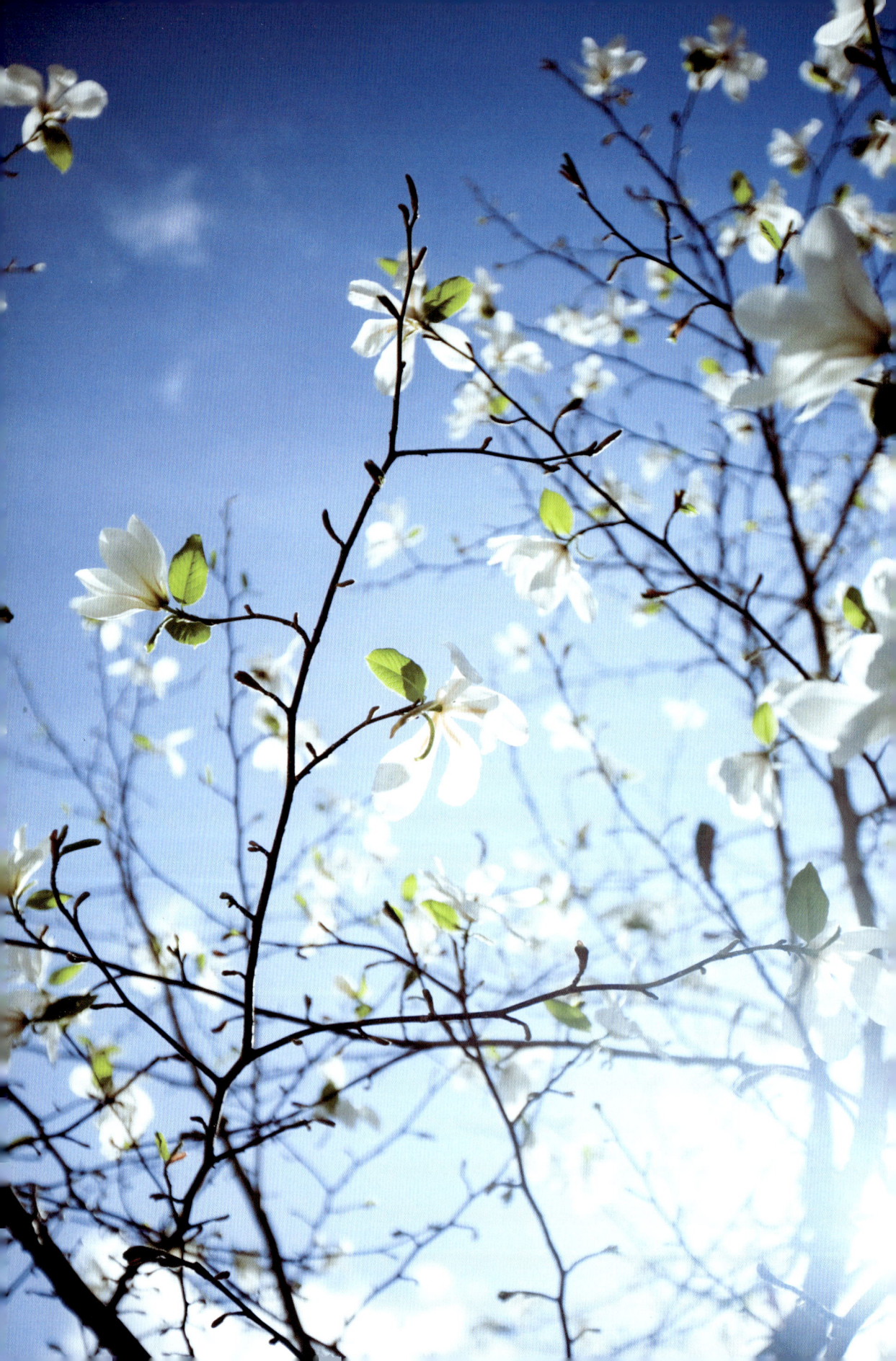

Case Study 2
The gardens at Plaisir Villa Ichikawa

Yuji Okubo

Green roof and façade greening in Japan

Securing green spaces within Japan's major cities and suburbs is problematic. As a result, there is insufficient area within which to grow trees, grass and flowers, and the problem of the 'heat-island' phenomenon[8] grows evermore serious year after year. Green roofs improve the urban environment and prevent buildings from retaining excess heat, and so demand for greening is heightening yearly. In Japan, the total national green area on rooftops and walls increased roughly tenfold between the years 2000 and 2005, and green roofing continues to expand primarily among major corporate and government buildings. On the other hand, the spread of green roofing among multi-tenant and multi-unit apartment buildings has lagged behind due to the sizeable burdens that start-up costs and maintenance impose.

With green roofing becoming obligatory in the Tokyo metropolitan area in 2001, local authorities have also recently endorsed green roofing and roof garden installations. Within major cities and suburbs, the 'Green Roof Grant-in-Aid' has been set up to encourage the green roofing of buildings, and the number of local authorities providing partial coverage of construction costs appears to be on the increase. The upper limit to these grants for a single building is roughly 500,000 yen (US $6400), though apparently applications for grants are increasing year by year.

Recently, the number of nursing homes constructing green roofs and rooftop gardens has also started to increase gradually. Rooftop gardens have become an important element in residential care, particularly for the nursing homes of major cities, as they allow elderly persons who have difficulty going outdoors to have some gentle contact with greenery, and are useful as healing spaces and for horticultural therapy.

Why green roof and roof gardens have increased

Reasons for the recent increase in green roof installations:

- root-resistant countermeasures are being administered so as to prevent root-damage to buildings
- it has become possible to secure water storage and a drainage layer to heighten the soil's air-permeability
- lightweight soil has been developed that is easy to use and puts less strain on buildings
- grant-in-aid systems for green roofing have been established.

These multiple factors have made the installation of roof gardens possible.

However, there are several hurdles relating to the maintenance and management of rooftop gardens that must be overcome. The nursing homes and group homes that I visited unanimously complained of the difficulties involved in maintaining and managing rooftop gardens.

---

8 The urban heat island phenomenon traps heat in thermal mass like concrete and black roads, which absorb, store and then re-emit this heat to the urban air at night. Temperatures of urban air domes can range up to 10-16C (50-60F) warmer than the surrounding countryside. Ref: http://www.urban-climate-energy.com

These difficulties were, more specifically, issues of who would care for the plants and how such costs would be covered. Of the facilities I visited, those that were overcoming such issues were either large-scale nursing homes which have more than a hundred staff, fee-charging homes, or homes in even a small-scale, yet able to secure volunteers to assist with horticulture.

Though a comparatively small-scale example, at this point I will introduce the case of Plaisir Villa Ichikawa which boasts a splendid Japanese-style garden and rooftop garden.

Japanese-style garden of Plaisir Villa Ichikawa

Plaisir Villa Ichikawa is about 20 minutes away from Tokyo in Ichikawa Suwada of Chiba Prefecture. Suwada, where the home is located, is an historic town having formerly served the region as a political and cultural hub. As a result, many historic artefacts (buildings, temples and literary inscriptions) can still be found close to the home, as well as many high schools and universities.

Plaisir Villa Ichikawa was constructed in 2005 as a fee-charging nursing home totally outfitted with individual rooms.

The home is a three-storey reinforced concrete structure, which houses 60 residents of which around 20 residents currently require care for dementia.

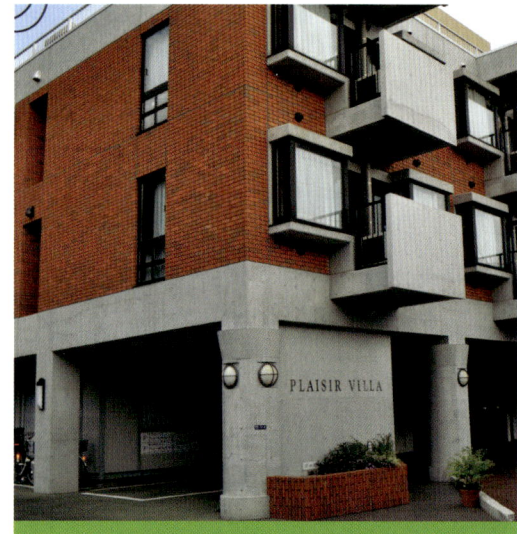

Fig. 17 The home is a three-storey reinforced concrete structure, which houses 60 residents of which around 20 residents currently require care for dementia

One of the wonderful aspects of the institution is that it is home to a garden and rooftop garden created by Hirokazu Kaku of the Japan Branch of the Royal Horticultural Society. Once through the entranceway, the lobby opens out before you and leads through to a combined restaurant and multi-purpose hall. The hall overlooks a beautiful Japanese-style garden that makes use of green slopes.

ROOF GARDEN

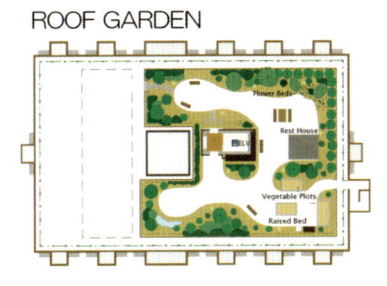

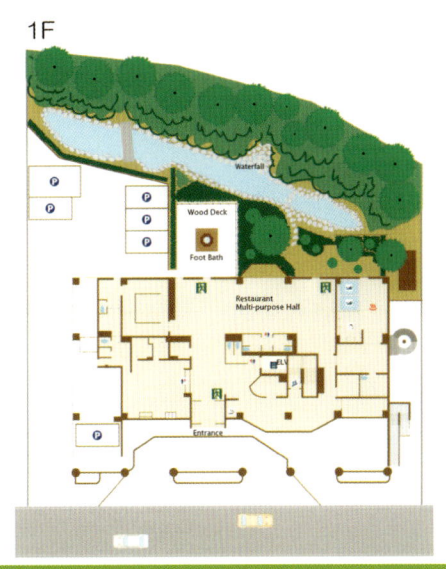

1F

Fig. 18 The garden layout (refer to appendix 1 on page 212 for enlarged version)

Fig. 19 Rehabilitation using the footbath is performed every morning

The garden is accessible from the hall, as there is no boundary between the two, and setting foot onto the wooden decking outside, one can feel the colours of the all-seasons garden in one's very skin. The deck is also installed with a footbath, and the sight of the turning leaves and snow-scenes can be enjoyed during the cold of autumn and winter while warming ones feet in hot water. The footbath stimulates blood flow, and has a rehabilitative effect while relaxing the spirit. Rehabilitation using the footbath is performed every morning.

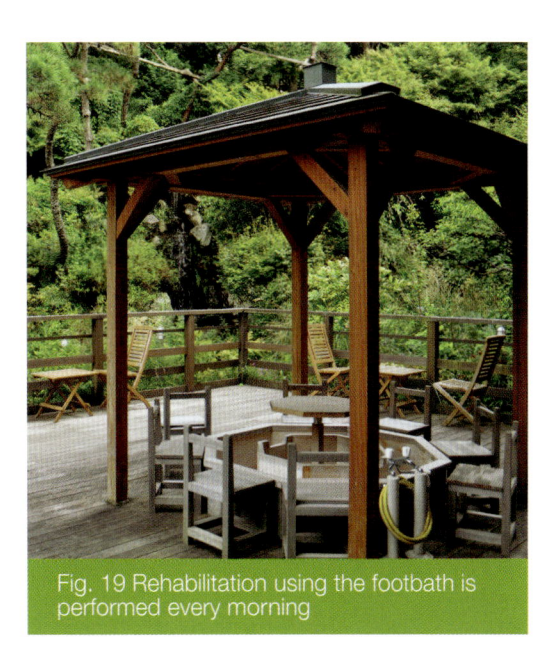

A stream about one metre in width flows through the centre of the garden, into which water pours from a waterfall constructed on a green slope, about 5 metres high. Surprisingly, this artificial waterfall was created and appreciated by the owner who formerly lived on the land. The waterfall circulates water to the stream, and provides oxygen to the vividly coloured koi carp therein. The feeling the view instills is truly akin to that of gazing at a Kyoto garden.

The rooftop garden of Plaisir Villa Ichikawa

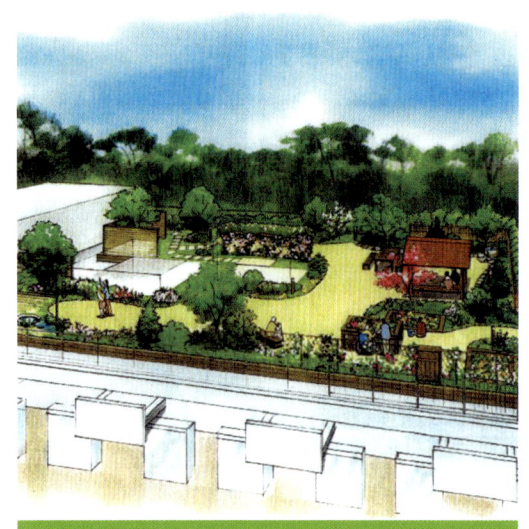

Fig. 20 The rooftop garden

The area of rooftop garden managed on the roof of the home even now is approximately 500m². I venture to say 'even now' because there are many facilities that do not manage their rooftop garden after its initial construction, however splendid it may be. I saw many facilities while gathering material for this book, but saw few that were being adequately managed and maintained. I sense that budgeting for the costs of garden management and maintenance is particularly problematic for long-term care insurance facilities. While I myself am a manager of a care insurance home, securing a budget to manage and maintain a garden is very difficult.

Even among such facilities as these, those that are comparatively well managed are those managed and maintained by horticulturalist volunteers, home staff and able-bodied residents.

At Plaisir Villa Ichikawa, management of the garden is outsourced to a maintenance company, though students from a nearby school for the disabled also volunteer for horticultural work. Though there are some costs involved, maintenance twice a month is indispensable so as to avoid the garden falling into disrepair, which would harm the image of the home and have an unsettling effect on residents.

Since the owner employed a landscaping firm to consult with from the initial phases of planning the garden, a 'true-to-the-concept' and ideal garden and rooftop garden were created. The rooftop garden is clearly differentiated as a section created for ornamental purposes and a section for residents and staff to grow flowers and vegetables.

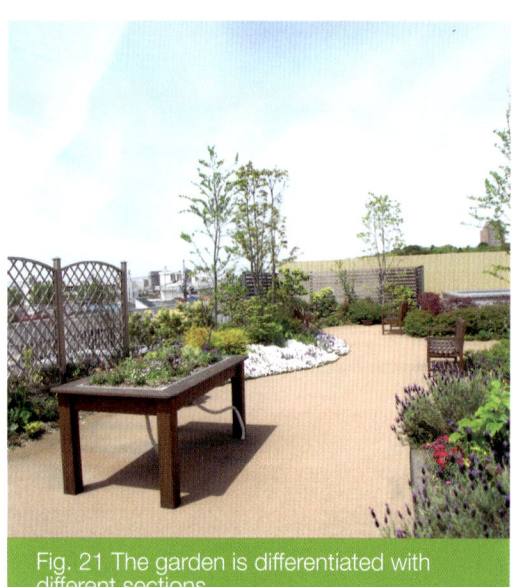

Fig. 21 The garden is differentiated with different sections

As can be seen from the photographs, raised beds have been placed in the garden so that residents can even work from wheelchairs, and on the edge of which are vegetable plots so that seasonal vegetables can be harvested. Of course, such horticultural work is carried out systematically throughout the year according to various programs. Similarly, in the ornamental section of the garden, flowers bloom throughout the seasons, instilling a feeling of peace in residents and helping them to have a sense of the different seasons. A quarter of the entire rooftop garden can be managed by residents. The pavement on which residents walk is well drained, and is reassuringly made from rubber chips in case any of the elderly were to have a fall.

The flowerbeds are not surrounded by raised kerbs, which makes planting easier for those in wheelchairs, and they have the look of borderless, natural flowerbeds. There are no special measures in place to provide protection from the wind and rain, though there is good drainage and the structure prevents the collection of excess moisture. Watering is carried out regularly by an automatic water-sprinkler system.

Gazing at the rooftop garden against the background of the green slopes, the scenery overlaps and is well integrated, which creates a sense of depth greater than the actual area. This is precisely the reason it is known as the garden in the sky.

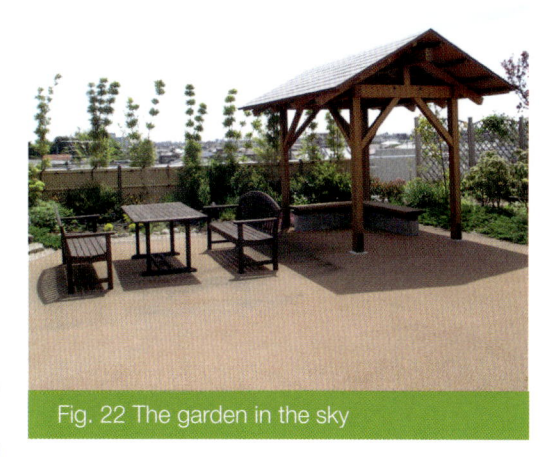

Fig. 22 The garden in the sky

The concept of the gardens

Mr Hirokazu Kaku, who designed the home's gardens and rooftop garden, describes the planning concept as follows:

"The Japanese garden and rooftop garden – named 'the garden in the sky' – make effective use of local natural resources. They were not created simply to be appreciated and enjoyed, but also as a space to be used and enjoyed. I hope that the garden becomes a place for practising horticultural well-being, and one that is enjoyed using all five senses through actually touching the earth, while planting, cultivating and harvesting flowers and crops. I hope that residents will draw energy from the plants, and that they will become healthy in body and spirit. I think that it will be a communal space where residents and their families can have a relaxing time amidst the flowers and greenery."

I could see that the garden was both created for and is currently being used in a manner true to this concept.

Events at the roof garden and the kinds of flowers and vegetables

In the roof garden, seasonal seedlings are planted and vegetables are harvested by the residents, their families and staff together. Various events are also held using the rooftop garden's blooming flowers. Around 25 residents – primarily those with dementia – participate in these events.

The main events that use the rooftop garden and its blooming flowers are as below:

- **April:** planting flower and vegetable seedlings
- **June:** flower arrangement
- **August:** making fans from pressed flowers
- **November:** planting tulips and pansies
- **December:** making Christmas wreaths
- **February:** flower arrangement.

Below are the main types of flowers and vegetables planted in the Plaisir Villa Ichikawa rooftop garden:

- **seasonal flowers:** snapdragon, scarlet sage, pansy, geranium, blue salvia, tulip, etc
- **seasonal vegetables:** lettuce, cucumber, aubergine, tomatoes, spinach, parsley, peas, red and yellow capsicum, peppers, etc
- **fruits:** blueberries, chocolate vine, quince, etc
- **herbs:** sage, jasmine, rosemary, mint, etc.

These flowers and vegetables colour the roof garden of Plaisir Villa Ichikawa every season, and bring enjoyment to residents.

Effectiveness of the roof garden

The roof garden is accessible to all via an elevator that calls at all floors. Naturally, residents with dementia are accompanied by staff or their families, and enjoy sitting in the sun with their families at weekends, while the able-bodied residents can enjoy reading, and appreciate the flowers in this perfect place to unwind. In the summertime, the fireworks of the famous Tokyo summer festivals can also be enjoyed from the rooftop. It is also an important place for the facility staff, as they sit and eat lunch on the benches and relax during break times.

Ms Endo, the Director of the home, says of the effects of the garden:

"The rooftop garden is a very useful place for calming the confusion experienced by residents with dementia. On leading them to the garden, they remember a past entwined with plants, and their expressions clearly become peaceful. I have the feeling that communing with greenery alleviates the symptoms of dementia."

Touching the earth and cultivating plants seems to conjure up some primordial human sensation. Of all the various types of care for dementia, that which utilises plants can be thought of as stimulating all five senses of those who have the condition.

Plaisir Villa Ichikawa is an example of a successfully managed and maintained garden at a small-scale home for the aged. One aspect of this success has been the clear division of the section of the garden that requires specialist-managed planting from that which can be managed by the residents and staff. Compared with other facilities, it is a fact that maintaining the garden takes funds and time. However, it is only due to precisely this kind of thorough planning concept and management policy that such a wonderful garden environment can be maintained.

No doubt new technological innovations to cut-costs and grant-in-aid systems from local authorities are necessary in order to adequately manage gardens and rooftop gardens at small-scale nursing homes in future. On the other hand, garden management and maintenance by volunteers must be carried out very carefully. This is because consistency and specialisation are indispensable in order to maintain a garden. While no doubt the circumstances surrounding horticultural volunteers differs from country to country, in Japan, either instruction from a horticultural specialist is required for a certain period of time, or planting must necessarily be carried out under specialist management. The creation of a mechanism able to carry out continuous management and maintenance is of the utmost importance. It is a sad occurrence when a garden that incurred a high start-up cost falls into disrepair and abandonment after years of under-maintenance.

While neatly kept gardens bring a sense of calm, those that have gone to waste are unsettling and risk damaging the home's image.

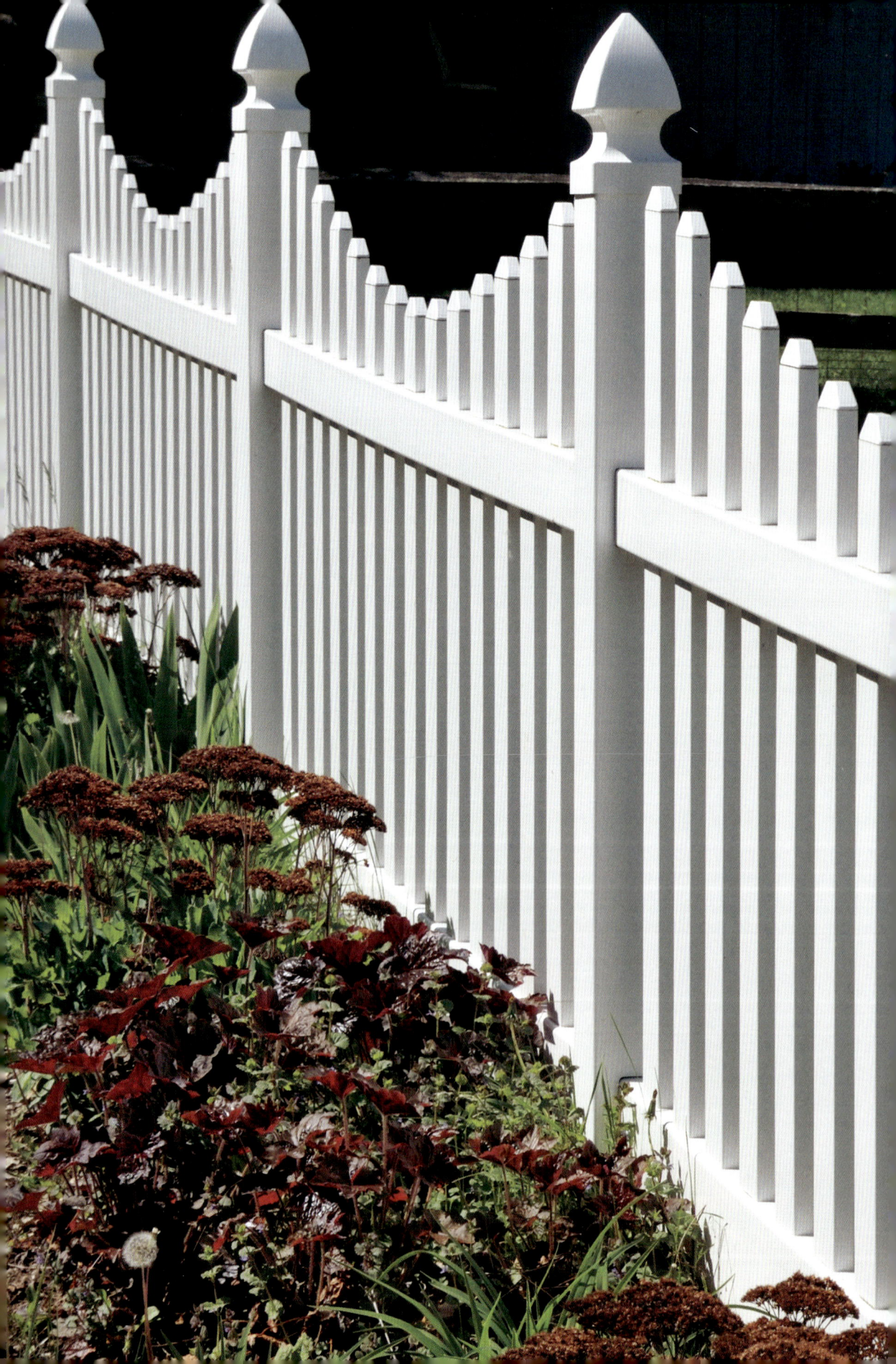

Chapter 4
Being outside 'down under'
Stephen Judd

Why outside?

Part 1 of this book looks at why being outside is important for the individual. Chapter 2 rightly notes that it was normal for most people to spend much of their childhood and adult years outside. And yet, far too many people with dementia spend far too little time outside.

This is particularly true for those who require residential care. Perhaps in the colder climates of the northern hemisphere this might be understandable. However, sadly, the same is true in Australia: older people in residential care in Australia spend far too little time outside. This is particularly ironic in Australia where, as a nation, we bask in the concept that we live in a country of 'the Great Outdoors'. Notwithstanding some exceptionally hot days in the height of summer, much of Australia has a temperate climate, which most Australians can happily and regularly enjoy.

The outside in the Australian experience

However, for Australians, the issue of being outside is not merely physical wellbeing. The outside has an important but ambiguous place in the Australian experience. The abundance of cheap and relatively flat land has meant that Australia, more than elsewhere, is the land of suburbia, of houses and gardens rather than dense networks of terraces or multi-storey tenements. In the 20th century, home ownership increased dramatically: after the Second World War, it increased from 50% to 70% in the fifteen years from 1947.

The dream of these new home owners was to own a house and garden. These home lots were large: the iconic 'quarter acre block' – about 1,000 square metres – and many lots were twice that size.

What distinguished this development of housing in Australia was the backyard. The houses were set back from the street and the front yards were typically unexceptional. But the backyards were large by international standards, taking up half of the entire lot of land. Such a large space meant that they served to function as "an integral domestic and child-rearing space" (Hall, 2010).

The backyard was home to the mandatory 'Hills Hoist', the rotary clothes line, airing and drying the flapping sheets and clothes amid a large expanse of lawn. The weekends produced a cacophony of competing lawnmowers as the men of the neighbourhood struggled year-round to keep the lawn in check. The backyard was the place where the chooks laid eggs; where the 'veggie' patch produced tomatoes that actually had flavour; where neighbouring children conducted epic football and cricket matches while mothers cooking in the kitchen had a grandstand view of proceedings and could occasionally referee to maintain good order, before calling grubby children in for dinner.

However, these domestic outside spaces were not just for the kids and for the family. While backyards could be a place of private enjoyment, particularly during the week – the cricket matches of children permitting – backyards are also the place to facilitate easy social interaction. Friends, relatives and neighbours gather in a backyard for the great Aussie barbeque and a few beers.

If the pub is the British venue to gather and socialise, then the vernacular venue for Australians to relax and unwind is the suburban backyard.

The great, hostile, outdoors

However, the Australian experience of 'the Great Outdoors' is not only that idyll. While, "collectively, backyards are a vivid part of suburban image and symbolise stability in an unpredictable urban environment" (Hall, 2010), the very character of the backyard is significantly shaped by the much harsher, Australian experience of the outdoors of the past 200 years.

It can be easily forgotten that the European experience of Australia has been comparatively short. Captain James Cook claimed the land for England in 1770 and Captain Arthur Phillip led the First Fleet to Botany Bay, hoisting the Union Jack in Sydney Cove in 1788; but planting the flag and claiming the land did not translate into European settlers feeling readily at ease with the physical nature of a dry Australian continent whose inland was at once vast and seemingly impenetrable, sparsely populated by a nomadic indigenous peoples who did not take kindly to being dispossessed by these white fellas. It is little wonder that Australia is one of the most urbanised nations on earth, with most of its population resolutely hugging the coast.

Also, the early non-indigenous settlers had no longstanding land title or generations of recognised ownership of the land. Indeed, for much of the 19th century, vast tracts of Australia were possessed by 'squatters', pastoralists who simply occupied large tracts of Crown land in order to graze sheep. They had no legal right to the land and simply took it over by being the first Europeans in the area. Often, the only expression of the Australian pastoralists' possession of their land was their fencing.

The challenge of the Australian fence

An integral part of Australia, and the Australian home, is the fence. The side and back fences of an Australian suburban property were typically six-foot high, wooden paling fences. In the past three decades, as backyard swimming pools have proliferated, tubular steel fences have also become more widespread. The common theme concerning these fences is that, far from keeping people in, they are designed to clearly define the space, assert ownership and keep people out! There is a strong sense of protection of the property, of signalling that you do not belong if you are not invited. The 'Australian Backyard' is not simply a fun and functional place for families to enjoy: the 'Australian Backyard' is a 'Claimed Compound', asserting the owner's possession of that land.

Many Australian, residential aged care homes reflect this normal suburban reality of an 'owned compound'. For example, Wintringham is a determined charitable organisation that focuses upon the aged who are homeless or at risk of homelessness. The design of Wintringham at Port Melbourne is defiantly non-institutional and its streetscape reflects the style of the neighbouring late Victorian houses. In keeping with its distinctive profile of its residents who have experienced homelessness, Wintringham has low picket fences around the perimeter to signal a defining spatial barrier.

Fig. 23 Low picket fences at Wintringham

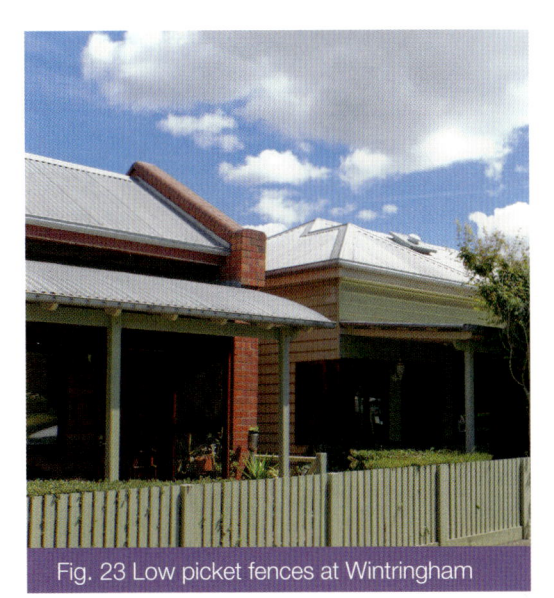

However, the design brief to the architect included a charge to make the hostel 'hostile' to visitors. Wintringham CEO Bryan Lipmann writes (2003):

"We were not trying to discourage residents from having visitors. It was more that we wanted to create an atmosphere which gave the residents power over their area and which clearly stated to everyone else that they were in someone else's home. You can't walk down the internal laneway (of Wintringham at Port Melbourne) without feeling that you are on someone else's property, that you are in fact 'running the gauntlet' as you pass by."

Kirsty Bennett, in Chapter 5, raises the issue of what fences mean to different cultures as a general consideration and, in particular, to the Anangu people. In Chapter 8, there is a photograph of the fence at Werruna, a classic Australian fence for a rural community.

HammondCare is a leading provider of dementia-specific services in Australia and over the past twenty years it has tried a variety of fences at its developments: it has installed wooden paling fences, fences with brick wall bases, as well as tubular 'pool' fencing.

Fig. 24 Different types of fencing tried at HammondCare

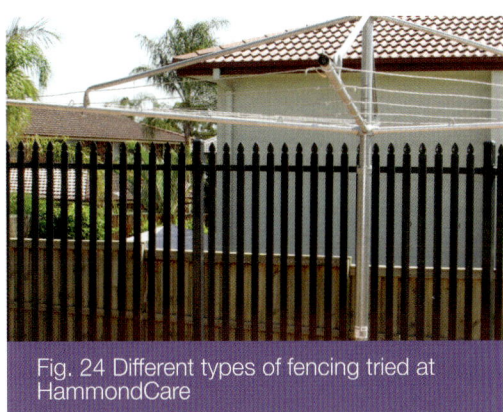

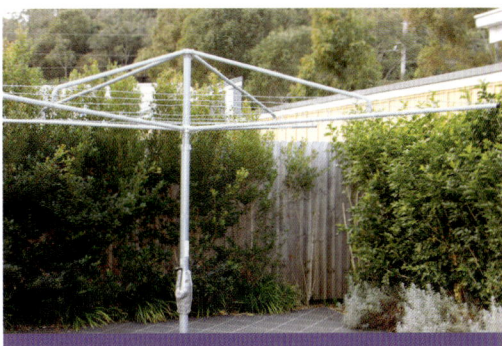

Fig. 25 Different types of fencing tried at HammondCare, including a hills hoist

Wooden paling fences? Fences with brick wall bases? Tubular 'pool' fencing? Which is most successful? The answer is simple: it depends on the individual resident. Some residents are content with an enclosed yard: a full, wooden paling fence satisfies them that they are in a defined space. Others encounter a pool fence and, seeing what is beyond, are content with that.

Still other residents are frustrated with either a pool or paling fence for the very fact that they *can see* what is outside.

Just like doors or many other objects, fences can sometimes promote frustration for someone with dementia. Their response can often be to say, "Open the door!" or "Open the fence gate!" At HammondCare in Southwood, a dementia-specific nursing home, one of the cottages is Linden, a special care cottage for eight people who would not otherwise be able to be supported within a nursing home. Like all the other cottages at Southwood, Linden has its own garden with rotary clothes line, lawn, plants and pergola with outdoor furniture, defined by tubular fencing. However, beyond this garden is another, much larger landscaped area with a pond and trees and a large expanse of lawn. If a resident wants to go beyond their own backyard, they can happily walk there, with or without company[9].

Some European visitors to Australia, (including one of the co-editors!) have been affronted by Australian fences. By contrast, the reaction of Australian relatives and visitors is resounding silence: relatives and residents think the fences are normal. These Australians are used to fenced backyards, which define the space, claim the area, and keep unwelcome people *out*.

What this means for outdoors dementia design in Australia

What is the purpose of the outdoor spaces in our aged care services? Surely our key goals for designing outdoor spaces for people with dementia is to have spaces that residents can readily access on their own that are familiar, domestic and 'normal'.

In that context, while the front garden might be more colourful, showing off to the street, the sheer plainness of the traditional, Aussie backyard is very limiting for the enthusiastic landscape architect. It is neither sophisticated nor formal. It is not complex. Its sensory features need not be contrived. It has lots of plain lawn! For a 'sensory' experience, nothing beats grass: to sit on, to lie down on, to walk barefoot on. There is good visual access between inside and outside: residents can see outside to the garden and then go there; from the garden they can see inside and readily return. This strong visual access in turn enables the staff to continue to support the residents (just as our mothers kept a casual eye over proceedings in the backyards of our (Australian) youth!).

A rotary clothes line, close to the domestic laundry, is a familiar iconic but practical feature. There are destinations such as open garden sheds and inviting shaded areas to sit and get some relief from the hot sun or enjoy a cooling breeze. There are choices as to what to do and where to go, but every choice is a right one. Pathways are simple while outdoor furniture faces back to the path and towards indoors in order not to disorient. There are garden beds, including vegetable gardens, perhaps in raised beds. While the front garden is open to the street, the backyard is fenced with a fence gate, which means that a resident can go beyond the fence, either independently or with company. These are simple elements, but they provide familiar, domestic and enabling outside spaces that older people with dementia can enjoy.

---

9 This area is primarily within a 100-year floodplain and is therefore not developed. Further, while this larger area is fenced where it meets neighbouring properties, that is not immediately obvious. Instead the plain looks like a broad expansive area with plenty of interest.

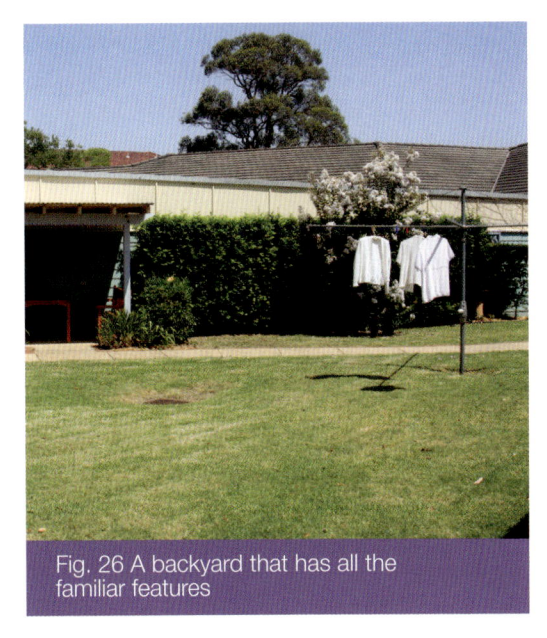

Fig. 26 A backyard that has all the familiar features

A regulatory regime that locks up unlawfully

If we know what these simple elements are, why are fewer older Australians, particularly those with dementia, enjoying 'the Great Outdoors'? One answer lies in the fear that has been engendered by an emerging regulatory regime that has developed in Australia. This regulatory regime is having the effect of preventing older residents – with or without dementia – from going outside. It is a regulatory regime intent on locking up residents unlawfully.

In May 2008, a man disappeared from his nursing home on the Central Coast of New South Wales. He was missing for four days, and died after suffering dehydration and hypothermia. Around the same period, a North Queensland resident also died after 'wandering' around for roughly the same time. In response, the then Australian Minister for Ageing, Justine Elliot, declared in June 2008 that the Government would require residential aged care services to report any cases of missing residents to the Australian Department of Health and Ageing (ADHA). This was for all residents, regardless of their condition or cognition. Further, although the idea was later rescinded, it was unofficially proposed that medi-tag bracelets should be *mandatory* for all residents with dementia.

The regulations to support this requirement of 'mandatory reporting to the Department when residents are missing' were introduced in December 2008. The new principles are carefully worded:

"An approved provider must tell the Secretary if:

(a) a care recipient is absent from a residential care service; and

(b) the absence is unexplained; and

(c) the absence has been reported to the police.

The Secretary must be told about the absence as soon as reasonably practicable, and in any case, within 24 hours after the provider reports the absence to the police[10]."

That sounds fair enough! It's a little like saying, "Listen, if you call the coppers about a missing resident can you give us at the Department a ring soon after? We get embarrassed hearing it first from the media."

Unfortunately, that is not how the Department has translated it. The Residential Care Manual, in which the ADHA describes the regulatory framework for the residential aged care in Australia, is prescriptive and threatening to providers of aged care:

10 Section 1.14A of the Accountability Principles 1998 of the Aged Care Act 1997 (as amended 2008)

"The Department (will) determine whether appropriate action has been taken by the approved provider in respect of the missing residents and whether there are adequate systems and processes in place to ensure other residents' safety. This reporting requirement is part of an approved provider's responsibility under the Act to provide a safe and secure environment."

"The Department's response to the notification will be to review the matter to establish whether there is an ongoing risk to residents. For example, it is unlikely further action will be taken where a missing resident turns up, having spent a day with family or friends. Whereas, if a resident is reported as missing without reasonable explanation and it is considered that the approved provider did not have adequate systems and processes in place to prevent the absence, then the Department can investigate and compliance action could be taken." (ADHA 2009)

The Manual and the related guidelines struggle briefly with the issue of the right of older people to move freely: "This measure in no way impinges on the basic human rights of older Australians" (ADHA 2008). It is as if by merely making such a statement, black will somehow become white. The Australian Government also implicitly acknowledges that these reporting requirements are at odds with the rights of older people:

"These requirements do not override an approved provider's responsibility to comply with the Charters of Residents' Rights and Responsibilities, which includes the resident's rights to move freely both inside and outside the service without undue restriction." (ADHA 2009)

What has happened is that the actual legislation, which says, "Give us a call if you happen to ring the coppers because you are worried about someone," has been perverted into guidelines that infer that "if one of your residents checks out and something bad happens, we'll come after you."

It is questionable whether, under administrative law, these guidelines and manuals would survive legal challenge. A fundamental principle in administrative law is that guidelines such as the Manual cannot go beyond the extent of what the legislation – Section 1.14A of the Accountability Principles of the Aged Care Act – actually says.

There are two points to be made here. First, the consequence of these developments has been profound. One of the fundamental rights of an Australian citizen who has not been imprisoned for a crime is the right of liberty, the right not to be restrained. That right is being ignored because residential aged care providers, threatened with action should residents go missing unaccountably, are actively keeping residents under lock and key. If the only way that residents can go missing is to go outside and 'wander' away, then proprietors of services are eliminating that risk by stopping them going outside. 'The Great Outdoors' is now a danger, not a delight. The rights of older people are being ignored with the full support – indeed the active urging – of a paternalistic Australian Government.

The second point to make is how vitally important it is to know what the legislation and regulations actually says, not what you are *told* they say. In this instance, the guidelines distort the very regulatory framework that they seek to interpret.

A protective disciplinary culture

How did we come to this? This regulatory regime has occurred with good intentions. No-one wants to see people die of hypothermia and dehydration. However, these regulations are part of a fast-developing 'protective disciplinary culture' within aged care[11]. In your own home, you have the right to smoke, the right to have pets, the right to get fat and even the right to have sex! You have the right to wander down to the shops. Yet far too many older Australians lose those rights when they enter residential aged care services. They become captive to a controlled environment, which dominates and imprisons them. It is an environment in which they are protectively disciplined for their own good, for their own health, for the peace of mind of their relative, to avoid the complaint. The result is that they do not belong; they do not feel in control.

This brings us to the question of 'wandering'. What is troubling about the discussion about 'wandering', missing residents and the security of residents is that the person with dementia is repeatedly presented as a subject, not as someone with a voice. Not a person, certainly not a citizen, but a voiceless subject. This is despite the fact that much research has concluded that so-called wandering is not so much a symptom or syndrome of dementia, but a sign of distress. Indeed, the very term 'wandering' suggests aimless walking, whereas it is more likely that the activity has some meaning for the person concerned. Walking is a normal human behaviour. In the context of dementia, it could be viewed as an activity used to adapt to living with dementia. As a person living with dementia so aptly put it, 'it must mean something because I do it naturally.' (Dewing, 2006)

Yet the focus is on stopping the person who is 'wandering' rather than stopping the distress that is causing the wandering! No-one seems to be looking at the plainly obvious: if you did not feel 'at home'; if you did not feel you belonged or were comfortable; if you were trapped in some nursing homes – let's be frank here – wanting to leave would be a perfectly sensible thing to do!

Key points

- being outdoors is part of Australian daily life: there is no more iconic Australian setting than an Australian backyard, with family and friends having a few drinks at an informal barbeque, with kids playing games and dodging the clothes line and the veggie patch

- the needs of outside spaces in an Australian aged care service are simple, domestic and familiar: they require attention to detail but not formal or stylised landscaping

- the protective disciplinary culture that has emerged in Australian aged care means that older Australians, and particularly those who dementia, are being denied ready and frequent access to this vital element of daily living

- it is unclear under what legal provision the freedom of older Australian citizens is being impaired. Perhaps it will only be a matter of time before an older Australian takes legal action against a service

---

11 I am grateful to John Braithwaite, Toni Makkai, Valerie Braithwaite, Regulating Aged Care, London 2008, for this phrase.

provider – and the Government – for unlawful restraint

- in the meantime, it will be up to passionate aged care providers to know the regulations – and the underlying legislation – better than the regulators; it will be up to passionate consumer groups to champion the rights of older residents with dementia, not just the concerns and fears of their loved ones

- and it will be up to all of us to lead by example so that all Australians can enjoy the Australian outdoors.

References

Australian Department of Health and Ageing. (2008). Notifying the department when residents are reported missing to police. In Guide to changes to the Regulatory Framework for Aged Care. (pp.21). Retrieved from http://www.health.gov.au/internet/main/publishing.nsf/Content/75A3796E08F4B81BCA257523007D16B3/$File/legislat%20guide.pdf

Australian Department of Health and Ageing. (2009). Providers' responsibilities and non-compliance. In *Residential care manual*. (Edition 1, Update 1, 234). Retrieved from http://www.health.gov.au/internet/main/publishing.nsf/Content/1CC3ACD213466762CA256F19000FC9A5/$File/RCMUpdates.pdf

Dewing, J. (2006). Wandering into the future: Reconceptualising wandering. *International Journal of Older People Nursing, 1*(4), 239-249.

Hall, T. (2010). *The life and death of the Australian backyard*. Melbourne: CSIRO Publishing.

Lipmann, B. (2003). Providing housing and care to elderly homeless men and women in Australia. *Care Management Journals, 4*(1), 23–30.

Case Study 3
Werruna: Creating an appropriate environment for rural Australians living with dementia

Peter Birkett

Hesse Rural Health Service, Winchelsea, Australia

Werruna is a rural Australian residential centre for persons with advanced memory loss and confusion. Its research and development stage started in 2004 and lasted five years. Werruna opened and accepted its first residents in September 2009.

The building is of contemporary design, based upon knowledge and understanding of the health and social needs of people with dementia. It reflects the value that people with dementia are entitled to live in high quality environments and is in keeping with local rural family cultures, retaining community integration.

Werruna promotes wellness and quality living, recognising that people in rural Australia spend much of their time outdoors. The facility comprises 500 square metres within two hectares of garden and farmland space and out buildings.

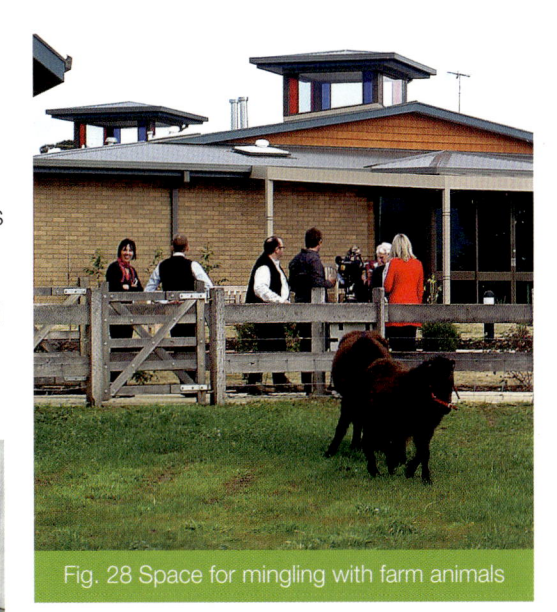

Fig. 28 Space for mingling with farm animals

The open-plan, spacious indoor and outdoor environments are unique in providing resident freedom and autonomy and provide a secure dementia care area for ten residents.

The internal layout is stimulating yet easy to find your way around. Bedrooms, with small private entrances, sit adjacent to lounge and dining spaces; this removes the need for confusing corridors or hallways. Immediately upon leaving their room, the resident is absorbed within a familiar point of social activity.

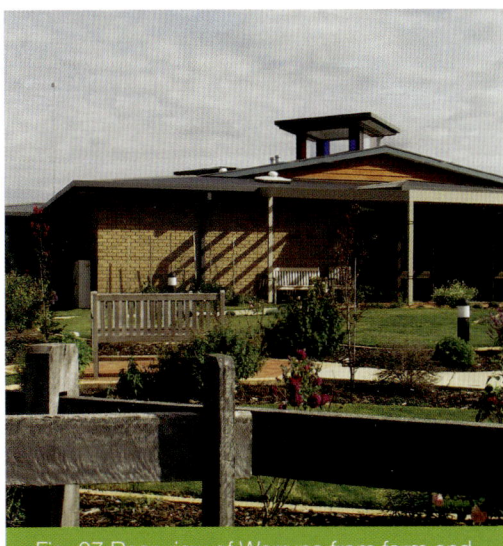

Fig. 27 Rear view of Werruna from farm and garden precinct

The open communal space is divided and contained by the design into recognisable, functional dining and living zones. A double-sided open fireplace forms the central feature. Familiar cedar panelling and solid blackwood cabinetry complement the internal tumbled brickwork. Alternative private breakaway points include a small formal glass conservatory, a kitchen and an artist's studio.

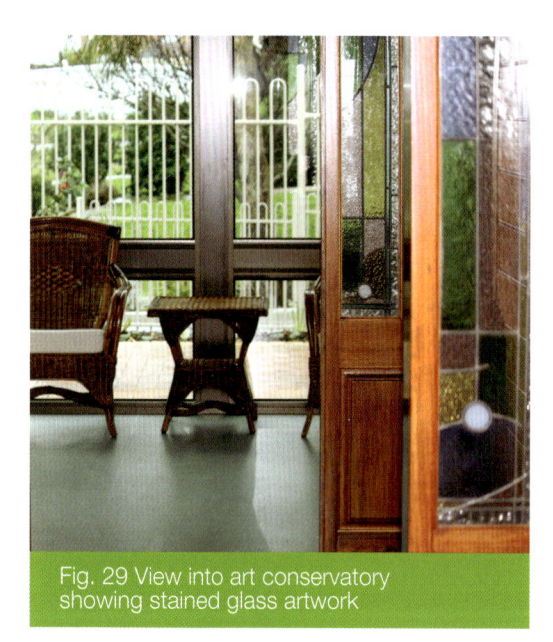

Fig. 29 View into art conservatory showing stained glass artwork

The high ceiling pitch, coloured leadlight glass and roof turrets cast a display of changing light streams across the floor providing a hint of spirituality. Coloured and textured glass has been incorporated into a series of panel doorways encased within blackwood surrounds. The stained glass is artistic, functional and therapeutic. The strong, natural colours have been inspired by the environment and perfectly encapsulate the essence of the development. The correct balance of light provides a sense of safety, control and improves mood.

The natural and introduced light entices residents away from the entrance to the large northern picture windows overlooking expansive and freely accessible garden and farm spaces.

The artist's studio, with exterior glass walls, overlooks tranquil garden spaces and caters for those residents who have developed an artistic flair as their condition changes. Locally produced fine art has been acquired to adorn the walls of the common areas. The art has been carefully selected based on an understanding that people with dementia connect with artwork containing people, children, animals and action.

Familiar gardens and traditional farming spaces offer great comfort for rural residents. The many exit doors remain unlocked, with hats and coats at the ready to encourage residents to walk outside at anytime to receive the important benefits of nature, sunlight and vitamin D. The residents get the opportunity to feel the summer sun, the cold winter chill, see the spring growth and watch the autumn leaves fall. Outdoor walking is encouraged either on the concrete pathways throughout the garden or through the uneven surface of the paddocks; this is a familiar unevenness that many of our farmers have been used to throughout their lives.

Pathways logically meander into gardens and the farming area, leading to points of meaningful interaction. Farm animals including sheep, alpacas, and chooks, and a farm machinery shed, with tractor, utility and a workbench, combines with a stockyard and an outhouse to mimic a typical Australian farm.

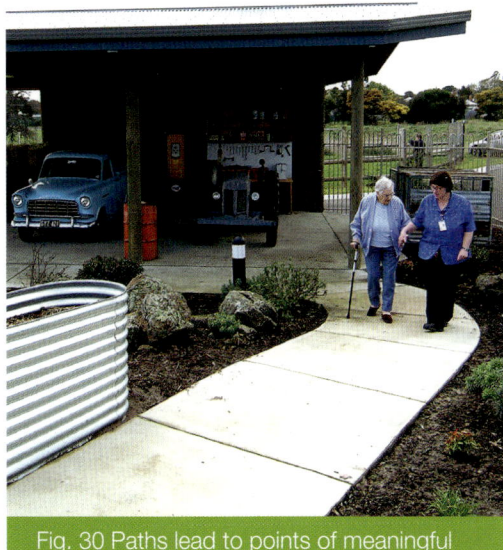

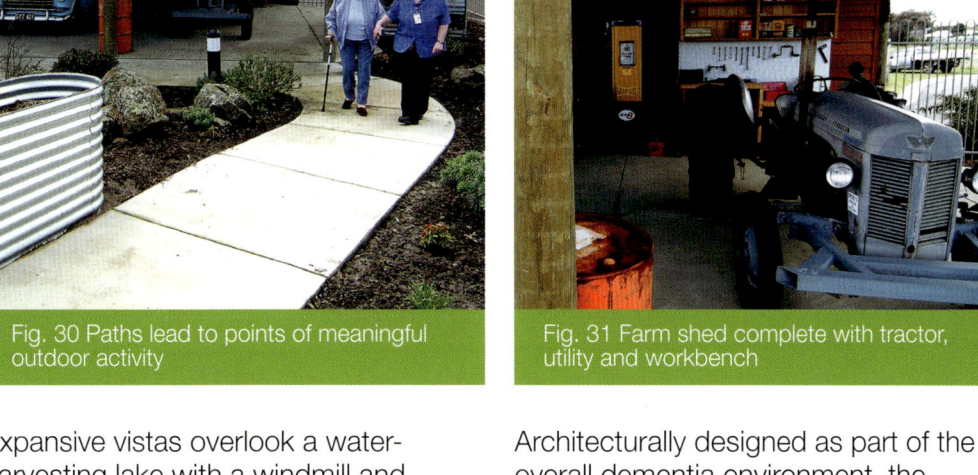

Fig. 30 Paths lead to points of meaningful outdoor activity

Fig. 31 Farm shed complete with tractor, utility and workbench

Expansive vistas overlook a water-harvesting lake with a windmill and community recreational spaces featuring a cricket ground with rural trains passing into the distance.

Farm gates open into the animal areas. Residents are free to walk amongst the animals, touch them, talk to them and feed them, or check they have enough water to drink in the trough. The chooks are fed the kitchen scraps and the residents delight in collecting the eggs. A traditional farming kelpie sheep dog visits each week. The farming shed has been equipped with tools, rabbit traps, horse harness, barrels and a petrol pump. Residents can open the door of the ute or sit on the tractor or enjoy a moment or two reflecting, or having a cuppa on the hay bales.

Architecturally designed as part of the overall dementia environment, the outdoor farm space is freely accessible to residents without staff assistance. The risks have been minimised through a series of familiar farm timber fences that deter climbing, which have been innovatively designed to roll and spin without points of leverage. Electronic cameras and outside, nurse call points, enable staff to monitor residents without the need to be beside them, allowing the residents to experience freedom and individuality.

"My mother has been a resident at Werrruna since shortly after it opened and it has afforded her a sense of peace and security that is very hard to achieve with a disease such as dementia. This is due to the wonderful surroundings and décor, which was thoroughly researched by the designers of the facility and the professionalism and kindness of the staff, which is second to none. There is a feeling of calm and warmth which is unlike anything I have ever felt in

an aged care facility… the outdoor rural setting is so appropriate for the location of the facility and the vocation of some of the residents who have come from farming backgrounds."

In addition to the positive feedback received from families, local doctors marvel at the change in the residents after a move into the Werruna environment. "I can't explain it. It just works. People seem to just settle."

Werruna is not typical, within the Australian landscape, of solutions to dementia residential care. It combines knowledge of the dementia condition with contemporary building design and translates it into the rural area, creating an environment that fosters the innovative use of space and meaningful points of interaction to enhance resident wellbeing.

Werruna offers rural people an environment that reflects the fabric of their life while maintaining connections with their families and local communities.

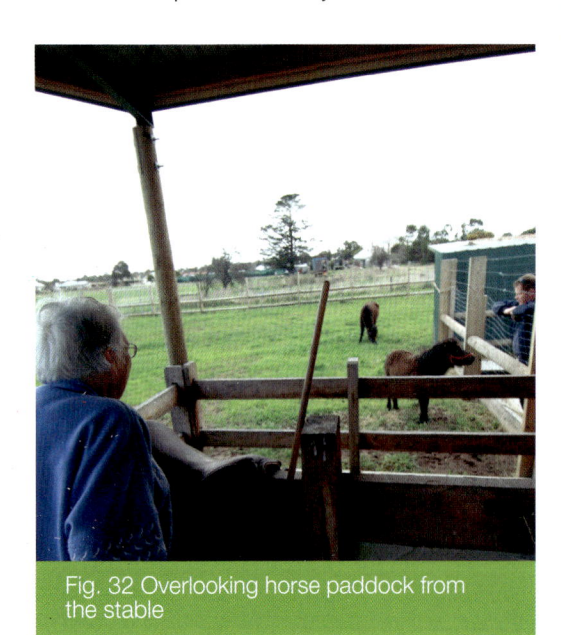

Fig. 32 Overlooking horse paddock from the stable

Chapter 5
Culturally appropriate design of outdoor spaces

Kirsty Bennett

One of the most important things we can do is realise the extent to which our cultural outlook shapes our needs and attitudes and therefore needs to inform any design response if it is to be appropriate. The way our cultural view affects us is something that we can be acutely aware of, or on the other hand, be oblivious to. When we think about designing outdoor spaces for other people we need to go back to first principles and try to set our own cultural view to the side. Assume nothing. There will be meaning in things that we do not expect. We may think we understand what we are looking at when in reality we don't. We need to stop and listen and observe.

This chapter will discuss some of the ways in which culture can influence the design of outdoor spaces: how we use them, how we live, and what can be meaningful in an outdoor space. It will do this by referring to a particular setting on the Anangu Pitjantjatjara Yankunytjatjara (APY) Lands.

The Anangu Pitjantjatjara Yankunytjatjara (APY) Lands are in northwest South Australia near the junction of the Northern Territory, Western Australia and South Australian borders and cover approximately 103,000 square kilometres. The APY Lands cover a large and remote area, and are owned by the Anangu Pitjantjatjara Yankunytjatjara. Water is scarce, and red dust is common. There are about 2500 people on the lands.

Introduction

Our cultural outlook affects many aspects of our lives and the design of outdoor spaces is no exception. Outdoor spaces can include built elements that are overtly related to a person's cultural background, such as a pagoda as a place of retreat in a garden, a toolshed or a 'milk house' (see Case study 4, Haugmotun). There are other design elements too, such as the interface between outdoors and indoors, which are perhaps less obvious but are also strongly influenced by culture.

Many of the Anangu come from homes where suitable housing is measured by the availability of running water, a functioning WC and a place to cook.

The residential aged care facility 'Tjilpi Pampaku Ngura' (TPN), meaning 'old men's, old women's place', was built at Pukatja on the APY Lands in 2000. It is home for up to 16 older Anangu and consists of four bedroom units, which each contain two bedrooms and an ensuite, and a central building, which houses social spaces, services areas (such as the laundry and kitchen) and administration areas. The separate buildings are connected by covered pathways. Three architects worked on the project: Adrian Welke of Troppo Architects who has experience in designing and building in remote areas, Paul Pholeros, an expert in indigenous housing who has worked on the Lands for many years, and Kirsty Bennett who has experience in designing for older people.

Fig. 33 Tjilpi Pampaku Ngura and its setting

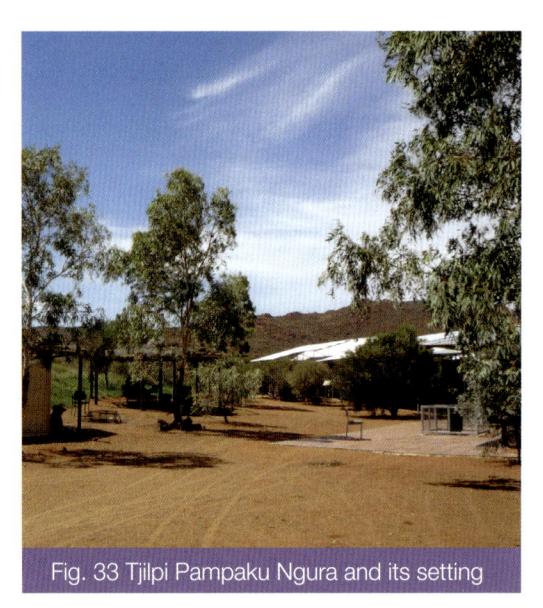

Culture was a guiding influence in all aspects of the design of TPN. While the design of this facility is very specific to the culture of the Anangu Pitjantjatjara Yankunytjatjara, the experiences that were gained from this project can offer valuable insights in other settings. Similar questions will need to be asked in every design of outdoor spaces. How do the people who will live there relate to outdoors? What do these people want to do? What is meaningful to them? How do they want to live?

It is hoped that the examples which follow from this culturally specific facility will remind us of the many ways in which culture can influence the design of outdoor settings, and encourage us to be open to explore the rich possibilities that are before us.

Attitude to outdoor spaces

Importance of outdoors

Culture affects the importance we give to outdoor spaces. We live our lives in quite distinct ways in different parts of the world.

In some places we focus on the indoors, in others on the outdoors. For some of us, gardening is an important pastime or hobby. For others, it is a vital part of life as the outdoors provides an essential source of food. For some people the external environment is crucial to their identity.

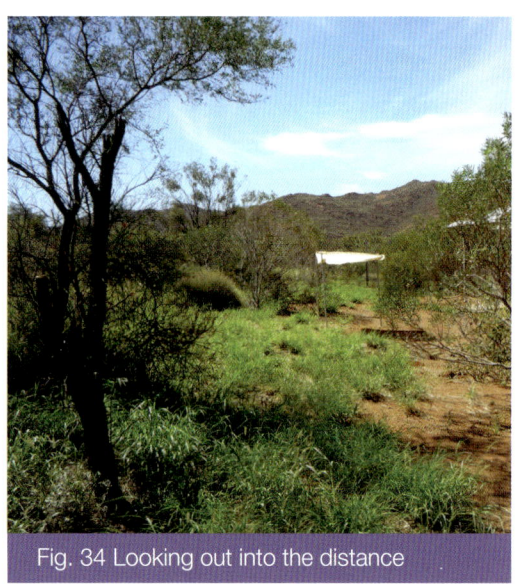

Fig. 34 Looking out into the distance

The Anangu refer to the land as their country. It is not an outdoor space. It is the place which is at the heart of life.

Country is integral to the wellbeing of the Anangu who live on the APY Lands. The strength of the Anangu's connection to the land is something which is perhaps hard for non-Anangu to understand. This connection is seen in many ways. It is important, for example, for Anangu to be able to look out far into the distance, and to be able to sit and watch the path of the sun and moon. Country governs the rhythms of life. Features in the landscape have significance and meaning that can go back for thousands of years.

Interface between indoors and outdoors

The interface between the indoor and outdoor environment is a key element in the design of an aged care facility. It will affect the selection of materials and finishes, the sizes of door and window openings, the locations of door and windows, the treatment of shading devices, the selection of interior decoration, and the use of blinds, curtains and outdoor screens. All of these areas can be varied and the design choices that are made can create an interface that is clearly defined and articulated, or one which is open and transparent.

The appropriate treatment of the interface between the indoor and outdoor environment will be strongly influenced by cultural considerations. When designing in Melbourne, a city in south-eastern Australia, for example, a common request is to 'bring the outdoors in'. In warmer climates such as Darwin in the Northern Territory, Australia, people will often take the inside out, as they eat around a table on a sundeck instead of in a dining room.

On the APY Lands we were told that people did not want to bring the outdoors into the building: if Anangu wanted to experience outside they would go outside!

When Anangu go into a building, they go to retreat from outdoors. The building offers them security, and a safe place. As a result, window openings at 'Tjilpi Pampaku Ngura' (TPN) are small, and the introduction of natural light is somewhat limited. The windows have perforated metal screens and wooden louvers that can be either fully closed to block out the light, or partially opened to suit residents' preferences. Curtains add colour and decoration to the bedrooms and provide another layer of flexibility to the space as they can be opened or closed.

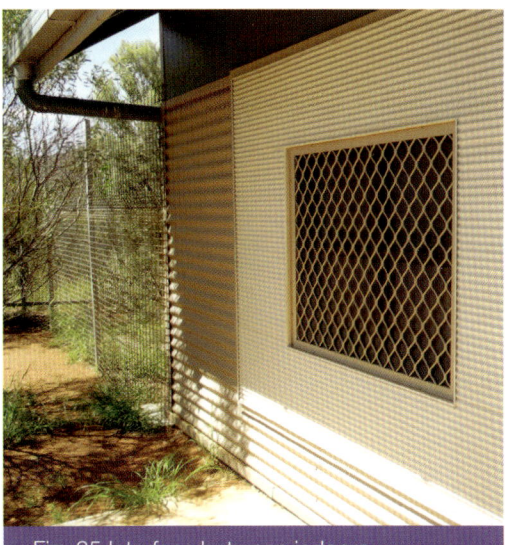

Fig. 35 Interface between indoors and outdoors

Fig. 36 Natural light in bedrooms can be adjusted to suit residents' preferences

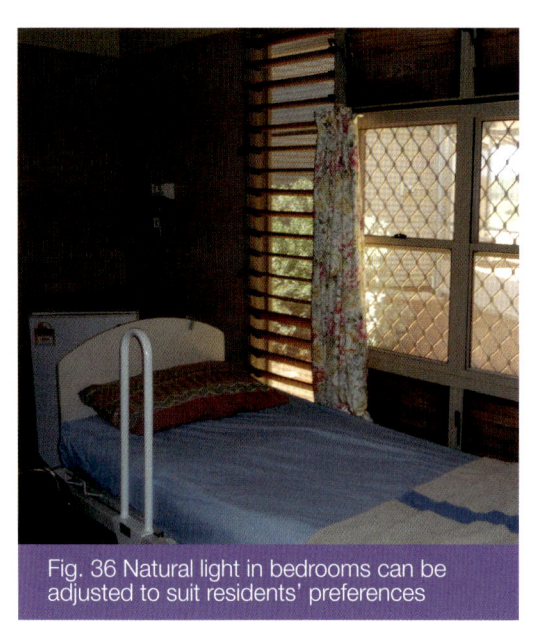

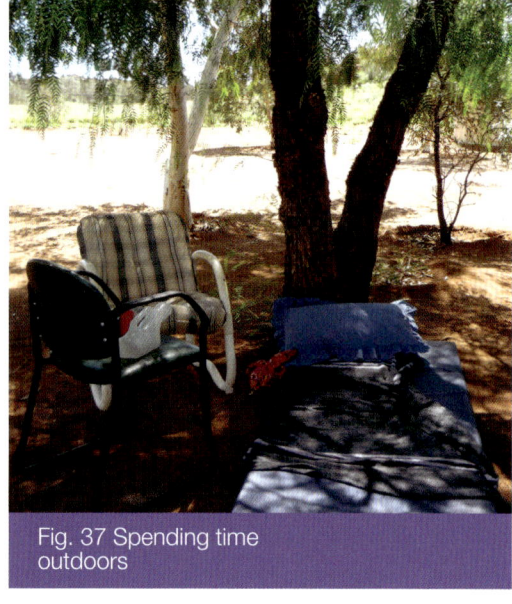

Fig. 37 Spending time outdoors

Approach to being indoors and outdoors

Our cultural outlook will influence how much time we spend indoors and how much time we spend outdoors. How we like to spend our time and our attitude to possessions will also be strongly formed by our cultural view.

A̲nangu can live happily with very limited belongings. They are not, therefore, looking to decorate a room with possessions that remind them of home and are not expecting to spend time indoors surrounded by things that make them feel at ease.

Instead, this sense of familiarity and wellbeing is gained by being outside, in a setting where vegetation and the features of the landscape offer meaning and significance. This means that a much greater emphasis was given to the design of outdoor places at Pukutja than in a setting for people of a different culture.

Use of outdoor spaces

Living outdoors rather than visiting outdoors

A key focus when designing environments for people with dementia is to create a domestic environment. This can best be described as designing a place where people can live as they wish to and do what they want to do. Attention often centres on creating an indoor setting which meets these needs. It is important to recognise that this is an area that is deeply affected by culture. In some cultures, people live outdoors, rather than visit outdoors. This then gives the outdoor environment a very different emphasis.

For Anangu, a domestic environment would mean having easy access to the outdoors (which includes being able to sit around, sleep and eat outside), and being able to see the surrounding country, with adequate shade and shelter.

At TPN, the buildings provide a backdrop, a place where people can go to receive key services. They are not where people live. Most older Anangu will live outside for much of the time and will sit on the ground. The buildings will mainly be used in bad weather, when a person is suffering from particularly bad health, and to store belongings.

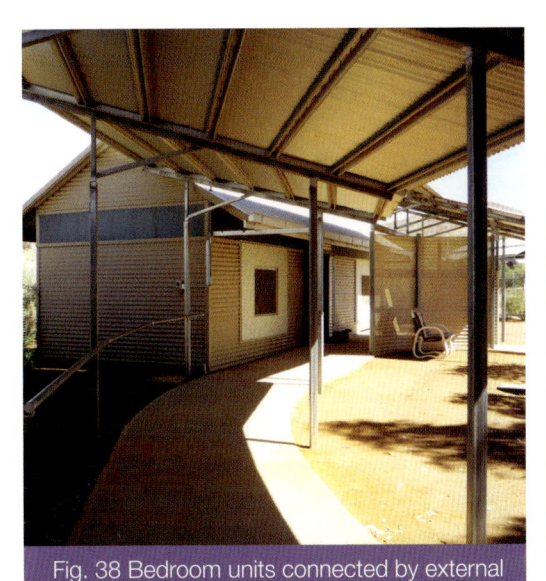

Fig. 38 Bedroom units connected by external walkway

In this place, the building is not the important part of the aged care facility. Instead it is the land, the country. Bedroom units are connected by external walkways which provide shelter but are open to the elements so that Anangu do not feel like they are inside. The buildings are designed to be small objects in a vast landscape, rather than be a significant presence.

What do people want to do outdoors?

The design of outdoor spaces is determined by what people want to do and how they wish to spend their time. How an outdoor area is used (and therefore what it needs to offer) is strongly influenced by our culture.

The design of the outdoors at TPN has been strongly influenced by the responses to the most fundamental question 'What do people want to do here?' Typically, older Anangu will want to go outside, no matter how sick he or she is, live close to or on the ground, and lie near fires. Anangu will want to be outdoors to practice traditional arts, and take part in singing, dancing and storytelling. They will want to be able to light a fire and sit by the fire with other Anangu.

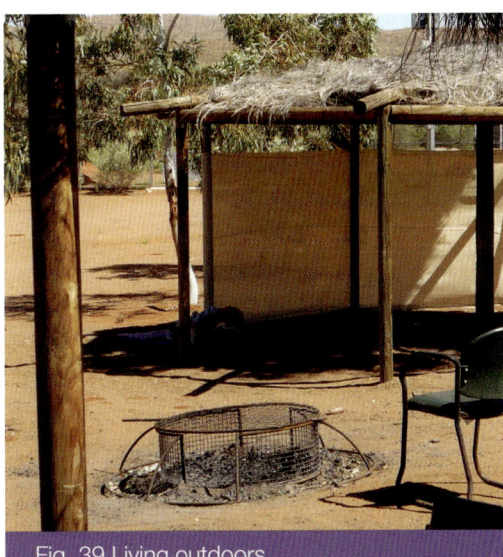

Fig. 39 Living outdoors

There are also other things that Anangu will wish to do outdoors which cannot be accommodated in the residential aged care facility but are important to be aware of. Anangu will wish to travel to participate in cultural business, maintain family and community links, socialise, and attend funerals and sorry business (this could involve leaving the facility and living in sorry camps). They will want to go hunting and gathering (and like to go on trips even if they can no longer physically hunt).

Designing outdoors

Selecting a site

Selecting a site is the first part of designing an outdoor environment. What natural features are important? Is it the view? Is it the type of vegetation? Is there access to public transport? Can car parking be provided? What is the desirable relationship between the site and the wider community?

On the APY Lands the location of TPN was more important than the design of the facility itself. This results from the cultural and spiritual significance that the land itself holds for the Anangu. The land is a source of identity for the Anangu and it shapes and nourishes people's lives.

Having determined on which part of the APY Lands TPN would be built (i.e. at Pukatja which is located centrally on the APY Lands), it was particularly important to select a site that was somewhat removed from the local township. This means that the site is not strongly identified with that particular community (this was important as the aged care facility is for people from all parts of the lands and so it is vital that all people feel welcome). Another reason for its distance from the township is to avoid humbug (or bother) from people within the community. The site selection then becomes an important part of providing a safe environment for older people. In this instance, it is about providing an environment where people feel safe from others.

How much to design?

Outdoor areas are often left incomplete on a new project. It is not unusual for them to be given the lowest budget, and in times of financial difficulty the scope of outdoor works is often reduced. This is because the works are seen to be easy to do later, whereas leaving a part of the building to complete later means that it is unlikely to be built. This situation can obscure the more important question: how much of the outdoor area should be designed? How much of the outdoor area can be designed by the people who will live there? Who has the appropriate expertise to design the outdoor areas? This is another matter that is influenced by our cultural view.

At TPN it was agreed that the design of the outside areas should be largely left for the Anangu to undertake once they had moved in. The focus was on designing for opportunities for the Anangu rather than designing an outdoor environment that was complete. This recognised that Anangu take a more active role in the outdoor environment than non-Anangu do. Consideration was therefore given to where water could be provided, where a wiltja (a small shelter) could be built, where sand could be laid, rather than providing these things. Others were then responsible for seeing that this happened if it was appropriate.

What to include?

The elements that should be included in a design will be determined by the people who will live there and their culture. As a designer it is vital to be open to suggestions and to observe how people live and what they wish to do so that the most appropriate elements are allowed for. At TPN, high priority was given to providing good sand to sit and lie on, which is not coarse. There also needed to be a good supply of firewood.

Shelter from the elements (extreme heat, extreme cold, dust and rain) was also important.

Each bedroom unit has a windbreak outside, so that people do not have far to go to reach a sheltered outdoor place.

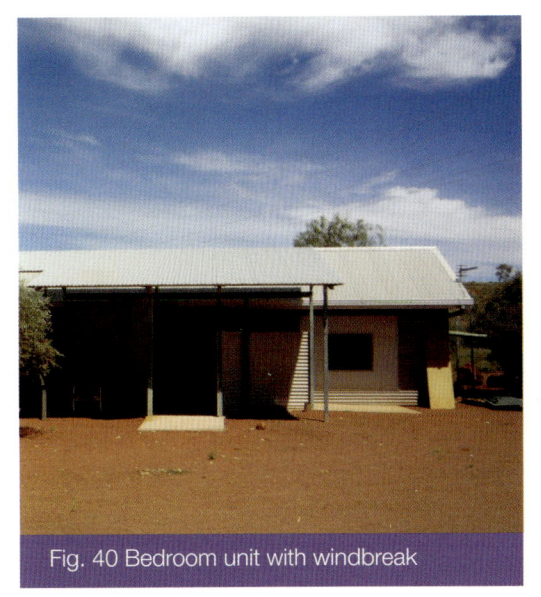

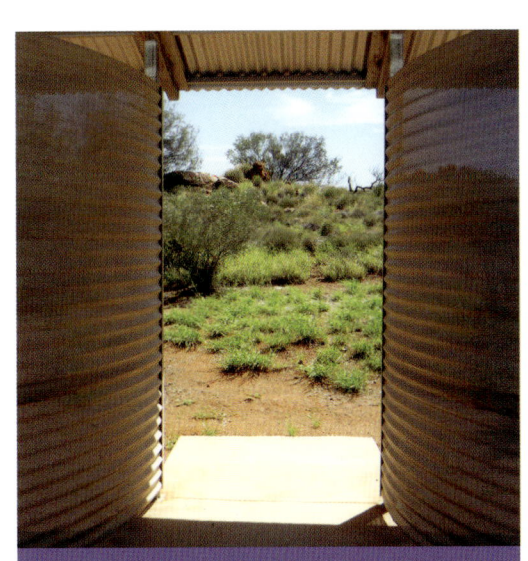

Fig. 40 Bedroom unit with windbreak

Fig. 41 View from bedroom unit past windbreak

It was important that there are shady, sheltered places, which have a view and a place to sit, where people can feel safe. There is a sharp contrast between the small shelter (wiltja) an Anangu will retreat to, and the large expanse of country that they are surrounded by. Anangu are used to either being in big country or in a small space.

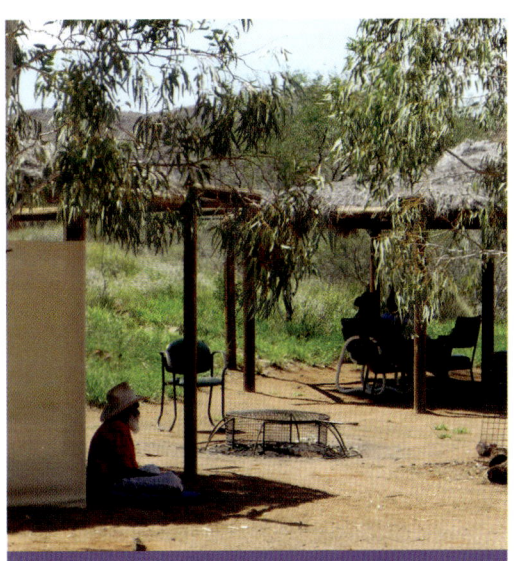

Fig. 42 Sheltered shady places are important

Fire is vital. It is needed for many things: for making cups of tea, for making spears, for dancing and singing, for making artefacts, for cooking and for warmth. Different types of fires are made for all these things, and the fires need to be able to be moved or lit in different places during the day to suit the sun and the wind. The provision of fire is an extremely difficult design request to respond to, as a fire can present a great risk to an older person. It is therefore recommended that fires are only lit when staff are present and that fire pits are appropriately fenced.

What cues and symbols are meaningful outdoors?

Landscapes and outdoor areas need to be familiar and recognisable if they are to be meaningful for people with dementia. It is important to recognise that our cultural outlook will play a strong part in determining what is meaningful and memorable.

Cues that are likely to be meaningful for Anangu are rocks, fire and views.

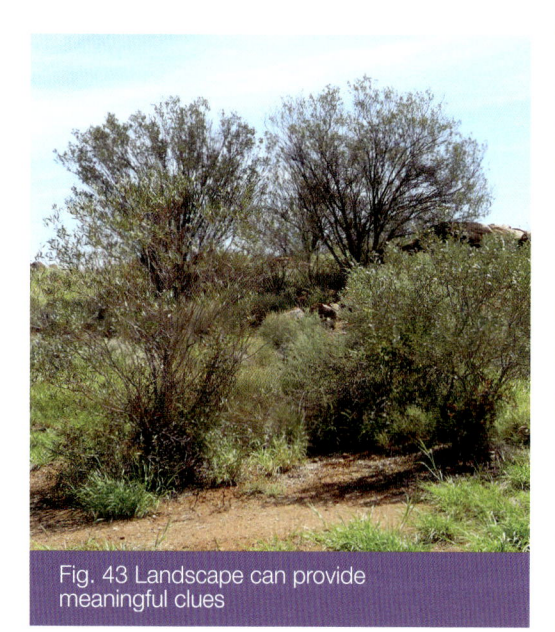

Fig. 43 Landscape can provide meaningful clues

It is also important not to assume that people will only like certain things because of their cultural outlook. Indigenous people like pretty flowers too!

Meaning of fences

Fences are a common feature of a facility for people with dementia. Much has been written about how a fence can be hidden and obscured when designing for people with dementia. It is important though to recognise that not all cultures see fences as a negative element. On the contrary, in some settings fences are seen as highly desirable.

At TPN, the perimeter of the site is clearly defined. Fences are seen as positive. Fences keep people out (rather than keeping the older people in) and stop other people from moving into the older person's place. Fences keep the troublemakers out and help stop the older people from being pestered.

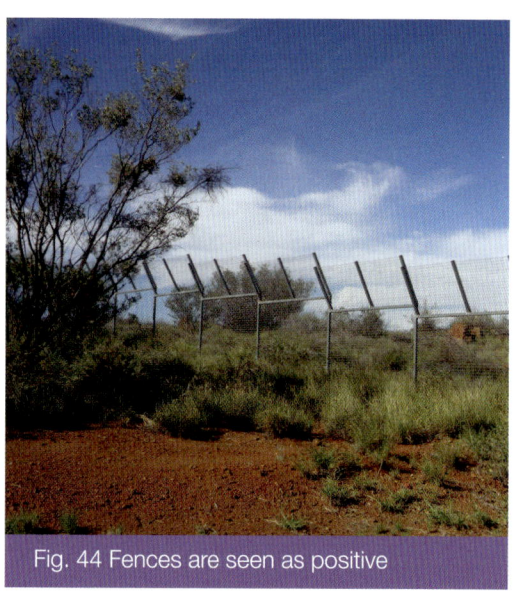

Fig. 44 Fences are seen as positive

Consulting effectively

In any project it is important to determine who are the best people to talk to and who is well-suited (and has the authority) to speak on behalf of others. It is also vital to then consider the best way to have these conversations with people. How many people should be present? Where should the conversations be held? How often should there be meetings? Is there a formal and an informal way to talk about things? How much time should be allowed for making decisions?

Prior to commencing the design of the facility, there was an intensive period of consultation with all the communities on the Lands. The types of service (and its location) were key topics for consideration, and Anangu often travelled great distances to participate in discussions.

Once a site had been selected, the consultant team was appointed and another series of conversations began. On the APY Lands there are strict rules about who can mix with another person according to gender and skin group. It would not have been appropriate for a non-Anangu to simply arrive and try to talk to Anangu (it would also have been extremely difficult due to our different language skills). To ensure that the information that was gathered was culturally appropriate and operationally meaningful, consultation was with senior Anangu and experienced non-Anangu aged care workers Maureen Arch and Douglas McManus who were living on the Lands. The non-Anangu workers were the key liaison point for visiting consultants. They then explored issues further with Anangu. Time was taken. The Anangu and non-Anangu aged care workers, along with architect Paul Pholeros, travelled to all parts of the Lands to meet with Anangu and talk about a model of the proposed facility.

The things we have heard

Outdoors is the place where Anangu live, rather than a place where they spend some time or go when the weather is good. It is vast. Views to the far distance are important, and the building is used to retreat from the land, rather than as a place that provides for people's wellbeing. Anangu feel at home outside, and look to be outside rather than inside. The key things that are important to Anangu (good sand, a fire in the right location and built with the right firewood, and a view to country) are not design elements, but things that are essential to their way of life.

For Anangu, the land is their country. It is not an outdoor space: it is the source of their being. The land is integral in the lives of the Anangu as it influences their way of life, their laws, their spiritually and their identity. Anangu see meaning in the land that non-Anangu cannot fully understand.

Key points

- our cultural outlook shapes our needs and attitudes: often without our even knowing this
- culture strongly influences the design of outdoor spaces as it affects the way we use outdoors and what is meaningful in an outdoor space
- culture affects the importance of outdoor spaces in our lives and how much time we spend in those spaces
- when designing outdoors, we especially need to consider site selection, how people live, how much we design, and how to consult effectively
- the design of outdoor spaces also needs to consider the interface between indoors and outdoors
- at Tjilpi Pampaku Ngura, we see a place where outdoors is a place to live, rather than a place to spend time or go when the weather is good
- for Anangu, the land is not an outdoor space: it is at the heart of life.

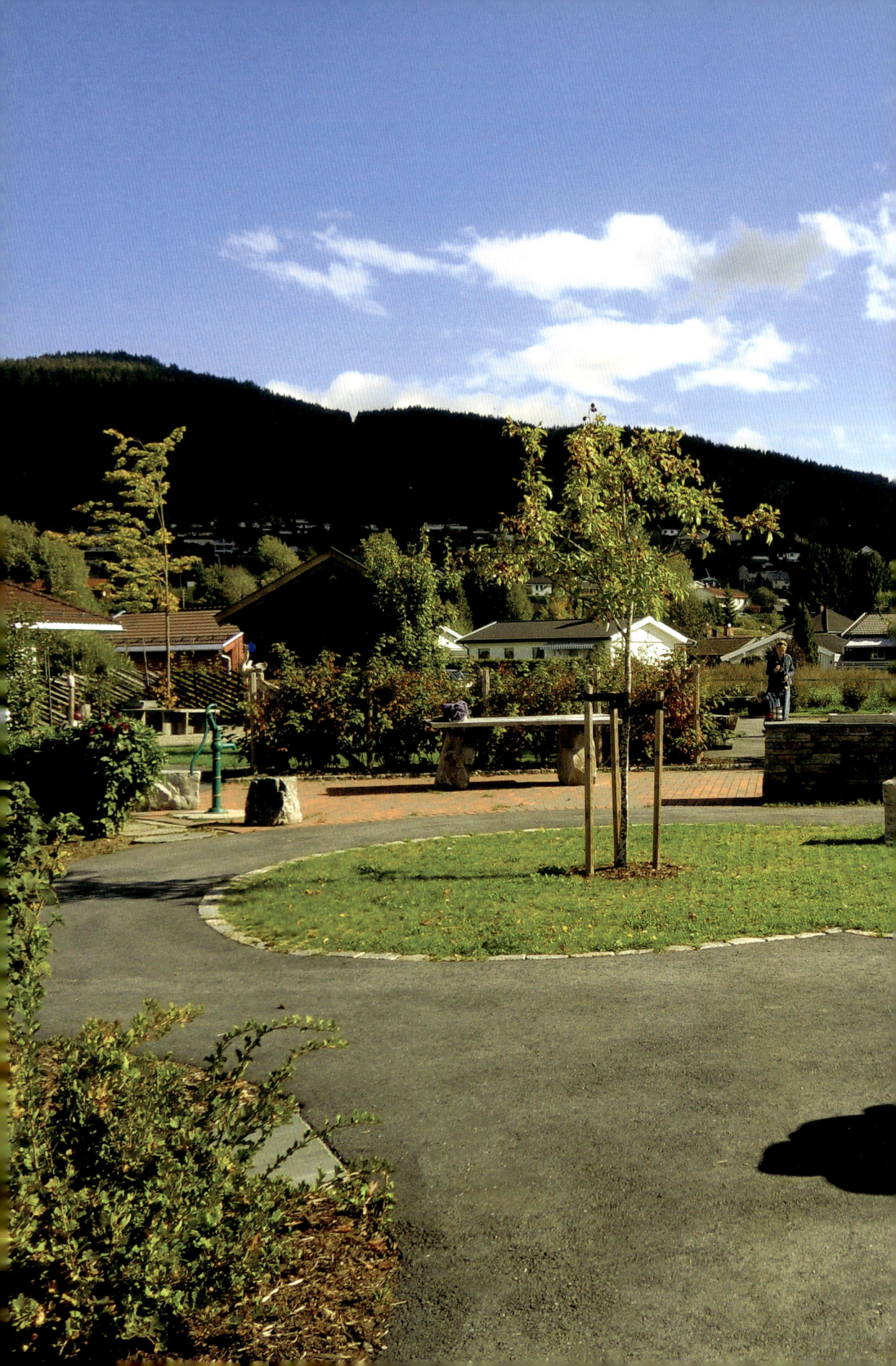

Case Study 4
Haugmotun Sensory Garden: a therapeutic garden for people with dementia

Ellen-Elisabeth Grefsrød and Nancy Gerlach-Spriggs

haug = small hill; mo = an area where it is difficult to grow plants because of bad soil conditions; tun = main part of a farm, the place where the farmhouse and other buildings are clustered

Haugmotun is a nursing home in the town of Notodden, Telemark County, Norway. The river Tinne whose name roughly translates 'the fishing place', bisects the town and is the site of one of Norway's first hydroelectric power plants. The people here have a close relationship with nature through traditional occupations of fishing and farming, and these legacies combine in the Haugmotun Sensory Garden designed in 2006 by Ellen-Elisabeth Grefsrød for the landscape architecture firm Nils Skaarer. The nearby river and typical farming activities inspired the garden's design. The impetus and funding for its construction came from Ole Holta, a wealthy power plant owner.

Holta's wife was diagnosed with dementia. After a period of stability, her condition quickly worsened and she needed to be institutionalised. She was lucky to have a husband who loved her so much and was able to fund a garden along with a new nursing home. This new construction was attached to a small house that previously hosted residents with Down's syndrome. Holta's only requirement was that this new institution should be built as soon as possible. The design was conceived and plans were drawn in February and March 2006 while the open site was covered in one meter of snow. The new nursing home and the garden were finished as planned in the autumn of that year, but

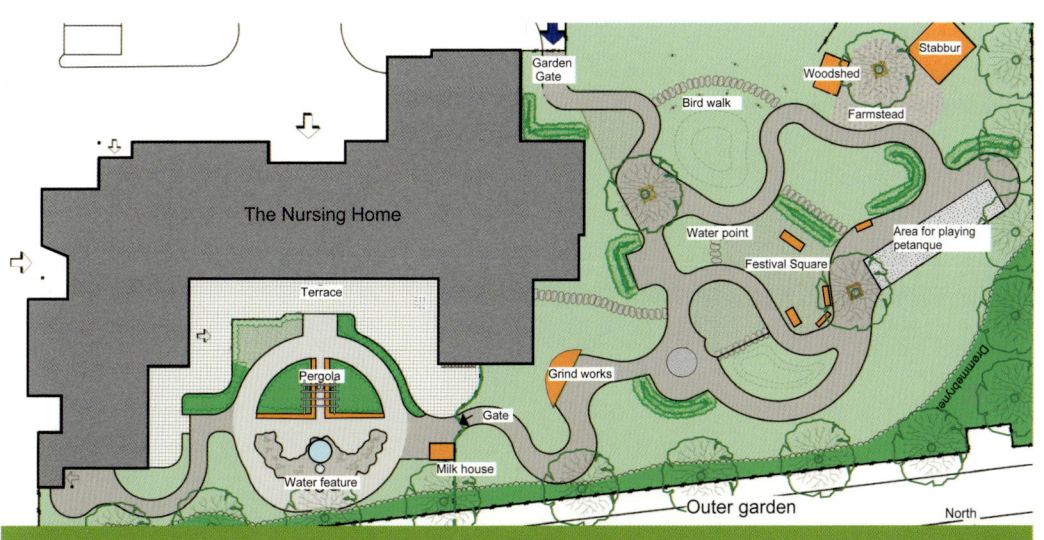

Fig. 45 Layout of garden showing the inner and outer gardens as described further in the case study (refer to appendix 1 on page 213 for enlarged version)

the town did not have the money to move patients there until spring of 2008. By then Holta's wife had died. This, of course, was a very sad start to a gift that was meant to give a much beloved wife the best possible last years of her life.

The growing season in this part of Norway is just over three months, yet the two-part garden is treasured both as a place to be in and a place to be viewed through the many windows of the facility during the long, cold winter. The inner garden, fenced for privacy and safety, is designed for 16 patients with dementia who need a serene and predictable space. The second outer garden is designed for 12 assisted living residents in flats next door. These residents are not diagnosed with dementia, but are elderly and can access nursing care as needed. This outer garden is designed for activity and is open to the public.

The inner garden is viewed from the living room of the dementia facility. A large terrace along the length of the building serves as a transition between the indoors and the garden.

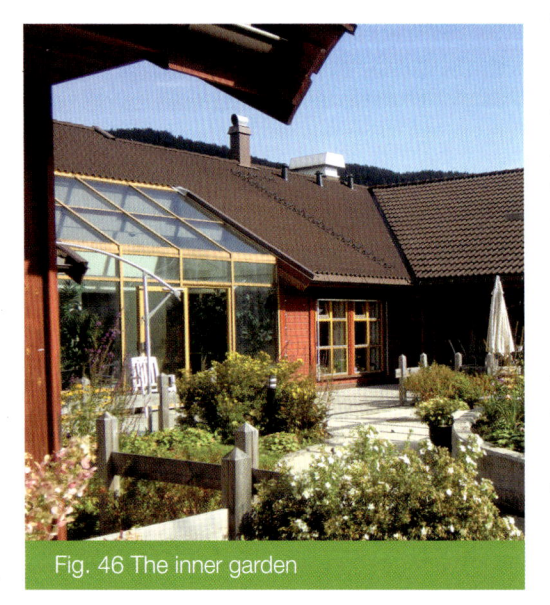

Fig. 46 The inner garden

This terrace offers choices of seating and is bounded by a railing that plays several roles. It defines the space as a 'safe' place to sit, rest and view the garden beyond. Patients can choose not to venture further, but the railing is a good place to pause, and because it is higher in some places, it is a good thing to lean against while standing. Patients can further survey the garden and eventually choose to take a walk to explore what it has to offer. Once in the garden, the railing provides a backdrop for colourful annuals.

The garden is filled with low-level sensory stimulation – visual, auditory, olfactory and tactile – intended to rekindle 'emotional memories' that may allow patients to engage with family and caregivers. It is designed to be used intuitively, with clear orienting features, a loop path that requires few decisions, and places to pause and sit as needed. The focal point of the inner garden can be seen from indoors and the terrace. It was inspired by the river that divides the northern part of Notodden and that is very much a part of the life of the community. The feature consists of a pergola and raised beds. It was originally planted with grasses reminiscent of the river and local vegetation but later amended by the nurses to include colourful flowers. This main focal point ends in a water feature also inspired by the river. A small waterfall and pond are surrounded by locally harvested, rounded river stones. It is a beautiful, quiet place with the sound of water trickling and the sunlight reflecting for those in the final stages of dementia.

The second, outer garden is connected to the inner garden with a gate hidden by a culturally familiar element – a 'milk house' or small structure where farmers stored the day's milk as it waited to be picked up by the cheese maker. If patients notice the gate and try to exit the inner garden, the milk house provides a topic of conversation and patients can be distracted away from the gate.

In contrast to the serene inner garden, the outer garden is a place of activity, choice and opportunity. Here, residents and guests can walk, feed and watch birds, garden, chop wood, have a party, barbeque, and even play sports.

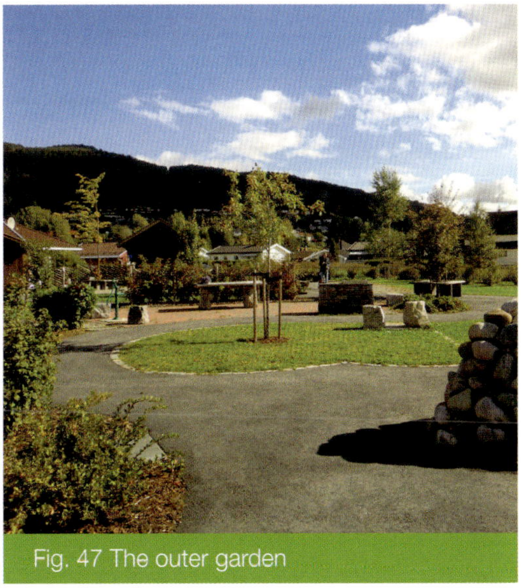

Fig. 47 The outer garden

The plant material was inspired by local flora, and traditional fruits and vegetables are grown – potatoes, strawberries, raspberries, black currants, apples and so on. Gardening tools are kept in a small traditional Norwegian structure.

Another classic Norwegian building, a stabbur or raised house, provides a place to chop, split and stack wood – important and well-known activities, which the male residents can engage in.

For residents who want less activity and who want to experience nature, there is seating under European mountain ash trees, which attract birds year round, but especially in autumn when they flock to eat the bright orange berries. There is also a 'bird walk', with bird sculptures made by local high school students and an area designed with native trees and shrubs that mimics the natural transition from the river's edge to the forest.

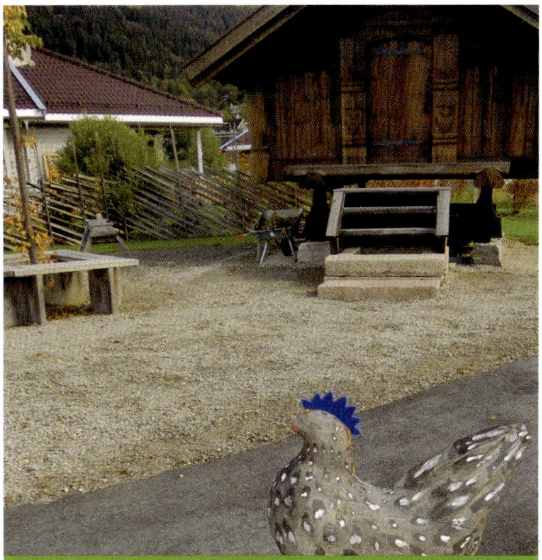

Fig. 48 The stabbur or raised house with bird sculpture

Not only residents enjoy this garden. The neighborhood school's 5th and 6th classes come once a week to garden, to walk, talk, or just be with the residents. The logo for Haugmoton, a sunburst with the words 'Sensory Garden' was a result of a competition between the pupils. The local garden society is also involved. Members come three times a year to start the garden in the spring, to host the important midsummer party and then to make ready the garden for winter. A retired man living in the neighborhood comes almost every day to work in the garden – on his own initiative.

The two gardens are deeply rooted in Norwegian culture and ecology. Patients and residents are surrounded by familiar landscape elements and as a result can engage in life-long activities and traditions.

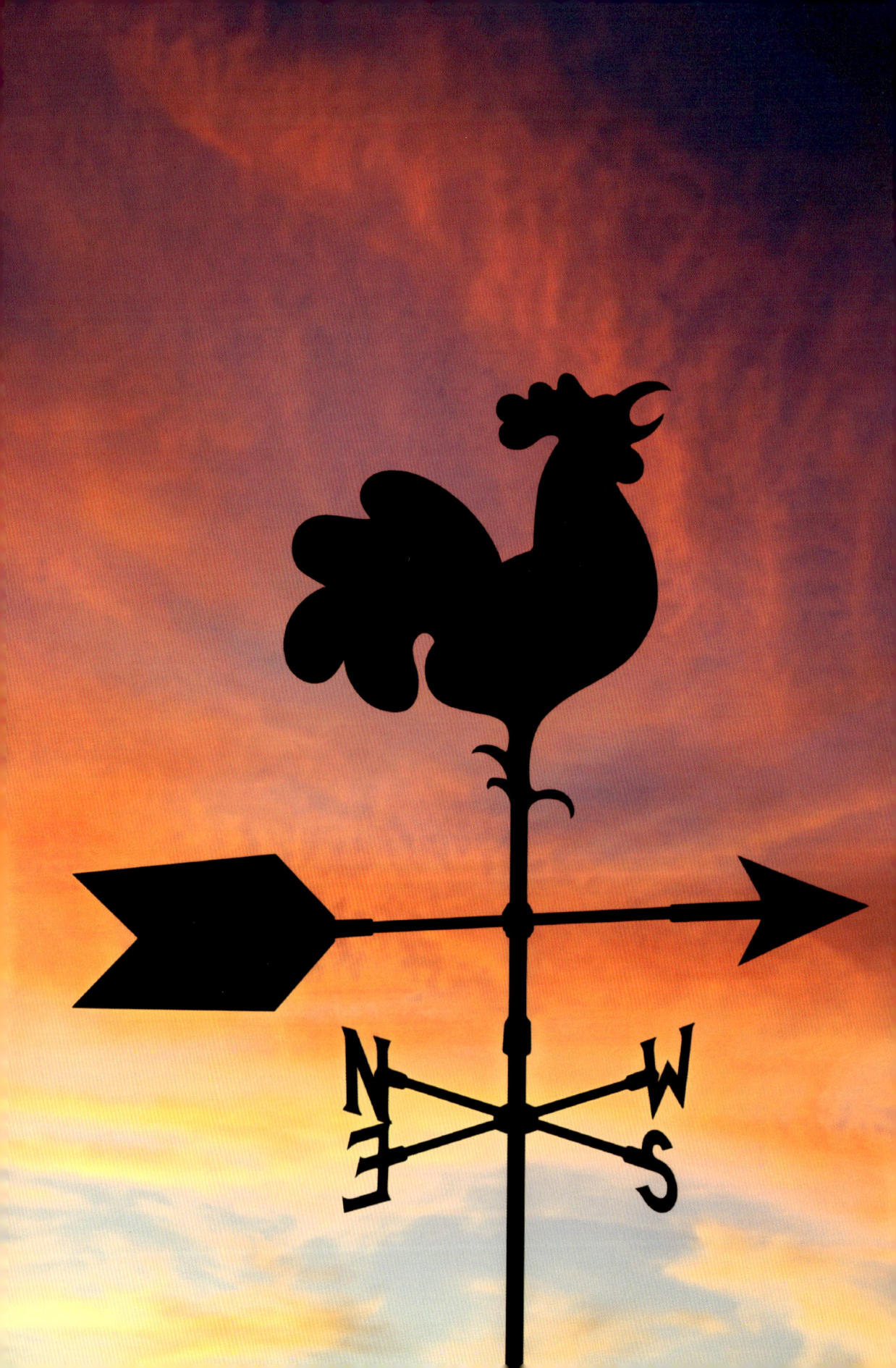

PART 3
DESIGN GUIDANCE

Chapter 6
Site and climate considerations

Annie Pollock, Richard Pollock, Clifford McClenaghan
Consultant: Fan Wang
Illustrations: Liz Fuggle

This chapter looks at environmental considerations in relation to the development of a site. These are relevant to all sites where the outside space is important, irrespective of the type of development. Everyone benefits from well-designed outdoor space, but for elderly people and in particular those with dementia, the external environment must be right, climatically as well as in detailed design terms, to encourage them to use it.

In a study in the USA of long-term care facilities with outdoor areas (Cohen-Mansfield, 2007) in response to the question, "Is the outdoor area used as much as it could be?" as many as 62% of the facilities responded "no". Over 30% noted "weather-related problems (e.g. too hot, too windy or too sunny)" as being a reason for non-use; of course in cool temperate climates, cold and rain are the more likely reasons for non-use.

Increasing pressure for land to be developed, especially in urban areas, means that available sites are often either considered as 'brownfield' (i.e. sites that have previously been developed for some use), or as land that has previously been considered undesirable to develop. Attractive, level 'greenfield' sites (i.e. sites that have never been developed) are few and far between. Land prices usually mean that the site has to be fairly densely developed; planning requirements for parking, fire access etc, often further reduce the areas of land that can be made into useful and recreational outdoor space.

The result of this is that architects are frequently faced with a difficult task in planning a site to maximise its use in terms of bed spaces. This makes it vital to assess the site at a very early stage to allot the best areas for outdoor use and areas that are large enough to provide viable 'outdoor rooms'.

The early involvement of a landscape architect will enable advice to be received on how best to ensure a good quality external site environment as the architect develops the building design. In assessing the site's attributes, the following will normally be looked at in detail, with sustainability as an overarching consideration:

- the building form and layout and its relationship to outdoor space
- climate and microclimate
- energy efficiency
- features within and outside the site that may affect it, e.g. buildings, trees, landform, noise
- flood risk, soil and drainage in relationship to getting plants grow healthily.

The following notes give basic advice, but do not take the place of detailed calculations to establish the microclimate around a proposed building and its open spaces. Further advice can be found in the references listed at the end of this chapter.

1. The building form and its relationship to outside space

To avoid confusion and repetition in this chapter, we deliberately avoid the use of 'north' or 'south' and instead use 'sun-facing' or 'not-sun-facing'. Therefore in the northern hemisphere, 'sun-facing' means south and 'not sun-facing' means north. Conversely in the southern hemisphere, 'sun-facing' means north and 'not sun-facing' means south.

The building footprint is often dictated, in part at least, by financial considerations and the need to put as much accommodation on the site as possible. Yet it should, ideally, arise out of equal consideration of the site, brief, use and user requirements, climate/microclimate and planning considerations as well as the business plan and funding model.

Each type of external space needs to be carefully considered in relation to its use and its microclimate. If the microclimate is not suitable, the space will not be successful. These external spaces include:

- **the public realm:** the 'public' environment around the care home, such as the roads, parking areas, the main entrance and any other 'public' landscaped space
- **courtyards:** internal open spaces surrounded by the building providing a safe secure environment
- **private and/or enclosed gardens:** partially enclosed by the development and walls or fencing
- **spaces at upper level:** balconies, terraces and roof gardens.

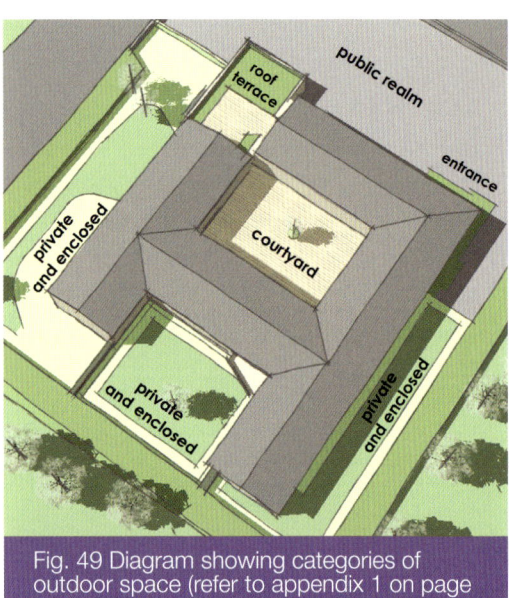

Fig. 49 Diagram showing categories of outdoor space (refer to appendix 1 on page 214 for enlarged version)

All of these open spaces associated with the built form provide an 'outdoor room' of some kind. The 'public realm' sets the scene for those arriving at the building and provides light to the rooms facing onto it. Courtyards, roof terraces, and gardens partly enclosed by the building will enable the building layout to accommodate more rooms with windows and attractive views facing into them, thereby allowing those who may be confined indoors to see out and feel closer to nature.

Well-designed 'outdoor rooms' can provide:

- warmth and sunlight, coolness and shade
- shelter from wind (particularly in colder climates where wind chill can lower ambient temperatures) and welcome breezes in hot climates

- daylight and an attractive outlook for the rooms surrounding or looking onto it
- space for activities and social events
- landscape in terms of plants, grass, trees and a setting for garden furnishings and sculptures
- an opportunity to experience the weather and change in seasons.

The site, and the layout of the building on it, must encourage the users to go outside by providing direct access from the building; it is essential that the outside space is easily usable, visible and safe. How the building is laid out on a site (which itself may have constraints of size, shape, and structure) will influence how well the external areas can be used.

Access from communal living areas to areas that are visible from within the building should be 'barrier free', through doors that are easy to use.

'Inside/outside' or intermediate spaces (e.g. lobbies, verandahs, conservatories) are particularly important in enabling easy use of the outdoors, as they allow:

- visibility of the outdoor area
- a sheltered space for people to sit and decide if they want to go out or not
- a space for undertaking 'outdoor' activities such as potting up plants if the weather is poor outside (e.g. too cold, too wet or too hot)
- a place where people can watch activities outside, even if they do not want to go out themselves
- a space to enjoy a meal or drink
- a space for putting on and taking off outdoor clothes and shoes.

Such spaces must be designed carefully so that they enable access to outdoor areas, rather than being a further barrier to going out (this is discussed in more detail in Chapter 9).

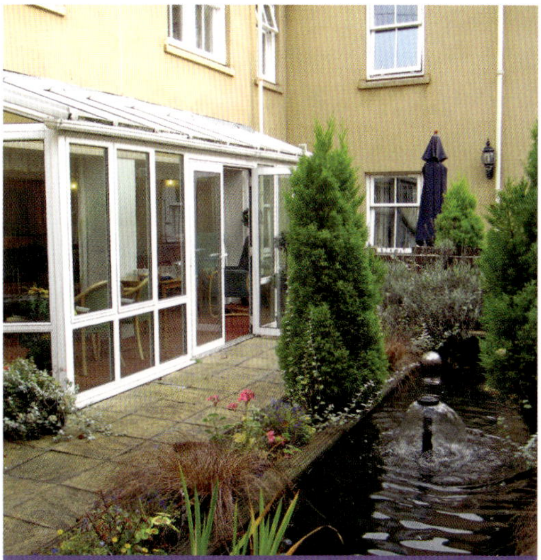

Fig. 50 Intermediate space enabling easy access to the outdoors

Sometimes atria are suggested as an alternative to outside space, particularly in the colder parts of the world where they can provide a bright space with plants when the weather is too poor to go out or on particularly tight, small sites where the provision of outdoor space is restricted.

However, apart from the fact that vitamin D cannot be gained from sunshine through glass (see Chapter 2), atria have some disadvantages that need to be carefully considered:

- additional fire and smoke risks necessitating fire separation and smoke barriers
- risk of overheating, necessitating specialised ventilation to ensure that the spaces stay cool in the summer and that odours are removed
- cost of glazing

- possible loss of daylight to rooms adjacent to them due to the roof structures causing shading
- the need for specialised lighting to ensure that plants within the atria can thrive.

General site planning principles

Large buildings on a site can often, by their form and shape, cause overshadowing and wind turbulence. Careful assessment of this is essential, whilst bearing in mind that climate change the world over is generally resulting in more extreme conditions such as drought, greater variation in temperature, more wind, fire, flooding and so on. This means that not only may open spaces require more upkeep, but they may be more challenging to use if the design does not take account of the building and its effect on the microclimate.

Some general principles of site planning are noted below for buildings in the northern and southern hemispheres. In making these recommendations, we make particular reference to P J Littlefair's books, published by the BRE press, and Brown and Gillespie's book *Microclimatic landscape design: creating thermal comfort and energy efficiency* (1995).

We have adapted diagrams from these references to illustrate our text.

- All key living spaces should, if at all possible, be 'sun-facing'; if a 'not-sun-facing' elevation is unavoidable, the buildings may need to be spaced further apart to allow penetration of sunlight to external spaces
- Sites that slope down away from the sun present even greater challenges to providing sun access; buildings will need to be spaced further apart to achieve this with the tallest buildings placed at the 'not-sun-facing' end of the site

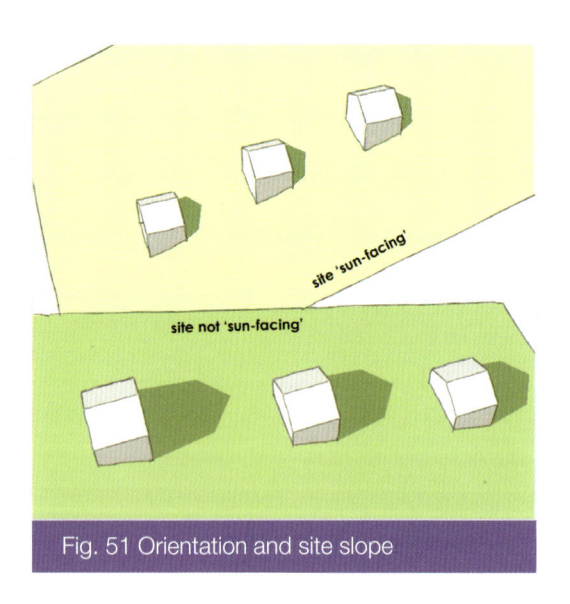

Fig. 51 Orientation and site slope

- Semi-enclosed spaces should be opened to the 'sun-facing' half of the sky; in a courtyard situation, ideally the 'sun-facing' part of the building should be lower to enable sun access

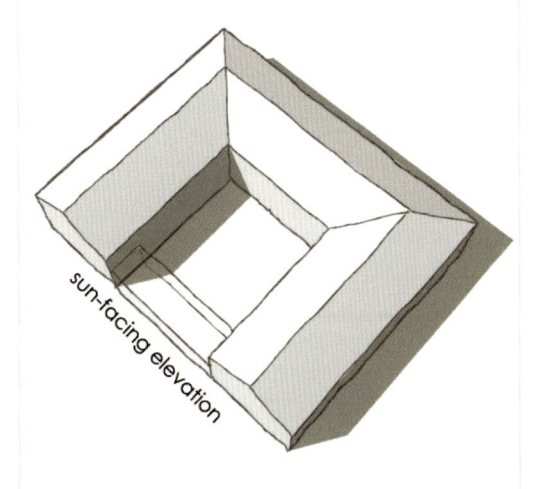

Fig. 52 Sun access and semi enclosed spaces

- Building extensions, building wings, garages etc, should be sited to the 'not-sun-facing' side of the main development to minimise overshadowing

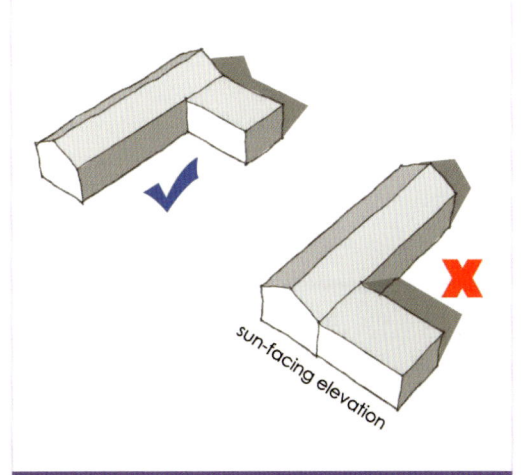

Fig. 54 Site extensions located to minimise overshadowing

- Terraced or slab buildings should be laid out on an east-west axis so that at least one elevation faces and accesses direct sunlight

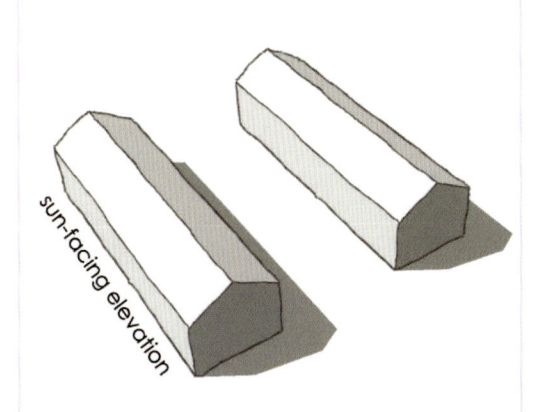

Fig. 53 Sun access to long elevation

- Bedrooms should ideally be east-facing, as this not only provides bright morning light to help rouse people from sleep but also prevents overheating during the afternoon and evening
- Wind modelling should be considered at an early stage to ensure built form provides shelter and avoids gusts of wind and wind chill, or in hotter climates, how cooling breezes can be directed into the living areas.

More detail on wind is provided later in this chapter.

Public realm

These areas form the approach to the building and will set the tone. They must not only 'feel' right, that is, be welcoming and comfortable to be in, but also be climatically successful. They should provide shelter from the wind, sun and glare, yet have sufficient sunlight to benefit the users and keep the planting and hard surfaces in a healthy state. Shady areas of the site can be utilised for service access and car parking. Further detail is provided later in this chapter under microclimatic considerations.

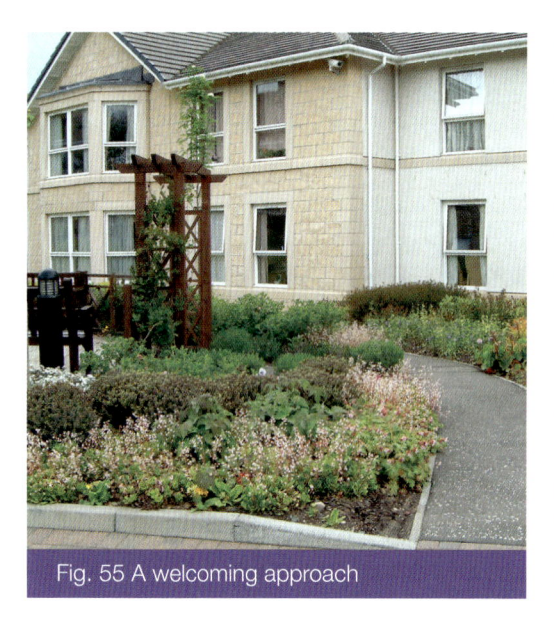

Fig. 55 A welcoming approach

Courtyards and private, enclosed gardens

In any social and people-orientated setting (and a care home is an example of this) courtyards and enclosed gardens may become the focus of communal life, since not only are they private but are also usually larger than any space inside the home. They provide 'neutral ground' and 'escape' from the busy internal environment.

Throughout history, courtyards in particular have been important architectural features, providing outdoor living spaces for family dwellings and public buildings alike. In hot countries they are designed to provide shade, often with water features to increase humidity and thereby cool the temperature; whereas in temperate climates, they are normally designed to provide warm, sunny and sheltered outdoor spaces without too much shade (means of providing shade can be added as required).

These fundamental differences are usually reflected in the size of the space. However, in a care-home setting, because the courtyard or enclosed garden may have bedrooms looking onto it, the need for privacy will also affect the size of the space.

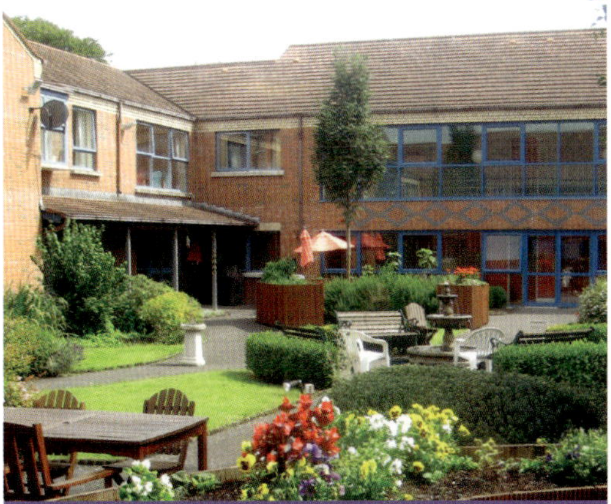

Fig. 56 Opportunities for activity whilst maintaining privacy for flats looking over it

The shape of a courtyard or enclosed garden can also affect wayfinding. For example, the internal corners of outdoor spaces, which are formed by the building, are usually shady and can seem gloomy. Consequently, the person with dementia could have difficulty in finding the door into the building in this location on a bright day.

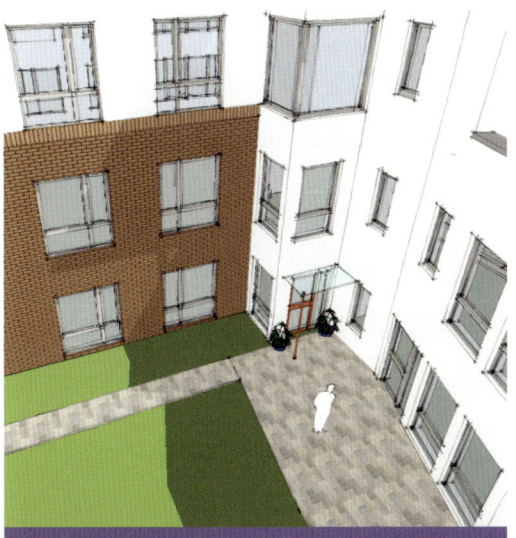

Fig. 57 Entrances in shady corners need to be made clearly visible

Terraces, roof gardens and balconies

These also have historically formed part of outdoor living spaces in both hot and temperate climates. Today, in care-home settings, features such as terraces, roof gardens and balconies are rarely included; this means that residents on upper floors have no easy access to outside space. It is so important for everyone to have ready access to the outdoors that consideration should always be given to providing terraces, roof gardens and balconies, to provide outdoor space at the upper levels (Marshall, 2010).

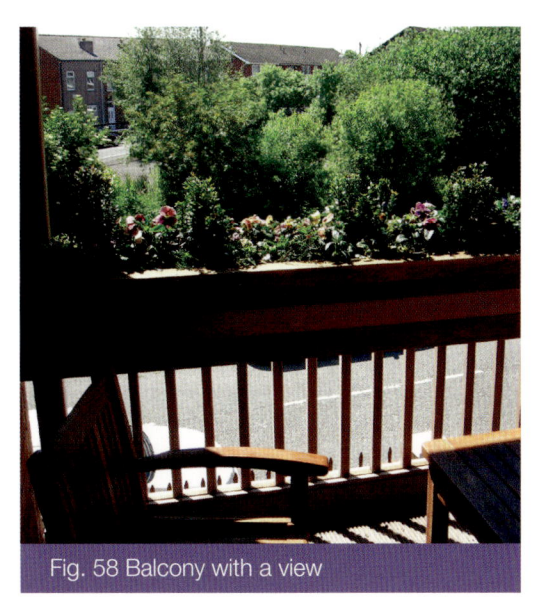

Fig. 58 Balcony with a view

The climatic considerations are generally the same as for other outdoor spaces. However, it must be noted that wind turbulence increases with altitude, therefore outdoor space at upper levels is likely to experience more wind and the design needs to take this into account.

Balconies may also provide both a means of shading in hot climates, to the rooms they lead from, and a degree of insulation for rooms in colder climates.

For example, in Finland there are balconies that can be enclosed by glass windows in the winter, thereby providing extra insulation to the room they lead off whilst retaining a bright semi-outdoor area to sit in on a sunny day; in Singapore, use is made of balconies with lots of planting to provide a cooler environment.

However, balconies and roof overhangs above windows will block sunlight, especially in the summer, and will also overshadow balconies of floors below. The design, therefore, should ideally stagger or set back balconies, as illustrated by this sketch adapted from P J Littlefairs's book (2011). However, in hot climates, this shade might be welcomed and/or shading devices incorporated into the design.

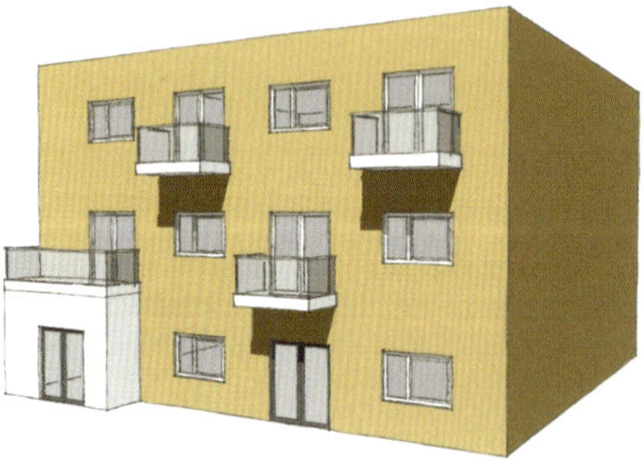

Fig. 59 Balconies should be staggered or set back

2. Climate and microclimate

The key issue in considering the climate and microclimate of a building in relation to its site, as noted by Brown and Gillespie (1995) is 'to create comfortable habitats for humans. Ultimately a landscape will not be well used by people if it does not provide a thermally comfortable environment.'

Surveys (Littlefair, 2011) have shown that people like sunny rooms.

"People like sunlight. In surveys, 90% of those asked said they appreciated having sunlight in their homes. The sun is seen as providing light and warmth, making rooms look bright and cheerful and also having a therapeutic, health giving affect."

Sun will warm up rooms. People with dementia may not be particularly active and in these circumstances an ambient temperature within the building of 21°-23°C (depending on your climate) is comfortable, whilst 25°C is too warm and 15°C is uncomfortably cool. However, if these internal spaces warm with the sun, this may inhibit activity and thereby make people less keen to venture outside.

Outside comfort depends not only on temperature but also on direct sun, wind, humidity and rainfall. A comfortable ambient temperature range inside the building may be uncomfortable in the external environment, depending on these other variables. Different climatic conditions will have different requirements for comfort; this will be further affected by the seasons. For example, in a cold northern climate, admitting sun is slightly more important than blocking wind, whereas in a hot southern climate, shade and breezes are essential.

This is precisely why consideration and manipulation of the external environment is so important if staff and people with dementia are to enjoy the outdoors.

Every site is unique in terms of its climatic and microclimatic considerations and so modelling in the design and planning stage is vital to explore issues of sunlight and wind. Expert advice is essential. This is discussed in more detail below under the following headings:

- Sun, sun angles and orientation
- Aspect ratio and solar shadow index
- Solar radiation
- Shelter from wind.

Sun, sun angles and orientation

In the UK alone, the length of daylight hours varies enormously from north to south. For example, in the Shetland Isles, there are almost 19 hours of daylight at midsummer and less than 6 hours in the winter. In contrast, in the south of England, there are approximately 15 hours of daylight in the summer and less than 8 hours in the winter.

The further south one goes, the less variable the length of day between summer and winter becomes, until at the equator they are equal in length. These same principles of shortening daylight hours apply with increasing latitude in the southern hemisphere.

Throughout northern Europe in particular, the need for sunshine after a long, dark winter is high for both mental and physical wellbeing. A survey of householders in Switzerland, Netherlands and the UK showed that over 75% of householders wanted plenty of sun in their homes, with less than 5% wanting little sun (Littlefair et al., 2000).

John Reynolds noted in his book (2002) that to someone living in an a northern temperate climate, low daylight levels are seen as a sign of deprivation of the sun's warmth, whereas to someone living in a hot, dry climate, an outdoor space with low daylight levels will often signify welcome coolness. Sunlight is vital for our very existence (see Chapter 2 for more detail) and site layout is the most important factor affecting the duration of sunlight in buildings and open spaces:

- direct sunlight makes vitamin D which promotes good health and maintains strong bones
- sunlight provides a high light intensity which maintains body rhythm and promotes alertness
- most garden plants need direct sunlight to thrive, many needing at least six hours of direct sunlight in the growing season
- sunlight can help kill germs and prevent hard surfaces developing green algal growth which can result from shaded damp conditions
- sunlight will melt frost and snow during the winter months.

The angle of the sun varies according to latitude, time of year and time of day; it will have a great influence on the amount of sun received.

In northern Europe (e.g. latitude 56°N), the sun's path is 270° wide at the summer solstice and the maximum solar altitude is 58°. At the winter solstice, the sun's path is 90° wide and the maximum solar altitude is 11°. There is no equivalent landmass in the southern hemisphere.

In southern Europe (e.g. latitude 36°N) and the southern hemisphere, e.g. South Australia (36°S), the sun's path is 240° wide at the summer solstice and the maximum solar altitude is 77°. At the winter solstice, the sun's path is 120° wide and the maximum solar altitude is 30°.

Sun-path diagrams, appropriate to the latitude, can be used to estimate when direct sunlight will reach the ground surface. The following diagrams are simplified to show the basic information.

Equally, the effect of a building on surrounding land and on enclosed garden areas can be plotted.

Most architectural offices now use computer software to plot sun and shade over the course of the day and in different seasons of the year. This is shown in the following diagrams, illustrating the solar envelope of a proposed care home in northern Europe at 8am, 11am, 2pm and 5pm in March and June and in Australia in September and December.

Fig. 60 Typical sun-path diagrams for northern hemisphere

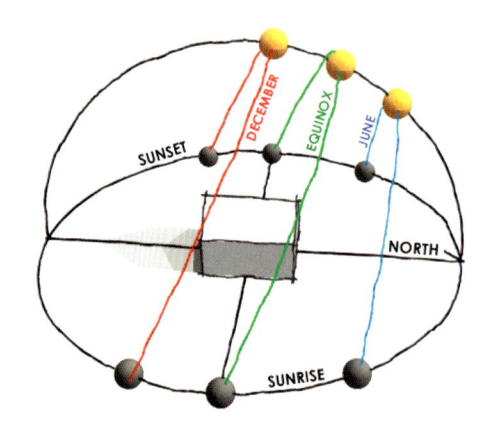

Fig. 61 Typical sun-path diagrams for southern hemisphere

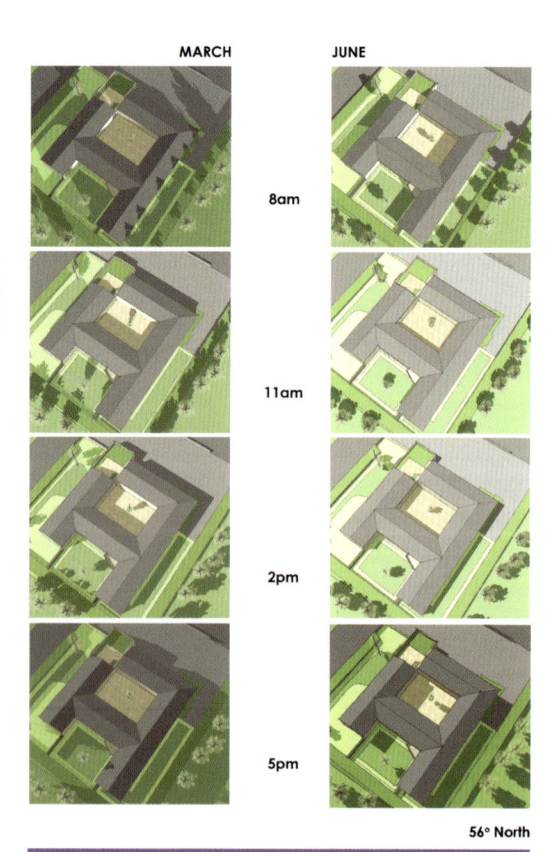

Fig. 62 Sun access throughout the day in the northern hemisphere (refer to appendix 1 on page 215 for enlarged version)

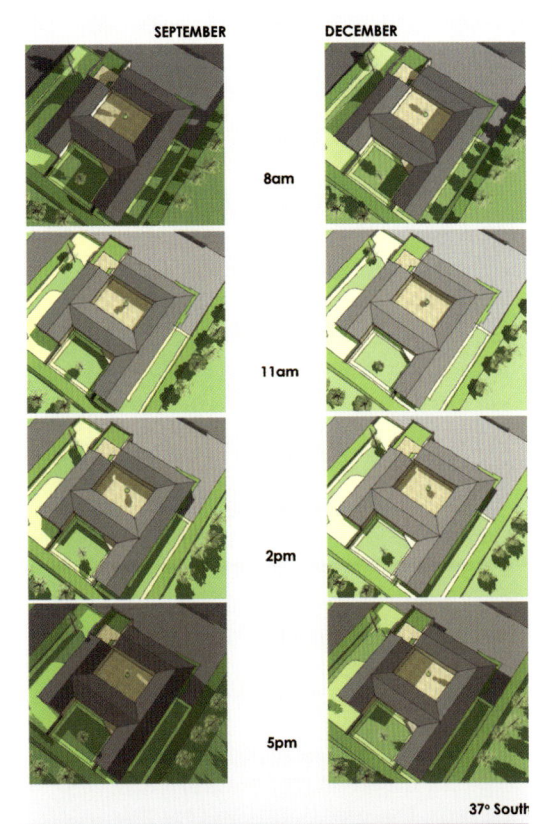

Fig. 63 Sun access throughout the day in the southern hemisphere (refer to appendix 1 on page 216 for enlarged version)

Any obstructions (i.e. existing site objects such as trees, buildings, or landform) should be incorporated into these diagrams to determine how they might affect the time of day and months of the year when sun will reach particular parts of the site. This will then inform the design to ensure that the spaces created are useful rather than just 'left over' from siting the building.

Key points

- in all proposals, the outdoor space for sun access should be carefully analysed, recognising that latitude and orientation will have a big affect on comfort

- a facility should ideally have several outdoor areas to maximise sun access at all times of the day; in the northern hemisphere, this means east-facing for morning use, south-facing for use during most of the day, and west and north-west-facing for evening use in the summer.

- in the southern hemisphere, east-facing spaces are good for morning use and north-facing spaces are good for use for most of the day

- west-facing spaces in hotter climates (e.g. latitudes 36°N and S) are generally too hot in the summer months

- sites furthest north and furthest south will need to maximise by design the daylight and sunlight reaching outdoor spaces during the winter months

- balcony design needs careful thought in respect of sun access and overshadowing when there are balconies on several floors.

Aspect ratio and solar shadow index

The amount of sun and shade a space receives is vital to its success and varies with the shape and size of the built form, enclosing walls, site slope and vegetation. This is referred to as 'aspect ratio' and 'solar shadow index'.

The ratio of height of surrounding buildings and width of space is a vital consideration, together with sun angle in summer and winter. Yoshinobu Ashihara, a Japanese architect, described the concept of 'aspect ratio' (1984). He noted that urban streets with a width (W) to height (H) ratio of greater than one lead to an open and spacious feeling whereas a ratio of less than one is likely to give occupants oppressive feelings.

The ideal is an outdoor space narrow enough to maintain a shaded area during the heat of a summer's day, yet wide enough to allow solar radiation in winter, probably a minimum W/H = 1.5 in a temperate climate.

From a climatic point of view, the size and degree of enclosure has a significant impact on its performance and indeed on that of the building enclosing it.

- if the enclosure is too wide relative to the height of the buildings surrounding it, it becomes a square or a park in character but the influence of the buildings on its microclimate diminishes (e.g. W/H = 3+)

- if the space becomes too narrow, it can become more of a ventilation shaft or light well. It may provide light and admit rain but its microclimate will be totally dominated by the building and anyone looking out of a window will not even be able to see the sky (e.g. W/H = 2/3" or less). This is particularly important when considering the design of courtyards, which are popular because they are 'secure', being internal to the building.

Reynolds (2002) also looked at aspect ratio, using another similar method of calculation: the area of the courtyard (rather than the width) divided by the average height of the surrounding walls. In addition, Reynolds also noted a 'solar shadow index', which, if used in conjunction with the aspect ratio will show the amount of sun that will reach ground level (solar shadow index = south wall height divided by north-south floor width). The greater the solar shadow index, the deeper the well formed by the courtyard and the less winter sun that will reach the floor and even the north wall of the space.

Aspect Ratios - Width/Height

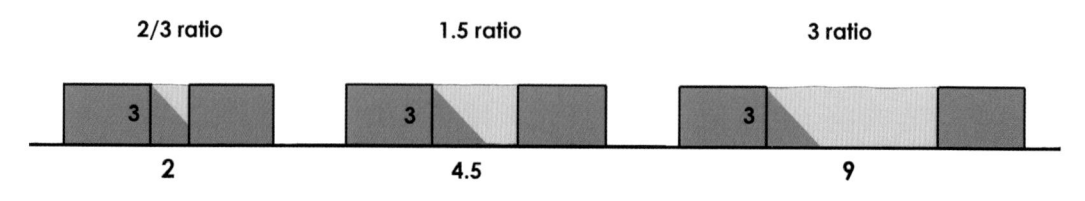

Fig. 64 Aspect ratio

Both of these methods could be used together with sun angle and slope of the site to determine sun access for a given location. The appropriate walls for sun entry (i.e. south-facing in the northern hemisphere and north-facing in the southern hemisphere) should be lower than the other sides and ideally single storey to minimise overshadowing.

The aim in the UK and other countries with temperate climates in the northern or southern hemispheres is to achieve outdoor spaces that receive sunshine. Items that create shade without relying on the built form can readily be added, such as parasols/umbrellas and awnings that can be easily erected and moved as required.

More permanent shade for very sunny sites and/or hotter climates can be created by the use of verandahs, roof overhangs or garden shelters such as summerhouses, gazebos or pergolas with climbing plants to grow over them. These can be included in the design from the start of a project or, in the case of summerhouses, gazebos and pergolas, added afterwards if required. With careful consideration of sun angles, overhanging roofs can provide shade from summer sun yet still allow penetration of winter sun into the area and the building to provide warmth (see Fig 66).

In very hot countries such as Australia, extreme weather conditions can restrict the use of gazebos, pergolas and other freestanding structures. For example, open roofed pergolas can be inviting in winter but unusable in summer and adding a permanent roof will make the structure 'season specific'. To overcome this, consideration should be given to include automated retractable roofs – let the structure adjust with the seasons!

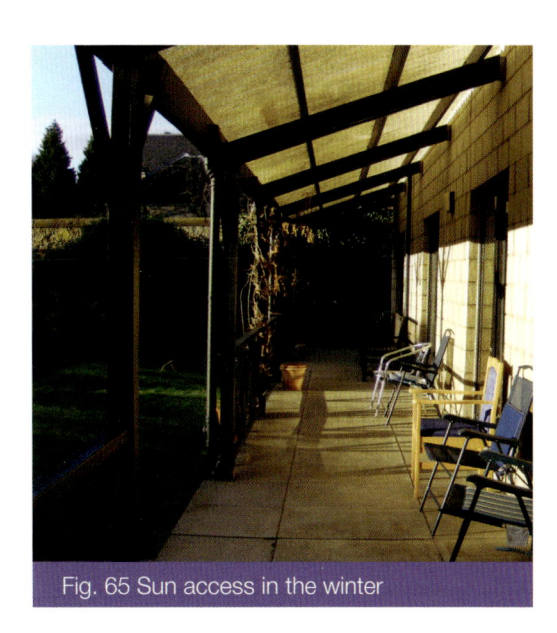

Fig. 65 Sun access in the winter

Outdoor spaces must be large enough for those using them not to feel overlooked or spied on by the windows looking out. It is equally important for those who live in the building to be able to look out of windows and see the sky so that they have a visual connection between their indoor space and the climate and outdoor world.

Key points:

- in the early design stages, the proportions of the outdoor spaces and their relation with the sun angles and sun access throughout the year should be carefully checked
- if the landform, neighbouring buildings, large trees on adjacent land or a requirement for high boundary walls will shade part of the site for most of the day; this should be considered at the outset of a project and a design approach developed to minimise their effect
- courtyards and semi-enclosed gardens or roof terraces must not be so small (i.e. with a high solar

shadow index) that they act only as a source of light to surrounding rooms; in addition to requirements for sun and shade, the need for privacy in an outdoor space should be considered, both for the users and for those in the rooms looking out

- in hot climates, where shade is needed, a tall narrow courtyard provides cool shady space; in colder climates where sun is needed, courtyards must be of a larger plan area surrounded by lower walls to allow sun access.

Solar radiation and solar gain

Solar radiation is the radiant energy emitted by the sun. Solar gain is the increase in surface and ambient temperatures resulting from solar radiation.

The colour of materials in the external environment is important to the amount of heat retained and subsequently radiated; light colours reflect heat, dark colours absorb heat.

Grass, trees and ground cover planting can also influence microclimate, keeping ground temperatures lower than most hard surfaces as a result of evapotranspiration and their ability to reduce the impact of solar radiation (Goulding, Lewis, & Steemers, 1992).

Outdoor 'rooms' can be comfortable in colder climates, even during the winter months, if the wind is blocked and sufficient solar radiation is available.

In terms of design for the older person and people with dementia, the following should be considered and a balance struck:

- very light colours are often used in building cladding and external paving in hot countries to prevent these structures absorbing too much heat from the sun and possibly being uncomfortable to touch or walk on; however, glare is a big issue for older eyes
- darker coloured materials may make evening use of outside areas more comfortable due to their ability to absorb solar radiation; however, they may get too hot to touch during the heat of the day and will cool quickly as temperatures drop
- sun-facing communal rooms may require shading devices to prevent the indoor environment becoming too hot in the summer
- bedrooms should ideally have an eastern aspect as any room facing due west is likely to be too hot in hot weather and shading devices may have to be so low due to afternoon and evening sun angles that they cut out daylight
- unglazed intermediate spaces, for example verandahs, arcades or courtyards can create their own microclimate. They will have a role in channeling wind and may be designed to provide protection from the sun for adjacent openings and surfaces in regions where the summers are hot; if designed carefully, they may also allow low-level winter sun to enter the building, thereby allowing heat gain in the building in the winter.

summer shadow line

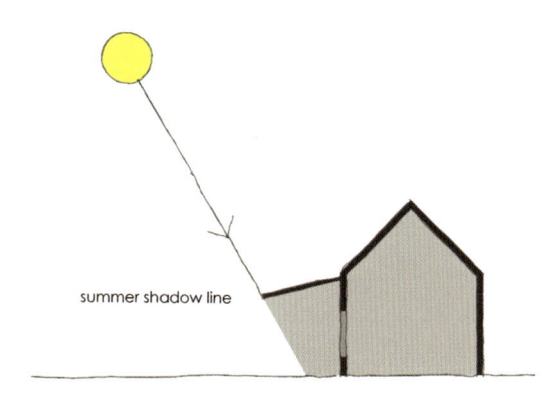

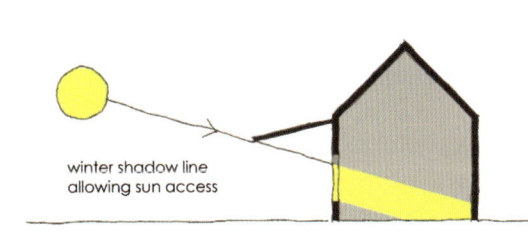

winter shadow line allowing sun access

Fig. 66 A covered verandah can help with both shade and sun access

- glare within the building due to low sun angles or bright external finishes needs to be addressed by blinds, awnings, tinted glass etc
- reflective surfacing can also be useful, not only to brighten a courtyard but also to augment the amount of solar radiation entering openings intended to allow sun access; care needs to be taken to avoid glare for users and for people with dementia it is vital not to provide a visual element they might not understand

- compensatory higher lighting levels on return to the building are essential to avoid momentary loss of vision and the possibility of falls on re-entering the building from a bright external environment. Good lighting design and control of adjacent glazing should compensate for this.

Key points:

- by understanding the wind and sun access for each site, it is possible to create a sunny outdoor environment that allows also for the provision of shade
- in cold climates, dark exterior surfaces are beneficial to absorb radiation, whereas in hot climates light surfaces are needed to reflect radiation; therefore consider carefully the heat absorbance and light reflective properties of the materials used externally, to maximise comfort and avoid glare
- minimise heat gain by using a balance of hard surfacing and grass and plants – a rule of thumb is 30:70 hard surface to soft landscape
- avoid strong differences between indoor and outdoor lighting levels.

Shelter from wind

In addition to maximising sun, shelter from wind is vital. The effect of the built environment on wind patterns needs to be clearly understood and appropriate measures incorporated to achieve shelter.

Wind is more complex and unpredictable than sun and solar exposure in site planning and consequently is much more difficult to deal with. Initially, a wind rose can be used to give an indication of the local conditions for any month or over the year in general.

Wind has a great effect on climate the world over. Wind chill, the air temperature felt on skin when exposed to wind, is always lower than the air temperature and therefore shelter is a serious consideration in cold climates. Conversely, in hot climates such as Australia, cooling winds off the sea are welcomed in the summer, whereas the impact of winds from the hot landmass need to minimised.

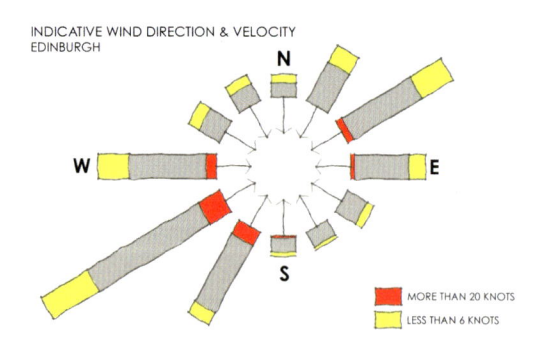

Fig. 67 Wind rose for Edinburgh, Scotland

According to what we see and hear, it is possible to estimate the windiness and decide what actions need to be taken.

- We feel wind physically by coolness, disturbance to hair, eyes, clothes and by its force; the effects range from pleasant breeze to nuisance, from discomfort to causing issues of safety.

- We 'see' wind by movement of tree leaves and branches, flags, plants, clothes on a clothes line.

- We hear wind due to the noise created by wind flow, the sound of wind in plants such as grasses, the rattling of building components and soon.

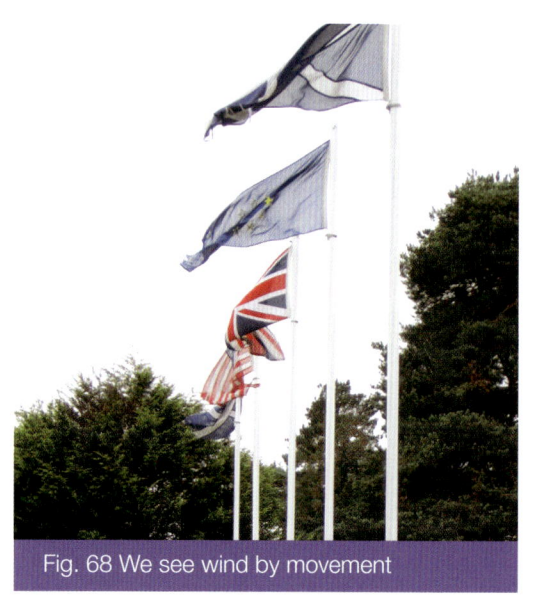

Fig. 68 We see wind by movement

When outside on a windy day, we can usually deal with the buffeting which gusts of wind cause; a few seconds in steady wind is often enough for the average person to adapt to windy conditions.

However, if the wind is sudden or unexpected this may be more difficult to deal with; our responses may not be fast enough and we may be blown over, blown off balance or blown out of position. For older people and people with dementia, this is far more difficult:

- they may not be able to understand the visuals and sound of wind and so the impact of it may be severe and confusing

- they are usually frailer and therefore less physically able to deal with wind; adjusting to gusts of wind requires strength (which they may not have) and learning (which they probably are unable to do)

- even if they do understand the signs of wind, they may be affected psychologically by its sound and a 'fear of falling'.

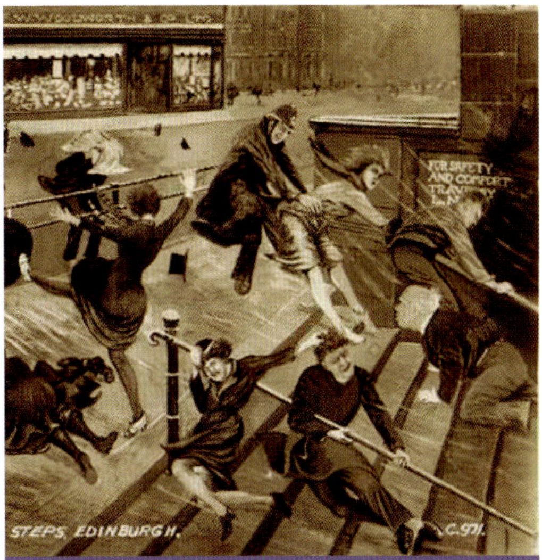

Fig. 69 Waverley Steps, Edinburgh, Scotland

Additionally, on a purely practical level, a gusty outdoor space will collect litter and leaf-fall and this will add to maintenance costs as well as causing issues for people with dementia.

Therefore, it is of the greatest importance to understand the effects of wind on buildings and how the built form may modify wind.

At site planning level, the main issues to note are:

- air flows from high pressure to low pressure; for example, when air meets an obstruction such as building or landform, it creates a high pressure zone of increased velocity on the windward side and a low pressure zone of lower velocity on the leeward side

- wind tends to flow round an obstruction rather than bounce off it in random directions, turbulence increases and velocity decreases behind the obstruction; certain building shapes are therefore preferable to avoid turbulence (see diagrams below)

- air speed is slower near the surface of the earth than higher in the atmosphere, therefore exposed buildings or sites at higher altitudes are likely to experience higher wind speed, which may affect balconies and roof terraces or gardens

- wind is accelerated when constricted, for example when it flows through a gap between two buildings

- near water, a breeze will tend to blow off water towards the land during the day; at night the flow is reversed

- in valleys, wind tends to blow uphill during the day and at night this reverses, with wind blowing back down into the valley; cool air will tend to collect in pockets formed by topography or vegetation.

Therefore, the shape of a building and its location are both important. They can affect normal wind patterns and create down drafts and eddies that could make, for example, a courtyard, semi-enclosed garden or the main entrance unusable in certain conditions. The text and sketches below show advice in respect to the shape of a building and wind (see also Brown & Gillespie, 1995 and P.J. Littlefair's books from which the following sketches have been adapted):

- orientate L-shaped buildings with the outside corner toward the prevailing wind

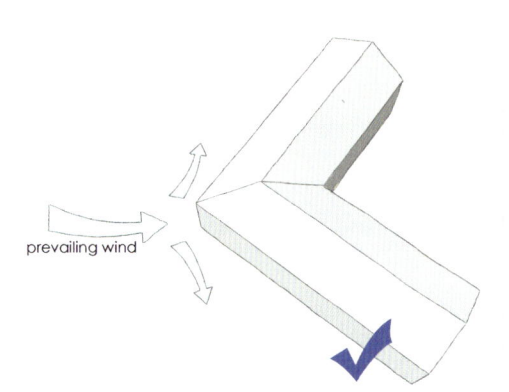

- in closed courtyards, note that the greatest shelter will be, on one side, dependent on the orientation of the courtyard in respect of the wind; the height of the courtyard buildings will extend the area of shelter (but will also create shadow)

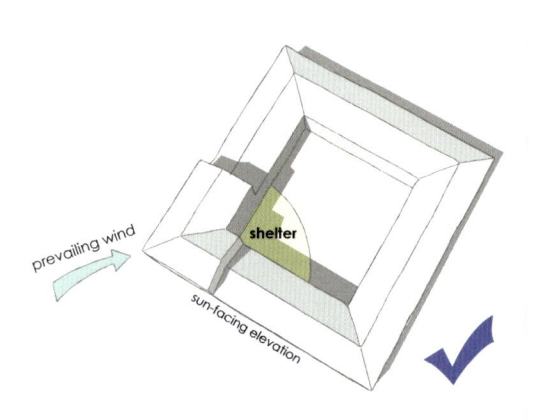

Fig. 70

Fig. 72

- orientate U-shaped buildings with the open side U facing leeward to provide more shelter

- don't create funnel-like gaps between buildings or narrow alleys (this can even occur with a joined building if the door is in the sharp corner)

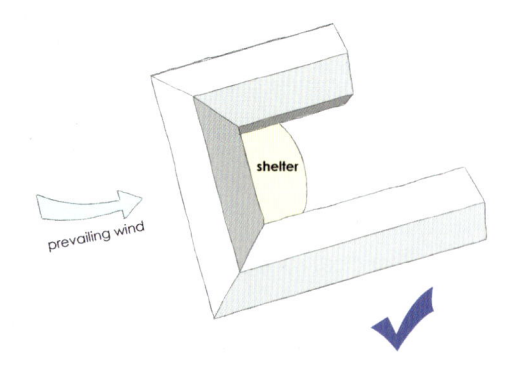

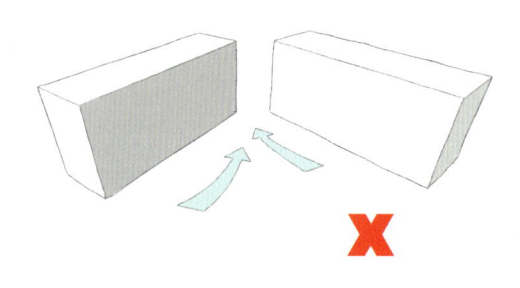

Fig. 71

Fig. 73

- orientate the long axis of a building parallel to the dominant wind; large side walls facing into the wind will create turbulence and eddies that may affect pedestrians adversely

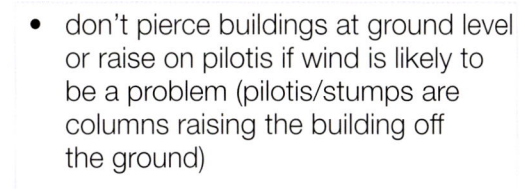

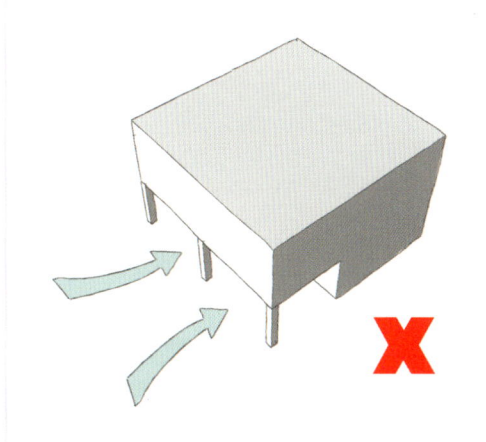

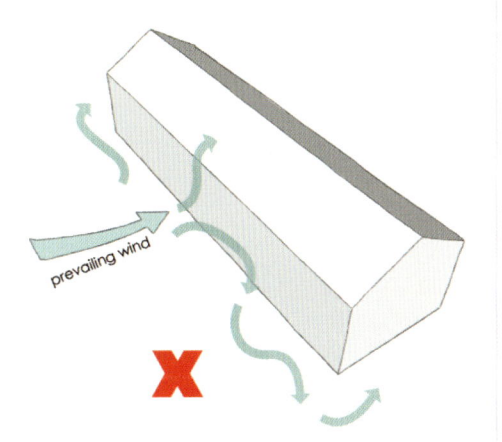

- don't pierce buildings at ground level or raise on pilotis if wind is likely to be a problem (pilotis/stumps are columns raising the building off the ground)

Fig. 75

- avoid creating large cube-shaped flat-roofed buildings (roof gardens will need careful consideration in this respect). A podium or raised base at ground level or a stepped, pyramidal or pitched-roofed building will help

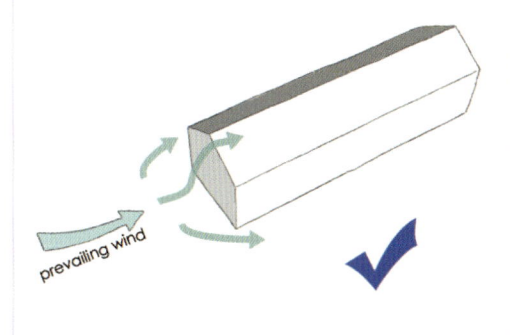

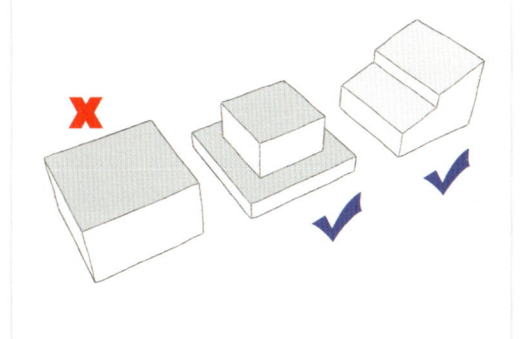

Fig. 74

Fig. 76

111

- avoid long, parallel rows of smooth faced buildings, as these will create turbulence.

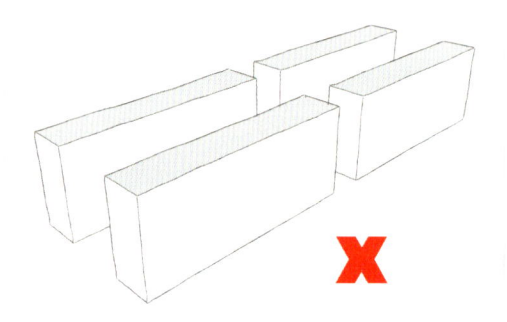

Fig. 77

Generally, tall buildings cause higher wind speeds at pavement level. If such a building is unavoidable, pavements and kerbs may need careful consideration to minimise people tripping off them when hit by gusty winds. Such issues are not usually part of the design approval process, yet gusty winds at ground level can be hazardous, as noted in the APS Digest (2011), where it was reported that gusts of wind had knocked pedestrians over at the base of the tallest tower in Yorkshire (England).

On a detailed design level, if people with dementia are to be encouraged to use an external space at will (garden, terrace, balcony, roof garden) the door to it needs to be easy to use. This in itself poses some challenges since, if use of the door affects the internal environment adversely (draught, cold, heat etc), there will be pressure to keep the door shut and even to lock it to prevent use. Consequently, thought must be given by the designer to minimise these aspects and, in particular, to providing 'intermediate space', which will allow a gradation of temperature, pressure, breeze etc, between the internal and external spaces.

Key points:

- wind is potentially hazardous for older people and people with dementia, who may no longer understand what it means
- landform and building shape should be considered from the outset as these can affect wind turbulence
- outdoor space at upper levels may need careful consideration to avoid wind turbulence – this may mean providing shelter by partial glazing or other means
- 'intermediate spaces' (e.g. lobby, verandah, sunroom) will provide shelter and maintain the thermal comfort of the building interior when easy access to the outside is provided.

How design can modify wind in the site context

Wind can be significantly modified by landscape elements, although the effect of the elements can rarely be accurately assessed since winds are so variable. There are two basic approaches:

- deflect wind flows to provide shelter
- dissipate wind energy by frictional processes to reduce wind velocity.

Trees, bushes, ground modelling as well as fences and walls can all help to provide shelter from wind as well as shade in the summer, however, this should be considered at the outset along with the building design, following the same principles outlined above.

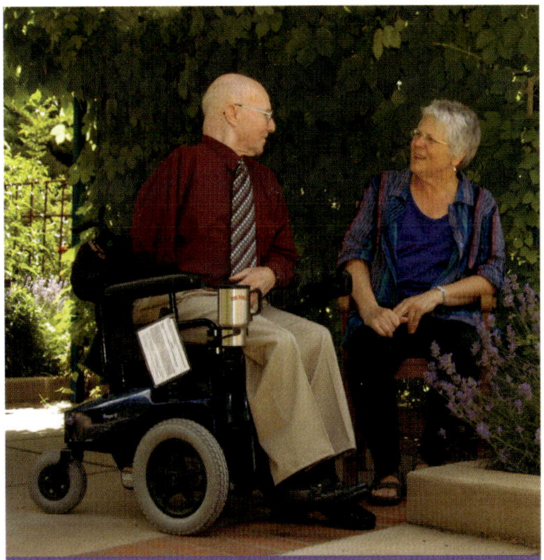

Fig. 78 A shady and sheltered spot

Generally the denser the shelter (i.e. less porous), the greater the effect on the wind speed, but the smaller the area affected. However, solid windbreaks are liable to generate excessive turbulence in their wake. The effect on the wind speed when using a more porous windbreak will be less but the area affected will be larger. Ideally, the permeability should decrease from top to bottom. However, sometimes these methods may have a contradictory impact on the quality of the space; for example, a screen to modify wind may also block precious sunlight, so a balance has to be struck.

Tree shelterbelts can be considered for the long-term, but the reduction in wind speed will depend on height, density, cross-sectional shape, width and length; expert advice will be needed to ensure the specification is correct. Their development takes time, and unless the shelterbelt contains a high proportion of evergreen trees, there will be seasonal variation with loss of leaf cover.

Key points:
- a combination of the permeable barrier and planting may well be the most effective solution, since visually the planting will not only 'soften' a fence and prevent an imprisoning appearance but also decrease the permeability
- the fence will also shelter the plants as they establish.

3. Energy efficiency

Many of the points noted in the climate and microclimate sections, and in particular the orientation of the building, will affect positively the building's energy efficiency. The aim is to control the internal environment by passive methods as far as possible and that means, in its simplest form, naturally controlling heat gain and heat loss, minimising drafts and maximising natural daylight.

This can include the following:

- use of draught lobbies to create air locks and reduce heat loss, which in turn will actually make the use of the outdoors easier
- use of verandahs and roof overhangs to prevent overheating of rooms facing the sun (i.e. west-facing rooms generally, and south-facing rooms in the northern hemisphere or north-facing rooms in the southern hemisphere)
- windows designed to control draughts, yet provide natural ventilation and natural light, views to the outdoors being an important part of their design

- avoiding planting large trees and shrubs directly outside windows where they can cut out light
- encouraging gardening activities such as recycling and composting to cut down waste.

4. Features within and outside the site that may affect it

Buildings, trees, landform

Loss of daylight can make a building dark and gloomy and the outside space unsuitable for use. Therefore, when a new building or extension is to be constructed, consideration should be given to both the way existing buildings, trees and landform may affect the proposed development as well as the affect of the new building or extension on adjacent buildings.

If some overshadowing of outdoor spaces at ground level is unavoidable, it may be necessary to consider whether a roof garden or upper level terrace should be provided, since this may access sunlight where the ground-level spaces are shaded.

Site slopes are covered earlier in this chapter and require careful design to maximise sun access.

> *Key points:*
> - Consider the physical obstructions within and outside the site at site analysis and design stages, including site slope
> - If sun access to ground floor outdoor spaces is limited, consider providing outdoor space at an upper level.

Noise

A recent planning advice note for Scotland, Planning Advice Note 1/2011: Planning and Noise, notes that noise is measured in decibels (dB) where zero dB is the lower limit of audibility and 140 dB is the level at which physical pain in the ear may be felt. However, noise is highly subjective and is affected by a range of factors, including non-acoustic matters such as attitude to noise source. Decibels measured on a sound-level meter, incorporating a frequency weighting that differentiates between sounds of different frequency (pitch) in a similar way to the human ear, are measured as dB(A).

Comfort levels may vary according to the time of day: at night we need quiet in order to sleep, a level of 20–35 dB(A), but during the day when there is general activity, a higher level of noise may be acceptable, such as 45 dB(A); ordinary conversation is around 50dB(A).

The Environmental Noise Directive (END) describes environmental noise as

*"unwanted or harmful outdoor sound created by public activities, including noise emitted by means of transport, road traffic, rail traffic, air traffic, and from sites of industrial activity."
(Directive 2002/49/EC, article 3)*

Noise levels from this kind of sound source are as follows:

- unsilenced pneumatic drill (at 7 m distance): 95dB(A)
- heavy diesel lorry (40 km/h at 7 m distance): 83dB(A)
- modern twin-engined jet (at take off at 152 m distance): 81dB(A)

- passenger car
  (60 km/h at 7 m distance):
  70dB(A)

(Figures taken from The Scottish Government's Planning Advice Note 1/2011)

Noise from extraneous sources is disturbing to everyone and particularly to people with dementia (McManus & McClenaghan, 2010). How many times have we heard people say, "Turn that noise off because I can't hear myself think"? People with dementia need to have the right environmental conditions to maximise their ability to think and carry out the activities of daily living.

Consequently, protection from external noise sources needs to be considered at the stages of site analysis and design for all projects involving care for people with dementia. This means:

- taking readings and surveys in areas where it is perceived that there will be excessive noise levels
- taking the necessary action to reduce the noise levels and provide better conditions of comfort for residents.

"Noise is the most significant environmental pollutant in the urban environment after exhaust fumes from vehicles." (Mommertz, 2009)

The following facts demonstrate the effects of certain levels of noise (European Commission, 2002):

- people living alongside roads where the average sound level during the day exceeds 65dB(A) have a 20% higher risk of suffering a heart attack
- a noise level of 55dB(A) measured on road and rail routes will impair communication and general wellbeing
- an average level of 45dB(A) of traffic noise will cause sleep disturbance.

Therefore, we can see that, when siting any residential building and in particular buildings for people with dementia, noise is an important consideration. Ideally such buildings should always be sited in a quiet area, but this is not always possible when land is expensive and in short supply. Urban sites are often chosen for economic and social considerations, for example, proximity to amenities and ease for visitors to reach.

Noise sources need to be dealt with to protect the living conditions of the residents and it is urban sites that are likely to need the most attention.

The simplest way to reduce the level of sound at the receiving end (i.e. the building and/or the outside space) is to increase the distance from the noise source, resulting in as much as a 3–6dB(A) reduction for each doubling of the distance. However, if this is not possible, screening measures can be used.

One way of dealing with external noise is to build an appropriate structure or structures between the source of the noise and the building or external space. Barriers, such as acoustic fences between the building and the source of the sound, can reduce the sound. Landform (hills, mounds) provides the most effective sound barrier against extraneous noise sources as this works due to its sheer mass.

The following diagrams illustrate these points:

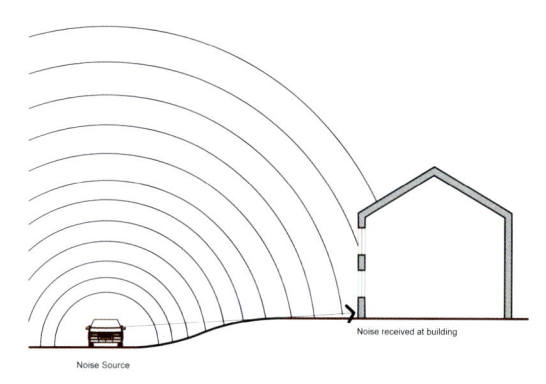

Fig. 79 External sound with no barrier

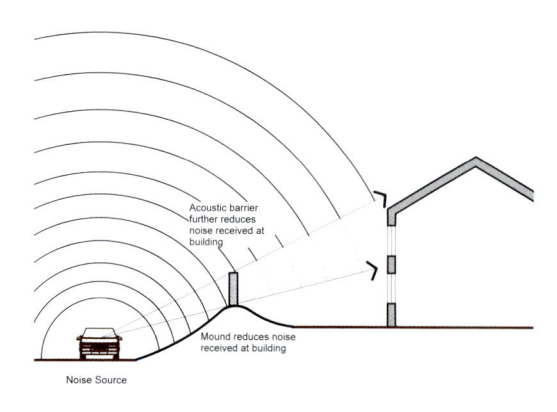

Fig. 80 External sound with a barrier

Although hedge planting or providing a shelterbelt or single rows of trees is ineffective in the reduction of sound, for many people and, in particular, people with dementia, visual barriers such as these can have a positive emotional effect.

Gabions (i.e. retaining walls made of stones within metal baskets) need sound insulating layers to prevent sound whistling through the gaps in the stones.

Roads and railway lines in cuttings cause less noise nuisance and a choice of site in such conditions will be more beneficial than one where roads and railways are level with or raised above the proposed site.

An 'inward-focussed' building can be designed as a noise barrier to enclose areas such as courtyards to provide a refuge from everyday hustle and bustle.

However, 1 in 7 people in the UK suffer from tinnitus (Dunmore, Riddiford & Tait, 2007) and background sounds e.g. distant traffic, the hubub of a busy office, wind in the trees, or waves breaking on the seashore, may make tinnitus less noticeable for them. At times, just opening a window may provide all the sound therapy they need (Handscomb & McKinney, 2010).

Therefore, a balanced approach, taking account of the needs of individuals, is required when dealing with the problems of background noise and stimulating sound.

Key points:

- consider external noise sources at stages of site analysis and design
- carry out readings and surveys
- site the building as far as possible away from noise sources
- where appropriate, utilise natural noise barriers on the site
- construct barriers between the source of the sound and the building/outside space

- use hedge planting or rows of trees for positive emotional effects, but realise that these will not reduce sound
- choose sites where nearby roads or railways are in cuttings
- use the building as a barrier to noise to provide quiet havens such as courtyards
- balance the importance of a degree of stimulation with a sense of calmness.

5. Flood risk, soil and site drainage assessment

Local planning authorities may ask for a 'flood risk assessment' as flooding incidents appear to be increasing in the UK and elsewhere with climate change; there may be a requirement to use Sustainable Urban Drainage Systems (SUDS) techniques. All of these requirements will have to be tied carefully with the overarching need to create an environment that is suitable for older people and for those with dementia.

Even if all the microclimatic aspects above work perfectly, the site soil (its makeup and drainage) may require modification for a garden to thrive.

An overly wet garden is hard for anyone to maintain: grass becomes filled with moss, water may lie after heavy rain, and plants will not thrive and may even die. Particularly for older people and people with dementia, good garden conditions are essential. Whilst these are partly due to the microclimatic considerations noted above in relation to the buildings, they are also affected by the site geology i.e. soil type, drainage patterns (which will relate to slope, watercourses and underground springs) and topography.

It is always worth obtaining a good site survey, soil analysis, and report at the outset of a project to ascertain its condition. Noting the existing plant locations, size and species that are on site will also provide a guide.

The following questions should be answered:

- is the soil pH acid, neutral or alkaline?
- is soil texture sandy, clay or a mixture?
- does the soil need fertiliser and other additives to provide a good growing medium?
- what are the site drainage patterns?
- when construction starts on site, it is vital to ensure the following:
- that the topsoil is stripped when dry enough, to prevent soil structure from being damaged, and stacked in soil heaps that are not too high
- that areas to be planted are protected from compaction by site machinery where possible
- where this is not possible, that these areas are ripped or ploughed when the site is dry, prior to the topsoil being spread, so that site drainage is not impeded
- that existing field drainage is researched and protected.

On sites where planting fails or does not thrive, it is usually for the following reasons:

- the topsoil is poor or has been damaged during storage and/or construction

- site drainage has been damaged during the construction process
- site levels have been adjusted without additional drainage measures being installed
- there is insufficient sunlight.

Existing trees should also be noted since they may be protected and, therefore, could be a constraint to development.

Key points:

- consider flood risk
- obtain a good site survey and survey of soil conditions before work starts i.e. location, size and species of trees, soil type, existing drainage patterns, analysis of fertility
- ensure that any building works are closely monitored, e.g. trees to be retained, soil handling, storage of materials, routes of heavy machinery
- ensure that imported soil comes with an analysis of fertility from a named location.

References

Association for Project Safety. (2011). Tower building wind effects: A health and safety design issue? *APS Digest*, 11, 15.

Ashihara, Y. (1984). *The aesthetic townscape*. Cambridge, MA: MIT Press.

Brown, R.D., & Gillespie, T.J. (1995). *Microclimatic landscape design: Creating thermal comfort and energy efficiency.* New York, NY: Wiley.

Cohen-Mansfield, J. (2007). Outdoor wandering parks for persons with dementia. In S. Rodiek & B. Schwarz (Eds.). *Outdoor environments for people with dementia*. Binghamton, NY: Haworth Press. 35–53.

Dunmore, K., Riddiford, G. & Tait, V. (2003). *Understanding Tinnitus: Managing the noises in your head*. London: Royal National Institute for Deaf People.

Goulding, J.R., Lewis, J.O., & Steemers, T.C. (Eds.) (1992). *Energy in architecture: The European passive solar handbook*. Retrieved from http://amergin.tippinst.ie/downloadsEnergyArchhtml.html

Handscomb, L., & McKinney, C. (2010). Sound therapy. Retrieved from http://www.tinnitus.org.uk/documents/56

Littlefair, P.J. (2011). *Site layout planning for daylight and sunlight: a guide to good practice*. Watford: IHS BRE Press.

Littlefair, P. J., Santamouris, M., Alvarez, S., Dupagne, A., Hall, D., Teller, J., & Papanikolaou, N. (2000). *Environmental site layout planning: Solar access, microclimate and passive cooling in urban areas*. Watford: IHS BRE Press.

Marshall, M. (2010). *Designing balconies, roof terraces, and roof gardens for people with dementia.* Stirling: Dementia Services Development Centre.

McManus, M., & McClenaghan, C. (2010). *Hearing, sound and the acoustic environment for people with dementia*. Stirling: Dementia Services Development Centre.

Mommertz, E. (2009). *Acoustics and sound insulation: principles, planning, examples*. Basel: Birkhäuser.

Reynolds, J.S. (2002). *Courtyards: Aesthetic, social and thermal delight*. New York, NY: Wiley.

European Commission. (2002).*The Environmental Noise Directive*. (2002/49/EC), article 3. Brussels: European Commission.

Scottish Government. (2011). *Planning advice note 1/2011: Planning and noise*. Edinburgh: Scottish Government.

Chapter 7
Dementia-friendly neighbourhoods – a step in the right direction

Lynne Mitchell and Elizabeth Burton

This chapter examines how older people with dementia use and experience their local streets and neighbourhoods and gives a set of preliminary recommendations for designing dementia-friendly neighbourhoods. The information comes from a three-year research project in which the authors interviewed older people with and without dementia and walked with them around their local neighbourhoods. The research was funded by the Engineering and Physical Research Council's Extending Quality Life (EPSRC EQUAL) programme. More information on the methodology can be found in the following publications: Mitchell, Burton and Raman (2004), Sheehan, Burton and Mitchell (2006), Mitchell and Burton (2006).

Why should neighbourhoods be dementia-friendly?

There are many reasons why it is important for older people with dementia to spend time outdoors. Access to sunlight is essential for the absorption of vitamin D, which helps regulate calcium and phosphate for healthy bones and teeth (as discussed in detail in Chapter 2). It is also important for the production of the mood-enhancing hormone, serotonin. Exposure to natural light and the cycle of day and night can help reduce increased agitation at dusk ('sundowning') and sleep disorders (Torrington & Tregenza, 2007; Marcus, 2009). While having a dementia-friendly home and garden is essential for helping people with dementia to lead good quality, active, independent lives, a supportive neighbourhood is just as important. Being able to do the shopping, post a letter, visit the GP or simply go for a walk has great benefits for physical and mental health and wellbeing and in prolonging people's abilities to do things for themselves.

Sadly, barriers in the built environment often restrict these abilities and make many people with dementia effectively housebound.

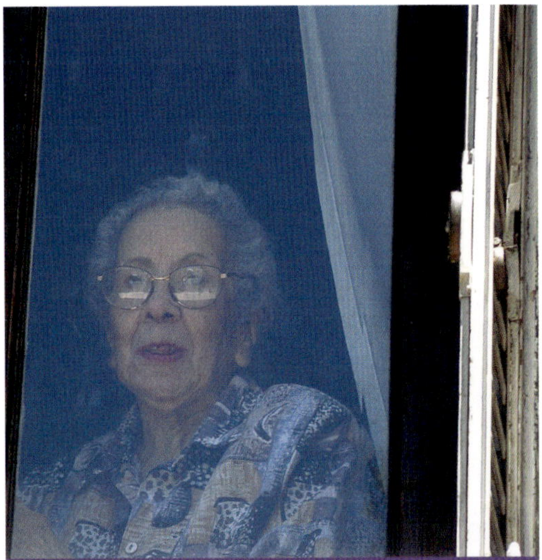

Fig. 81 Our research participants often described feelings of claustrophobia and loneliness if they could not get out, or as one participant put it "I enjoy going out, I feel ugh if I don't!"

Excessive walking has typically been seen as a negative symptom of dementia that should be controlled or discouraged (Marshall & Allan, 2006), yet recent research has shown that walking, as a physical activity, can improve and maintain general health, reduce the likelihood of becoming disabled or experiencing chronic illness, and improve cognitive function (Kennedy, 2007; Abbot et al., 2004; Larson et al., 2006; Weuve et al., 2004). Walking in familiar surroundings can help to ease anxiety and confusion, as Wilson, Hines, Sacre and Abbey (2007, p.49) explain: "Going down familiar streets means memories of happier times flood back, anxiety starts to decrease and they begin to feel more secure and more composed, spirits are uplifted." One of our participants pointed out that she had always enjoyed walking and saw no reason to stop now she had dementia.

Fig. 82 Walking is good for physical and mental health and wellbeing

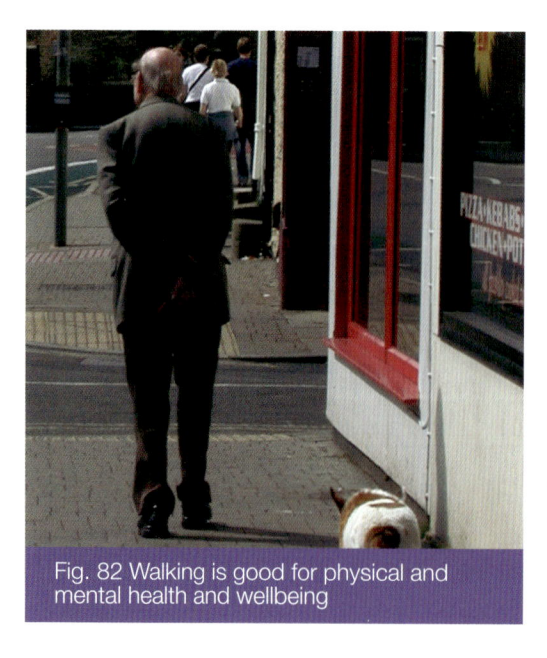

Local neighbourhoods that people with dementia can safely and comfortably access, use, enjoy and find their way around are supportive environments in which people can meet their own needs, enjoy fresh air and exercise, seek pleasure in attractive or stimulating environments and interact with others.

How our participants used and experienced their neighbourhoods

Most of our research participants went out alone and about half of these went out daily. Most said they enjoyed going out and that it greatly enhanced their sense of independence and self-respect, or as one participant put it: "The world belongs to me for that bit of time." They all went shopping and most also visited the local post office and park. However, we found that they generally visited just one place per trip and that they tended to avoid socially demanding destinations, such as the library, church, visiting friends, or visiting formal places such as large public squares with imposing buildings. They preferred relatively easy trips such as posting a letter, buying a newspaper or taking the dog for a walk, and seemed to feel much more comfortable and less intimidated in informal places such as streets, parks and small open spaces with plenty of activity. This is most likely because people with dementia often struggle to interpret the cues that signal the use of buildings or spaces, the location of entrances, the behaviour that is expected in different places, or the intentions of people around them. Their independent activities also tended to be restricted to within walking distance of home because they could no longer drive and were reluctant to use public transport alone. However, regular use of the same streets and places helped to reinforce their recognition and memories of those places.

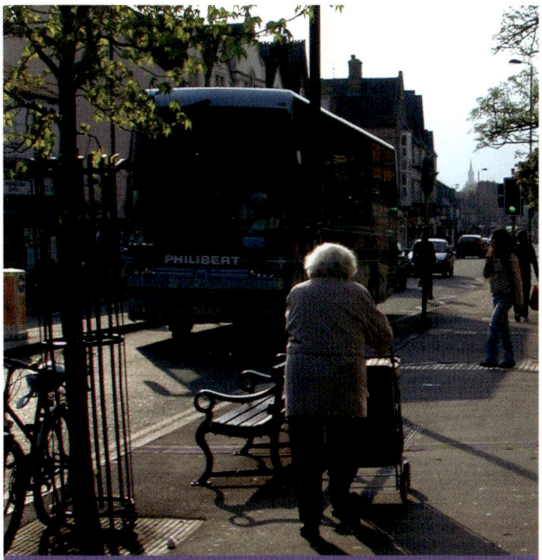

Fig. 83 A supportive local neighbourhood aids active ageing, independence and self-respect

Designing dementia-friendly neighbourhoods

From the research findings we identified six interdependent key design principles for making neighbourhoods dementia-friendly.

Familiarity

Familiar surroundings enable people to recognise and understand their surroundings. This prevents or alleviates spatial disorientation and confusion.

Legibility

People can understand where they are and identify which way they need to go, alleviating spatial disorientation, confusion and anxiety.

Distinctiveness

People's attention and concentration are captured by the distinctiveness of the different parts of the neighbourhood, which aids orientation and wayfinding.

Accessibility

People are able to reach, enter, use and move around the places and spaces they need or wish to visit, regardless of any physical, sensory or cognitive impairment.

Comfort

People feel at ease and are able to visit, use and enjoy places and spaces without physical or psychological discomfort.

Safety

People are able to use, enjoy and move around the neighbourhood without fear of coming to harm.

We identified 17 key design recommendations, relating to all scales from urban design to street furniture, which could be incorporated into new developments and/or refurbishment of existing neighbourhoods. The principle met by each recommendation is included in brackets.

1. Small blocks laid out on an irregular grid with minimal crossroads (legibility)

During the accompanied walks we found that participants who lost their way lived in neighbourhoods with few connecting streets (e.g. many cul-de-sacs), in areas where the streets were very similar in terms of length, shape and architecture, or where road junctions gave too many choices of direction. Although the uniform grid provides a pattern of well-connected streets, the layout of identical streets and crossroads can be as confusing as the 'lollipop' pattern of cul-de-sacs. The irregular grid creates a more interesting overall street pattern, provides direct, connected routes which are easy to understand and gives people a clearer view ahead than the 90° turns and blind bends created by uniform grids.

uniform grid pattern   'lollipop' pattern   irregular grid pattern

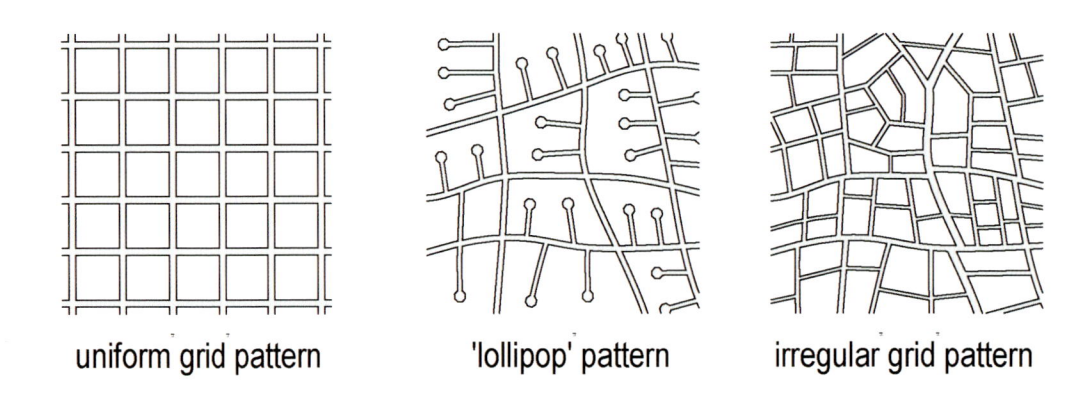

Fig. 84 The irregular grid pattern has small perimeter blocks and connected streets and provides a variety of block and street shapes and varied, less complex junctions, such as staggered, forked and T-junctions

2. A hierarchy of familiar types of streets, including high streets and residential side streets (familiarity)

Familiar environments and features that people have grown up with and understand help maintain orientation and memory. For example, high streets are usually wide and are lined with large buildings with shops on the ground floor and flats or offices above, while side streets are normally narrower, quieter and more residential. When streets meet these expectations they provide familiar, predictable and understandable environments, which help people to recognise where they are and what is expected in that setting.

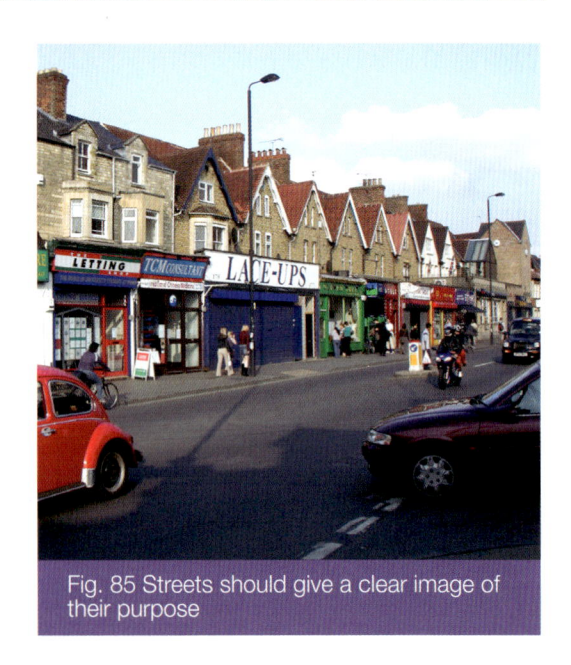

Fig. 85 Streets should give a clear image of their purpose

3. Gently winding streets (legibility)

Most participants preferred short, gently winding streets as, even though they may not reduce the length of the journey, they provide the interest and variety needed to maintain the concentration necessary to avoid becoming disoriented or confused.

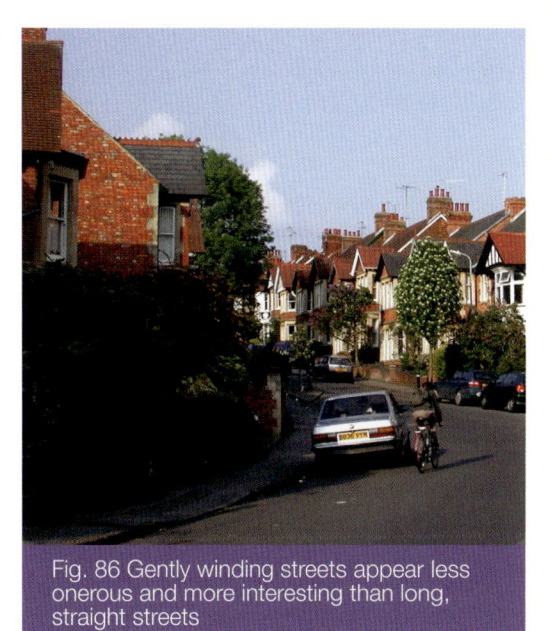

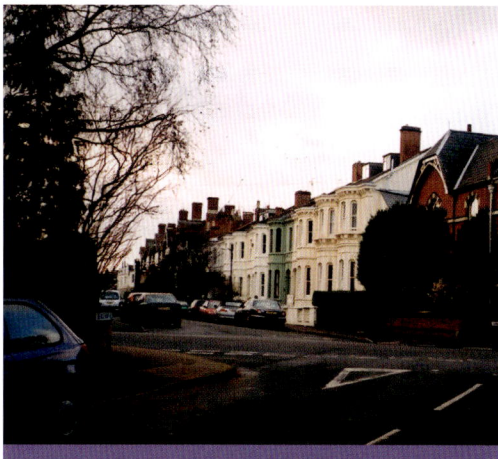

Fig. 86 Gently winding streets appear less onerous and more interesting than long, straight streets

Fig. 87 A variety of local designs, materials and features, rather than uniform streets, help maintain concentration and wayfinding

4. Varied urban form and architecture that reflects local character (distinctiveness)

On accompanied walks most participants chose uncomplicated routes with more variety of land use, building form and architectural features even when they were not the quickest routes. Participants explained saying, "I prefer the variation in architecture", "it's got more character about it" and "it's more interesting and colourful." Interestingly, varied features help maintain concentration.

5. A mix of uses, including plenty of services and facilities and open space (accessibility)

A mix of uses helps older people to access necessary facilities and services. People in their mid-70s will generally take around 10-20 minutes to walk 400-500 yards compared with younger adults (5-10 minutes over the same distance).

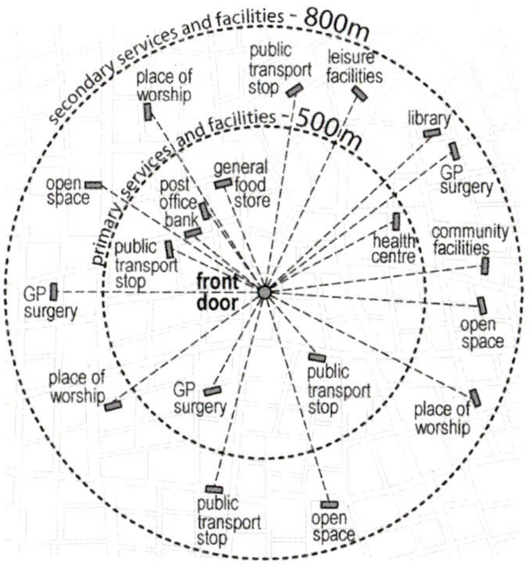

Fig. 88 Primary services and facilities should be within 500 metres of older people's housing and secondary services within 800 metres (refer to appendix 1 on page 217 for enlarged version)

Part 3 Chapter 7 Dementia-friendly neighborhoods - a step in the right direction

123

6. Permeable buffer zones between busy roads and footways e.g. trees, grass verge (comfort and safety)

Participants often lost concentration on accompanied walks if there was a lot of traffic noise or if they were startled by a sudden noise, such as an emergency vehicle siren.

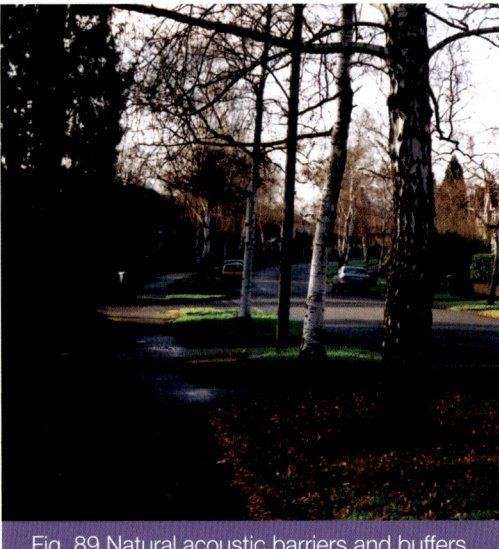

Fig. 89 Natural acoustic barriers and buffers can help reduce street and background noises, add greenery to the street scene and help shield pedestrians from traffic

7. Buildings/facilities designed to reflect uses (familiarity and legibility)

Just as people have expectations of what different types of places should look like, they also have a general idea of the visual images of different building usages, such as shops, offices and houses. When designs follow these familiar visual styles, people immediately recognise what they are for, but ambiguous or unfamiliar designs cause confusion and anxiety. Many of our participants did not recognise modern designs of street furniture, such as public benches, telephone boxes and automated 'superloos'. However, the important issue is not whether the design is traditional or modern but that the design clearly depicts the purpose of the building or feature.

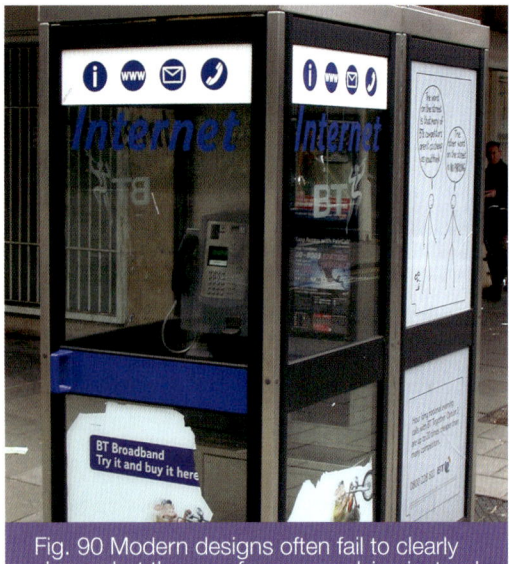

Fig. 90 Modern designs often fail to clearly show what they are for, some relying instead on signs that may or may not clarify the issue!

8. Obvious entrances to buildings (legibility and accessibility)

People with dementia often find it difficult to 'read' the nature and use of different spaces if the identity of these spaces is ambiguous, and they require buildings to face onto the street with the main entrance clearly visible at the front.

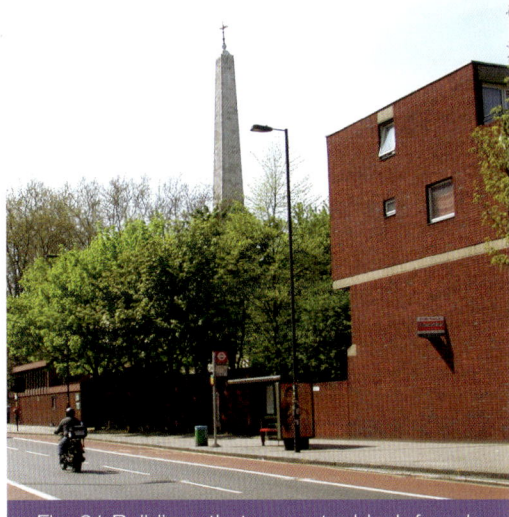

Fig. 91 Buildings that present a blank façade to the street give few clues as to what they are for or how to get into them. Buildings should face the street. Canopies and porches can help identify entrances

9. Landmarks and environmental cues (legibility and distinctiveness)

During the walks we found that participants commonly used both distant and nearby landmarks and other environmental features to help them identify where they were, and which way they needed to go to continue or to retrace their steps when they lost their way. The types of landmarks and cues used fall into three categories:

- historic, civic and distinctive buildings and structures, such as churches, memorials, town halls, bridges and towers

- places of interest and activity, such as parks, nature reserves and tennis courts

- unusual places, buildings or usages, particularly those with a distinctive local identity, such as some described by participants as "the toothpaste tube houses", "the witch's gingerbread house" and "the big ugly house at the end".

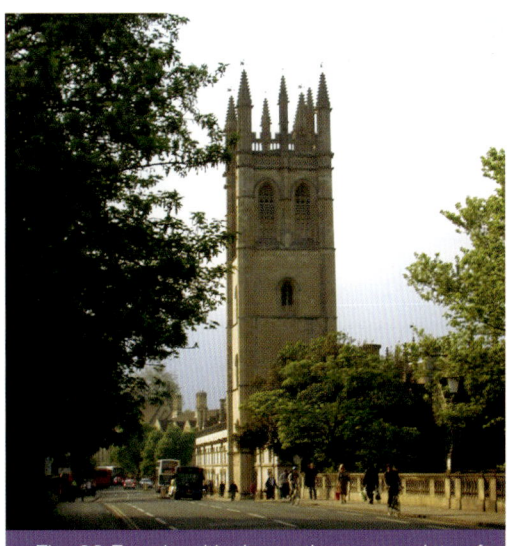

Fig. 92 People with dementia use a variety of landmarks

10. Special/distinctive features, e.g. street furniture and trees at junctions (legibility)

In addition to landmarks and environmental cues, participants also used aesthetic and practical features, such as fountains, ponds, trees, planters and street furniture as wayfinding cues.

Fig. 93 Distinctive features are particularly useful as wayfinding cues when they are at street junctions or when they break up the view along a straight or monotonous street

11. Wide, flat, smooth, plain, non-slip and non-reflective footways separate from cycle lanes (accessibility and safety)

People with dementia often feel anxious in crowded places and struggle to interpret the intentions of people coming towards them. Footways at least two metres wide help people with dementia and/or mobility problems to safely pass oncoming pedestrians. People with dementia often walk with a slow, unsteady shuffling gait so that coarse-textured or uneven paving materials are particularly difficult for them to walk along without tripping or stumbling. People with poor visual acuity or impaired depth perception often mistake sharp colour contrasts or paving patterns for steps or holes. Busy patterns, such as chessboard squares or repetitive lines can also cause dizziness and shiny or reflective surfaces are seen at wet and slippery. Paving should, therefore, be plain and in clear colour contrast to kerbs.

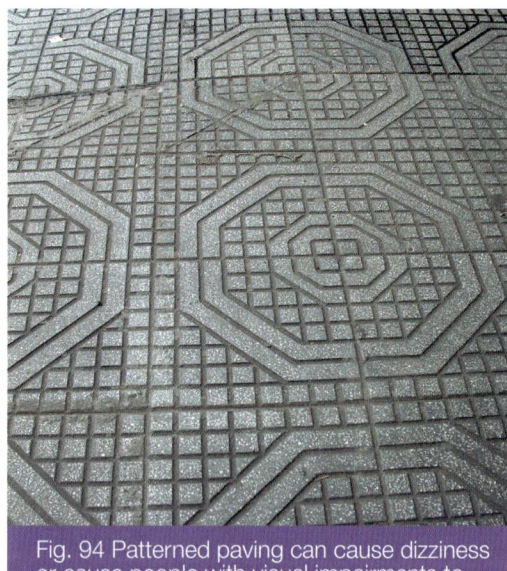

Fig. 94 Patterned paving can cause dizziness or cause people with visual impairments to perceive patterns as steps or holes

Many participants were very anxious about being knocked over by cyclists on the footway, even when footways were divided into pedestrian and cycle lanes. One participant explained that "it's difficult to remember which side to walk on and I've got enough to think about making sure I don't get lost", while many complained that cyclists ride too fast and they were frightened of being unbalanced by a bicycle suddenly passing them.

12. Frequent pedestrian crossings with audible and visual signals suitable for older people (safety)

Crossing a wide or busy road can be difficult for anyone but for people with slow reactions, reduced cognitive abilities and/or mobility problems it can be very frightening. Participants complained that drivers often do not stop at zebra crossings nor wait long enough for them to cross over safely. Puffin crossings (pedestrian user-friendly intelligent crossing) were not considered user-friendly by our participants who disliked not having a visual signal on the far side of the road and were not aware that the crossing would stay in their favour until they reached the other side. Pelican crossings (pedestrian light-controlled crossing) were considered to be the safest crossing as they are familiar, participants felt confident that vehicles would stop, and felt safer being able to watch the visual signal as they crossed over.

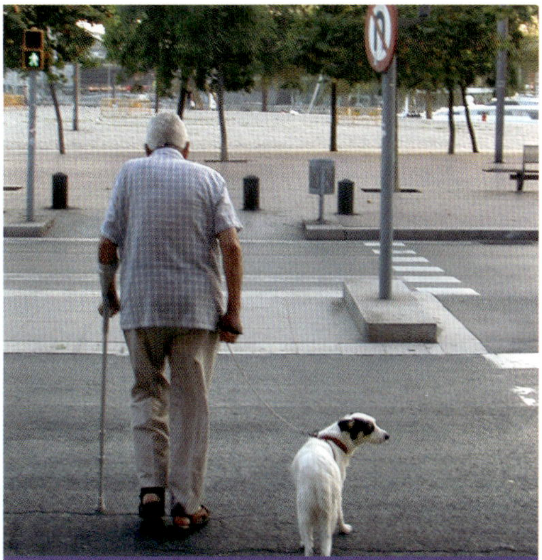

Fig. 95 Combining the familiarity of the Pelican crossing with the Puffin's ability to detect when a person is still on the crossing and providing audible signals at a low pitch would be preferable

13. Level changes only when unavoidable (accessibility)

Accessible streets should avoid changes in level wherever possible but, when very small changes in level are unavoidable, gentle slopes are easier for older people to see and negotiate than one or two small steps. For greater inclines both a ramp, with a maximum gradient of 1:15, and steps are necessary for people with different needs.

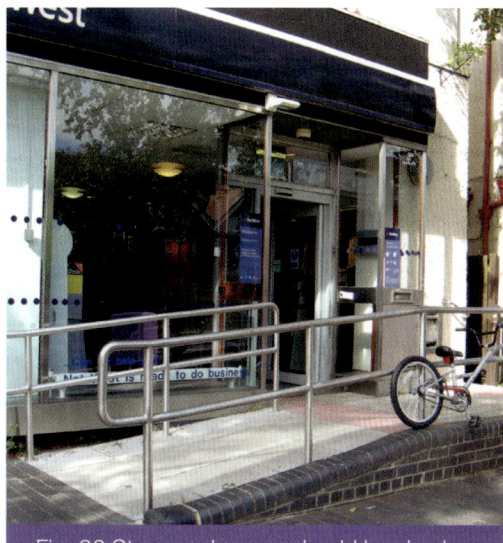

Fig. 96 Steps and ramps should be clearly marked and well lit with handrails and non-slip, non-glare surfaces

Part 3 Chapter 7 Dementia-friendly neighborhoods - a step in the right direction

127

14. Clear signs throughout (legibility)

People with dementia find signs increasingly difficult to cope with: they struggle to interpret the information on the signs and will sometimes follow the instructions regardless of where they actually want to go. Our participants found clusters of signs difficult to read and signs crowded with information too complicated to make sense of. Stylised signs were generally too ambiguous to be easily interpreted. Pedestrian post-and-multiple pointers were distrusted as "they can be confusing which way they are pointing and kids turn them round" and the graphics were criticised for being difficult to read either because they were too small or the colour of the graphics were not in a clear colour contrast to the background.

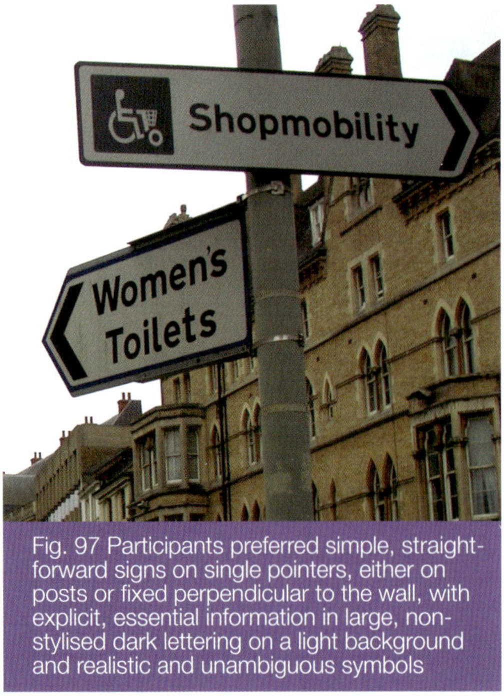

Fig. 97 Participants preferred simple, straight-forward signs on single pointers, either on posts or fixed perpendicular to the wall, with explicit, essential information in large, non-stylised dark lettering on a light background and realistic and unambiguous symbols

15. Sturdy public seating with back rests and preferably arm rests (comfort)

A lack of seating was often mentioned by participants as a deterrent to going to certain places. Many older people cannot walk for longer than 10 minutes without resting and so public seating should be provided at regular intervals, preferably every 100–125 m.

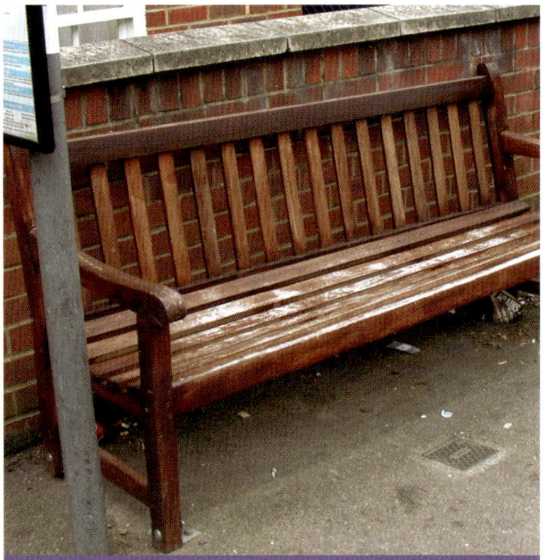

Fig. 98 Seats should be made from warm materials, such as wood, with back and arm rests for comfort and support

16. Ground level toilets (accessibility, comfort and safety)

Many older people need to visit the toilet more often than younger adults and the lack of safe, clean, easily accessible toilets often prevented our participants from going to certain places or from staying out for as long as they would have liked. Participants were distrustful of modern automated toilets or failed to recognise what they were, while underground toilets were seen as onerous or impossible to access.

Underground toilets were also considered dangerous in terms of both fear of attack and fear of falling. Public toilets should, therefore, be conventional and at ground level.

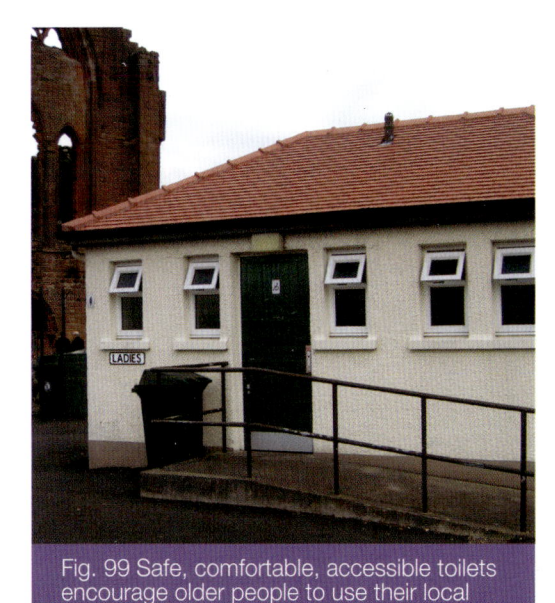

Fig. 99 Safe, comfortable, accessible toilets encourage older people to use their local neighbourhood

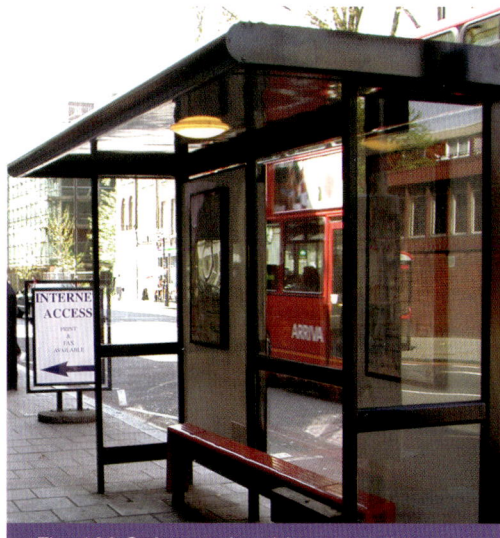

Fig. 100 Safe, comfortable, accessible shelters encourage older people to use their local neighbourhood

17. Enclosed bus shelters, with seating and transparent walls or large clear windows (comfort)

Whenever possible, bus stops should provide some form of shelter from the weather, preferably at least semi-enclosed with large, clear windows so that people can see who is already in the shelter and can watch for the bus in comfort. They should also have wide, flat seats made on non-slippery materials that do not conduct heat or cold.

Dementia-friendly neighbourhoods in practice

Where and when?

We developed the recommendations for a wide variety of situations. Ideally they should be incorporated within all new development. However, urban areas tend to be modified slowly over time, and the rate of change of the built environment is small. So the recommendations can also be used when redeveloping or regenerating urban areas, or even for improving the dementia-friendliness of an area when no other changes are planned.

Where no development or adaptation is planned, the following improvements are likely to be helpful for people with dementia:

- add landmarks, distinctive structures, open spaces or places of activity
- add special features (e.g. postboxes, telephone boxes, trees, statues) at junctions, particularly complex ones

- add porches, canopies and clear signs to make entrances to public buildings obvious
- increase the widths of footways (e.g. by reducing the widths of roads)
- on busy roads, create a green buffer zone between pedestrians and cars
- move cycle lanes from footways to roads
- increase the frequency of pedestrian crossings
- where there are steps, provide a slope or ramp (no more than a gradient of 1 in 15) as well
- add handrails to steps or ramps, if they don't have them
- fix clear signs and symbols (where existing ones are poor) to publicly accessible buildings, preferably perpendicular to walls
- remove all unclear and unnecessary signs
- replace all unclear road and directional signs with clear ones
- increase variety in the existing built form (e.g. by painting doors and windows different colours and adding details such as window boxes)
- add trees and street furniture where possible
- only use seats, telephone boxes, bus shelters and toilets that are suitable for older people
- replace gates and doors where necessary so that they require no more than 2 kg of pressure to open and have lever handles
- improve audible cues at pedestrian crossings where necessary to increase crossing time
- replace cobbled, rough or patterned footways with smooth, plain ones
- reduce street clutter (e.g. boards, adverts, signs)
- increase the amount of street lighting where necessary.

All or nothing?

Each design recommendation is of value in its own right in helping to create streets that are easy and enjoyable to use as we grow older in our neighbourhoods. Some are clearly more fundamental than others, and some will be of benefit to nearly all older people while others are of particular benefit to those with dementia. We would perhaps recommend first the importance of a mix of uses because facilities, services and open space need to be within easy reach for those who often find walking difficult. Next, we would list the recommendations that help older people to walk safely and comfortably to the places they want to visit: wide, smooth, non-slip footways are very important, as are adequate seating, toilets and handrails. It is also important that older people can walk relatively directly to their destinations, through a street network that is well connected in a grid pattern, which gives the person lots of choices of routes and avoids the lengthy walks and confusion often created by cul-de-sac patterns. The remaining recommendations are more relevant for people with dementia, helping them to find their way around. Their focus is ensuring variety in the environment and having plenty of landmarks and features.

Back to principles

It is important to point out that our principles, criteria or objectives for designing dementia-friendly streets are as important as our recommendations. The recommendations are drawn from just one research project focusing on a limited number of older people and there may be many other ways of achieving the six principles of familiarity, legibility, distinctiveness, accessibility, comfort and safety. Those wanting to create dementia-friendly streets should look at older people's needs and requirements. Good designers may well come up with new solutions, ones we have not thought of.

Putting it all together

Designers are faced with enormous challenges when designing outdoor environments because of the many different requirements placed on those environments. Urban environments are complex because they have so many different users and so many different uses, which change over time. Dementia-friendly streets should be considered along with other requirements, and it is possible there may be conflicts. The issues that take priority will vary from situation to situation. There are many issues to consider when producing or maintaining streets and neighbourhoods, including:

- conservation of heritage
- environmental sustainability
- needs of other users (e.g. those of different ages and abilities, visitors as well as residents)
- designers' requirements (e.g. aesthetic objectives)
- developers' requirements (e.g. cost, profitability, ease of maintenance).

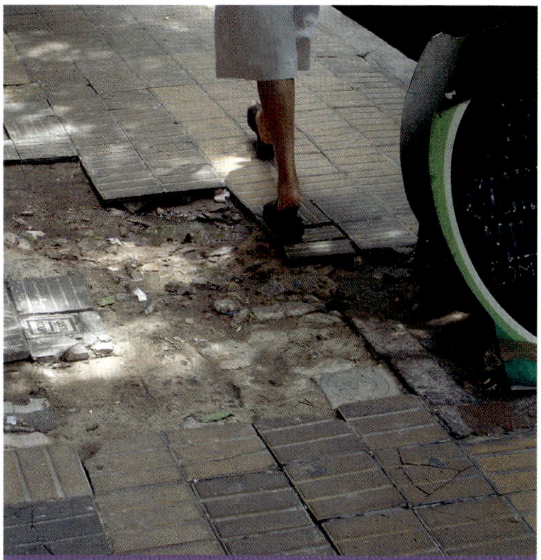

Fig. 101 The needs of all users must be considered

Seamless design for life

Ideally, our recommendations should be used alongside guidance for other aspects of lifetime design. There will be little advantage in creating accessible streets if older people's homes are no longer suitable. Further, older people need transport, whether private or public, to be accessible and comfortable for them. And for a good quality of life they need open spaces and parks that are easy to enjoy. It is also important that they can enter and use shops, libraries, healthcare buildings, places of worship and other facilities. We intend dementia-friendly streets to form one important part of a whole new inclusive approach to design, from the armchair to the home, street and neighbourhood.

Key points

- getting outdoors is important for physical and mental health

- barriers in the outdoor environment make many people with dementia effectively housebound

- walking in familiar surroundings can help to ease anxiety and confusion

- promotion of the new concept of dementia-friendly neighbourhoods should help people, with and without dementia, to access safely and comfortably, use, enjoy and find their way around their local areas

- dementia-friendly neighbourhoods should be designed according to the six key design principles of familiarity, legibility, distinctiveness, accessibility, comfort and safety

- the most important recommendations for designing dementia-friendly neighbourhoods are:

    - a mix of uses
    - wide, flat, plain, non-slip footways
    - adequate seating, toilets, pedestrian crossings, shelters and handrails
    - a hierarchy of familiar streets laid out on an irregular grid pattern
    - buildings, facilities and street furniture designed to clearly reflect uses
    - a variety of distinctive landmarks and environmental cues.

References

Abbott, R., White, L., Ross, G., Masaki, K., Curb, D., & Petrovitch, H. (2004). Walking and dementia in physically capable elderly men. *Journal of the American Medical Association, 292*(12), 1447-1453.

Burton, E., & Mitchell, L. (2006). *Inclusive urban design: Streets for life.* Oxford: Architectural Press.

Marcus, C.C. (2009). *Landscape design: Patient-specific healing gardens.* Retrieved from http://www.worldhealthdesign.com/Patient-specific-Healing-Gardens.aspx

Kennedy, G. (2007). Exercise, aging, and mental health. *Primary Psychiatry, 14*(4), 23-28.

Larson, E., Wang, L., Bowen, J., McCormick, W., Teri, L., Crane, P., & Kukull, W. (2006). Exercise is associated with reduced risk for incident dementia among persons 65 years of age and older. *Annals of Internal Medicine, 144*, 73-81.

Marshall, M., & Allan, K. (2006). (Eds.) *Dementia: Walking not wandering.* London: Hawker.

Mitchell, L., & Burton, E. (2006). Neighbourhoods for life: Designing dementia-friendly outdoor environments. *Quality in Ageing - Policy, Practice and Research, 7*(1), March, 26–33.

Mitchell, L., Burton, E., & Raman, S. (2004). Dementia-friendly cities: Designing intelligible neighbourhoods for life. *Journal of Urban Design, 9*(1), 89-101.

Sheehan, B., Burton, E., & Mitchell, L. (2006). Outdoor wayfinding in dementia. *Dementia: International Journal of Social Research and Practice, 5*(2), 271-281.

Torrington, J., & Tregenza, P. (2007). Lighting for people with dementia. *Lighting Research and Technology, 39*(1), 81-97.

Weuve, J., Hee Kang, J., Manson, J., Breteler, M., Ware, J., & Grodstein, F. (2004). Physical activity, including walking, and cognitive function in older women. *Journal of the American Medical Association, 292*(12), 1454-1461.

Wilson, J., Hines, S., Sacre, S., & Abbey, J. (2007) Appropriateness of using a symbol to identify dementia and/or delirium: A systematic review. *Queensland: Dementia Collaborative Research Centre.*

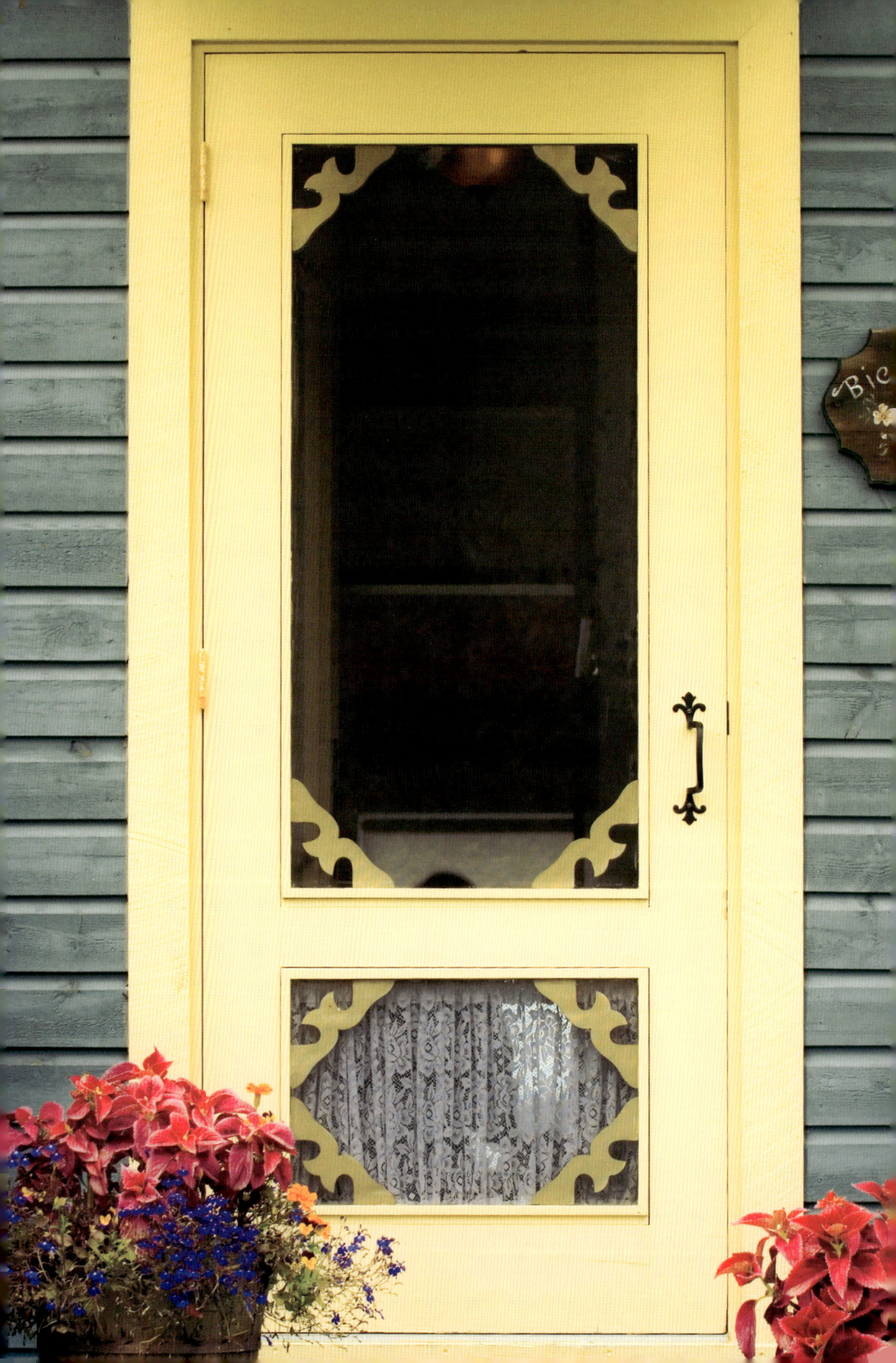

Case Study 5
Back Porch Garden, Medford Leas, Medford, New Jersey, USA

Jack Carman

"I like to think it is Mother Nature that gives everyone an equal space to be in the garden," said Jane Weston, Director of Marketing and Community relations at Medford Leas.

Medford Leas, a Quaker-related, accredited, continuing care retirement community, was founded in 1971. The retirement community is comprised of 168 acres and located in southern New Jersey near Philadelphia. It offers a broad range of residential housing options from independent living, to assisted living, to skilled nursing and dementia care.

The residential community has also been developed as an arboretum, the Lewis W Barton Arboretum, which is one of the first of its kind. The arboretum is comprised of landscaped grounds, courtyard and patio gardens, wildflower meadows, and natural woodlands, which are administered by the residents of the community.

Access to the outdoors has been an essential part of the community and the residents are very focused upon nature and the environment. Gerry Stride, Resident Life Coordinator at Medford Leas noted the aims of the project:

"The area outside of the nursing and assisted living units was a brown rubber roof. To convert that area into something that enticed residents to go outside or enjoy nature from their patios and windows and provide a safe, accessible and beautiful area, which involved all their senses. To also use flowers, plants and vegetables to stir up memories since many of our residents had been farmers."

Development of the Back Porch Garden.

The creation of a special outdoor setting for elders with special needs was the primary thinking behind the development of the Back Porch Garden.

The garden is located in the healthcare section of the community between Estaugh Assisted Living to the south and Woolman Skilled Nursing and Dementia Care to the north.

An activities and multi-purpose recreation room is located to the east and a covered walkway to the west encloses the garden. The eastern half of the garden, closest to the recreation room, is a rooftop and the surfaces here have been painted green: the walking path is dark green and the areas to either side are light green. The surfaces to the west are light tan concrete.

The elders residing in the assisted living, skilled nursing and dementia residences are the primary users of the Back Porch Garden because they are not as physically able to visit the outer areas of the arboretum. The development of a nature-filled, outdoor living environment between the buildings was vital for the residents in order to continue to participate in activities outdoors.

Initially, the garden area was underutilized and a design for the area was solicited in 1999. Exposed air-condition equipment and vents, the lack of plants, a shiny rooftop surface and other conditions made the area unpleasant and infrequently used.

A landscape plan for the outdoor area was developed by Design for Generations, LLC.

Representatives from the care staff, administration staff and residents attended all the briefing meetings to discuss the uses for the garden area. Conceptual plans for the garden area were developed and reviewed by all of the stakeholders. The need for shade, plants to help 'soften' the area, reducing the glare from the hard surfaces and creating 'rooms' for various programs were some of the components of the design equation.

Familiar garden elements that were typically a part a person's yard were sought. Water features, a barbeque grill, a small pond, a vegetable garden, fruit trees, bird feeders, potted plants, and similar garden features were all important elements to be added to the garden.

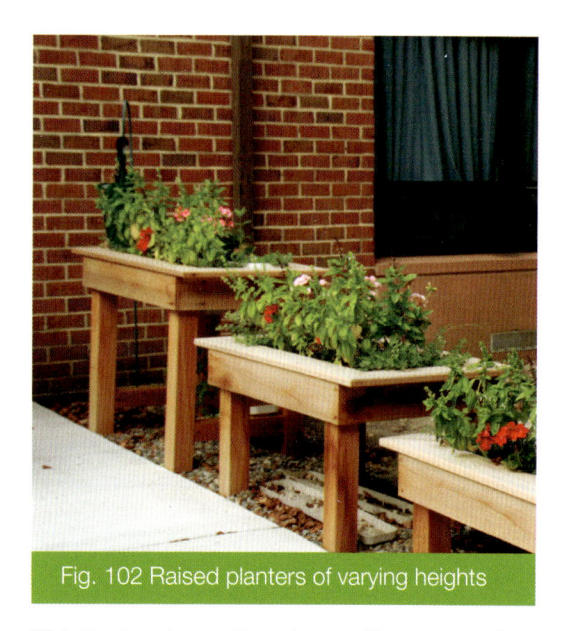

Fig. 102 Raised planters of varying heights

Thistle feeders attract specific types of birds to the garden.

One of the residents who owned an apple orchard selected the apple trees to be planted in the garden.

Raised planters of varying heights would provide opportunities for residents to continue to garden.

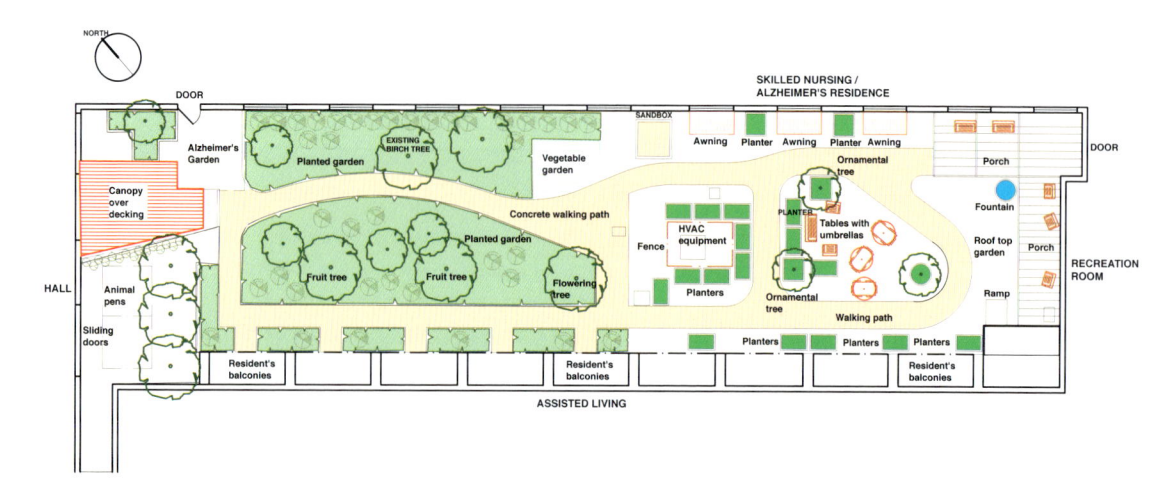

Fig. 103 Layout of garden (refer to appendix 1 on page 218 for enlarged version)

According to Gerry Stride, Resident Life Coordinator at Medford Leas:

"The flowers, plants and vegetables stir up memories, since many of our residents had been gardeners and farmers."

Constructing a back porch for residents to sit outside under a canopy was an essential component of the garden. This offers residents, staff and guests an opportunity to sit on a real porch, which is an iconic architectural element familiar to almost everyone.

Staff are very involved in scheduling activities within the garden from spring to fall. There is a wide range of events, including Easter parades with children from the neighborhood, holiday parties, fashion shows, barbeques and picnics, to name a few. There are weekly evening concerts and everyone from the retirement community attends.

The residents with dementia living in Woolman have a special patio area within the western section of the Back Porch Garden.

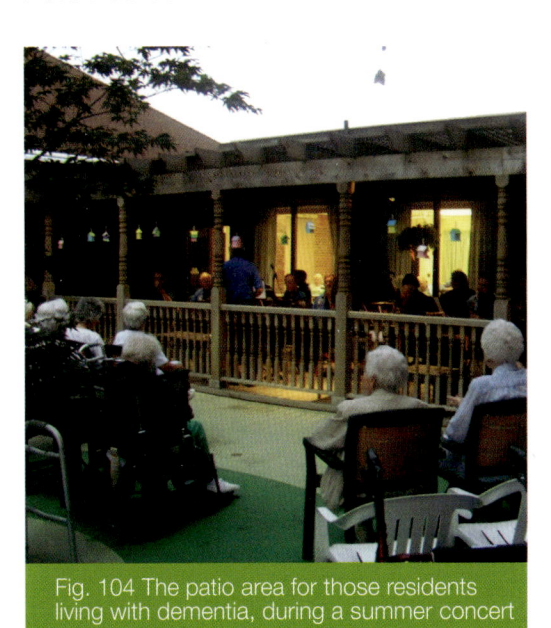

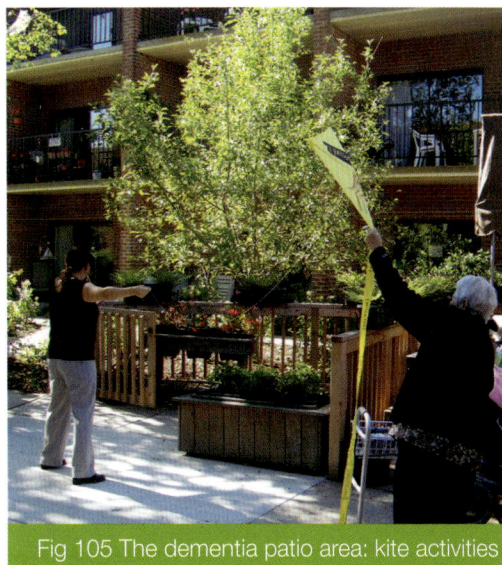

Fig 105 The dementia patio area: kite activities

This is their area where they can be in a quieter setting, yet still be close to the main events. The area is covered in part by an awning and enclosed by a low fence. Because this smaller garden area is located within the larger courtyard area, elopement is not a concern. The residents of Woolman are able to enjoy the overall garden, with assistance, as many of the residents are confined to wheel chairs and participate in many of the larger group activities, such as concerts, when it is appropriate.

One of the special features of the Back Porch Garden is the interaction of all of the residents of the community.

Fig. 104 The patio area for those residents living with dementia, during a summer concert

Fig. 106 Many events are open to all of the residents within the senior community

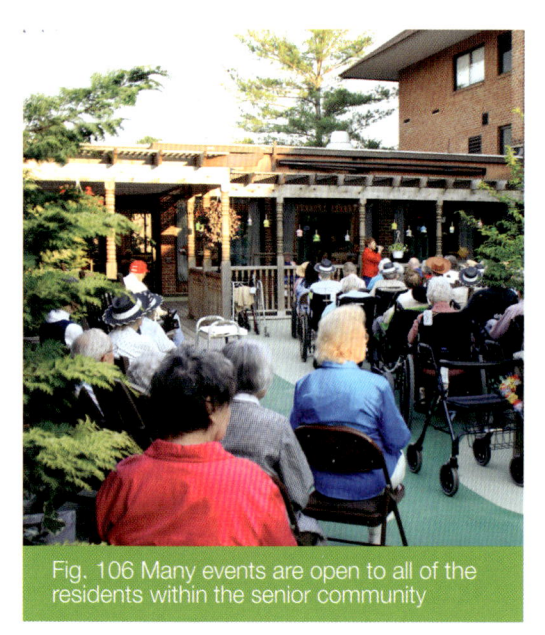

Many of the events are open to all of the residents within the senior community. Visitors to the community also participate.

Residents living in the healthcare sections of a continuing care retirement development are often physically separated from the rest of the community, but this is not the case at Medford Leas. The location of the recreation room and the Back Porch Garden helps to bring the entire community together. The elders who are living in the independent residences participate in horticultural activities, special events and other activities. The Alzheimer's Garden is a part of the overall garden setting and has not been created as a separate entity. This is important because individuals with dementia need to be able to participate in programs and activities within the community-at-large and are able to access the larger garden at will.

"The Back Porch Garden warms my heart in many ways – to see residents who live in our licensed areas connect with nature is wonderful to witness on a regular basis. And, on another level, one of the greatest gifts that I have seen is that this special garden enables all members of our community to come together in a lovely garden setting to enjoy our Summer Series of Concerts on the Back Porch. The music, combined with the garden setting, creates a space where all individuals come together to enjoy an event, regardless of their physical and cognitive abilities."

Jane Weston, Director of Marketing and Community Relations at Medford Leas.

Chapter 8
Design principles that apply to all outside spaces

Clare Cooper Marcus, Mary Marshall, Annie Pollock, Richard Pollock

This chapter looks at the characteristics of an outside space and offers some suggestions and guidance on its design, specifically for older people and people with dementia.

Much of this design guidance will apply to all types of outside spaces, i.e. gardens, courtyards, balconies, roof terraces or roof gardens. Although this chapter is specifically concerned with design, there is obviously a degree of overlap both within this chapter and with others. The most significant of these overlaps is to do with outdoor activities; these are only touched on in this chapter as they are fully covered in Chapter 9: Activities and outside space.

1. General visibility

Ideally, the whole of the outside space that is accessible to residents should be visible to staff within the building. In many situations where this is not the case, studies show that staff keep the exterior door locked to prevent people going outside when they, the staff, cannot keep an eye on them, thus precluding patients from the benefits of spending time outdoors (Grant, 2003).

It is also important for the person with dementia to see the outside areas, to find the way there and to be able to observe activities going on outside – as all these will provide great encouragement to going outside as Clare Cooper Marcus illustrates in Case study 1.

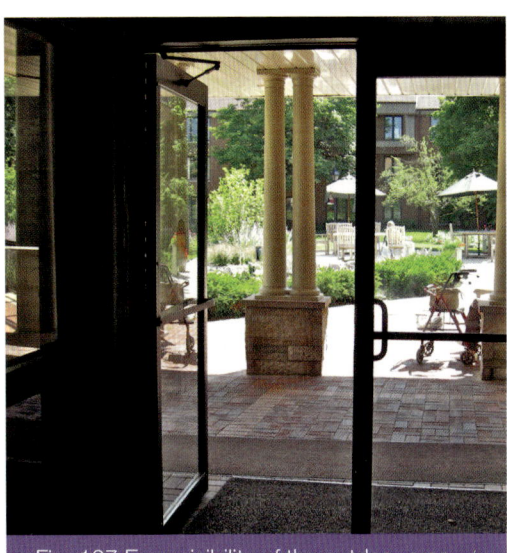

Fig. 107 Easy visibility of the outdoor area

Key points:

- visibility encourages use of outside spaces
- visibility aids wayfinding.

2. A safe and secure perimeter

People with dementia do not always have the ability to work out what is safe and secure and what is not, so it is important that any outside spaces for their use should be both unobtrusively safe and secure. In the most basic sense, this means that people should not be able to escape to a potentially unsafe or unsuitable area.

As in all dementia design, the skill is in providing a safe environment without hurting the feelings of the person with dementia, without demeaning them and, as far as possible, without depriving them of their basic human rights. It is also vital that staff should feel relaxed and comfortable in encouraging those that they care for to go outdoors; this can only be achieved if they know there is no possibility of people with dementia escaping or coming to harm.

Zeisel (2011) emphasises that staff will only allow people with dementia to go outdoors whenever they want to if they, the staff, are confident that the space is completely safe.

There are two things that need to be borne in mind:

- **civil liberties:** these issues are addressed in Part 2, Chapters 3 and 4, although there are no easy answers. Stephen Judd looks at it from an Australian viewpoint and Donny Lyons suggests ways to approach it from a Scottish viewpoint
- **feeling of imprisonment:** making people feel imprisoned is a likely way of encouraging them to escape, and this is particularly true of people with dementia. The height and design of fencing and other barriers are critical factors in this feeling of imprisonment and careful consideration needs to be given to their design.

The height of buildings and fencing also affects the microclimate within the garden. Very high fencing may cast a lot of shadow thereby creating a space that is cold and where plants will not thrive. On balconies, roof terraces or roof gardens, a solid balustrade will cast shadows over the floor area whereas a glazed balustrade or one constructed of open mesh or metal bars will allow light through.

For most people with dementia the visual impact of enclosure can be minimised by drawing their attention away from the perimeter. The fence or wall can usually be concealed with planting so that it is not obviously a barrier. This is also beneficial for shelter (see Chapter 6). If it is a roof garden, balcony or terrace, the balustrade can be made to look normal, even if it has an inward slope or a curved top to make it very difficult to climb (Marshall, 2010).

It is also possible to obtain fencing that has a low visual impact, with fine mesh that allows views through, and there are situations where this would be beneficial.

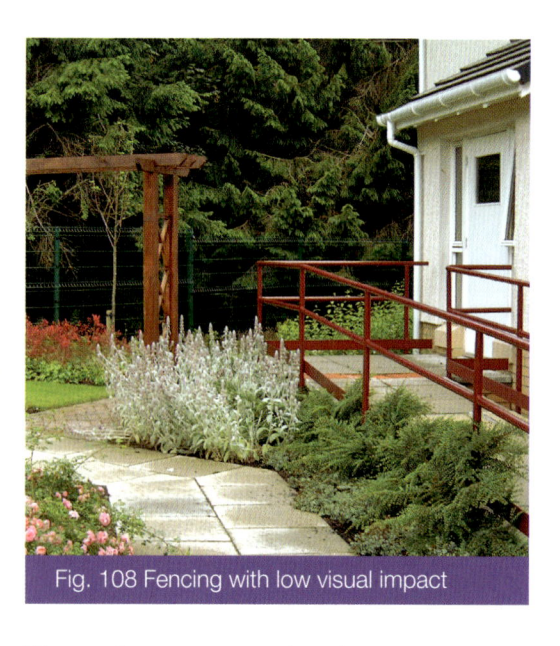

Fig. 108 Fencing with low visual impact

There also are exceptional circumstances when a simple railing is normal and acceptable, for example, when there is a lot to watch on the other side such as a school playground or a busy street. Then a railing is somehow perceived to benefit the people on the other side as much as the people behind it.

In some cultures, a railing to keep out animals is normal (much of Australia, for example, see Chapter 4) so the person with dementia would feel safe rather than imprisoned.

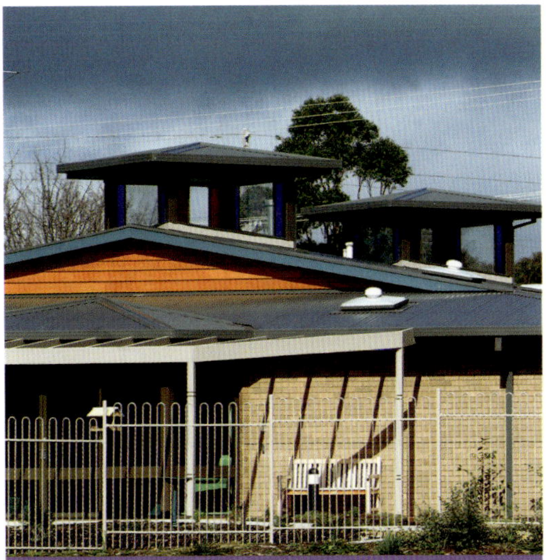

Another factor to be aware of is the visual effect of the sun's rays coming through any sort of barrier and making shadows on the ground or flooring, which can potentially be confusing and alarming for the person with dementia.

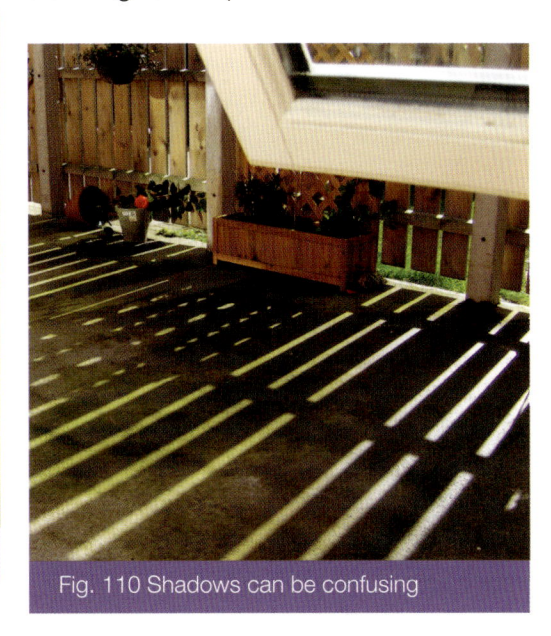

Fig. 109 Railing at Werruna, Australia

Fig. 110 Shadows can be confusing

Impeding climbing is important for any kind of barrier. For a balustrade, an inward curve at the top has already been mentioned. For a garden fence it is important to avoid any potential foothold on the garden side.

Gates that are locked need to be concealed to look like a continuation of the fence.

A path leading to a visible locked gate is guaranteed to cause frustration and confusion and this should be avoided by design. This is no different from the design guidance for interiors (Pollock, 2003), which recommends that doors not intended to be accessible to people with dementia should be designed to be invisible.

Again this can be minimised by screen planting in front of the barrier.

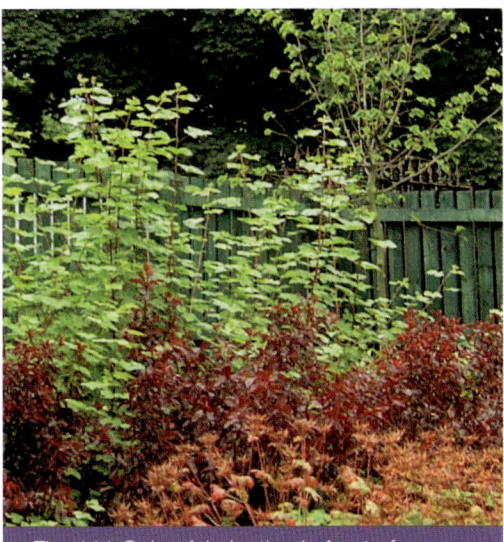

Fig. 111 Colourful planting in front of the fence

141

Key points:

- the perimeter fence should be very hard to climb but as low as possible – of the minimum acceptable for safety to avoid feeling imprisoned
- each site will impose different constraints and it is important that each facility manager undertakes a risk assessment regarding enclosure
- the perimeter fence should be concealed with planting so people do not feel imprisoned
- gates should be disguised unless the person with dementia can pass through them at will
- overshadowing due to the form and orientation of the barrier may cause confusing shadows on the ground or flooring.

3. Access

Free access to outside space is very helpful in reducing frustration and aggression in people with dementia (Namazi & Johnson, 1992) so every effort needs to be made to make access to outside spaces as easy as possible. A study in the USA (Kearney & Winterbottom, 2005) noted that the most prominent barrier to going outside was the inability to access it, both because of physical limitations and lack of assistance.

Doors

Easy access starts with the door, which normally should be off a communal area and be highly visible. A fully glazed door, with glazing to one or both sides of the door, will help the person with dementia to see the outside space as well as enabling staff to keep an eye on those who are outside. Care must be taken in the design, however, to ensure that the door is clearly distinguishable from the glazing to either side.

Outside spaces are sometimes accessed off a corridor, often using the fire escape door. This is rarely satisfactory since it does not provide easy visual contact with the garden and informal supervision by staff of those in the garden. It also confuses two types of access, but sadly is an all too common unsatisfactory solution.

Doors should be very easy to understand and the door handles clearly visible and easy to operate both for the resident and the staff, particularly if they are bringing someone out who is in a wheelchair.

Doors could be self-opening, but some people with dementia might not understand how a particular type of automatic door works, and in any case they may not be affordable. It should therefore at least be possible for doors to be held open or to have an overhead door closer which will stop the door shutting too quickly. If the door is open, people with dementia are more likely to go out.

Fig. 112 If the door is open, people with dementia are more likely to go out

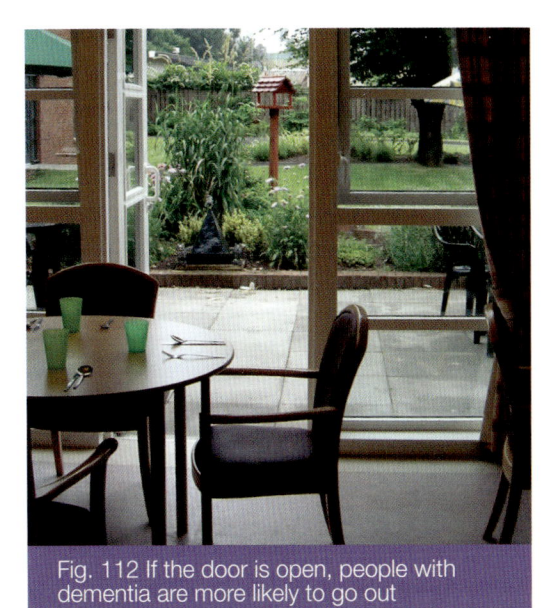

In a recent USA study of many facilities for older people, the door to the outside was a significant complaint of many residents and "in places where residents could easily cross the door threshold, residents spent 195 more minutes per week outdoors." (Rodiek, 2009)

Some designs allow outside spaces to be accessed directly from bedrooms, which is clearly much appreciated by some people.

However, providing this without any visual access for staff can add to their burden of care as without appropriate assistive technologies, staff may not know when someone has gone outside. People with dementia may also go back into the wrong door if all the doors look the same. Therefore, making sure that as much of the garden, courtyard, balcony or roof terrace is visible from a communal area where staff are likely to be can be very helpful whatever the access.

Cameras monitoring the garden can also be useful, if gardens are not easily monitored at all times by busy staff.

Signage

It is important to have clear signage, indicating the way to the garden, on or pointing towards the exit door. In addition, there should be signage indicating the route back from the outdoors to the room from which the resident came. This should say what the room function is, e.g. living room or dining room.

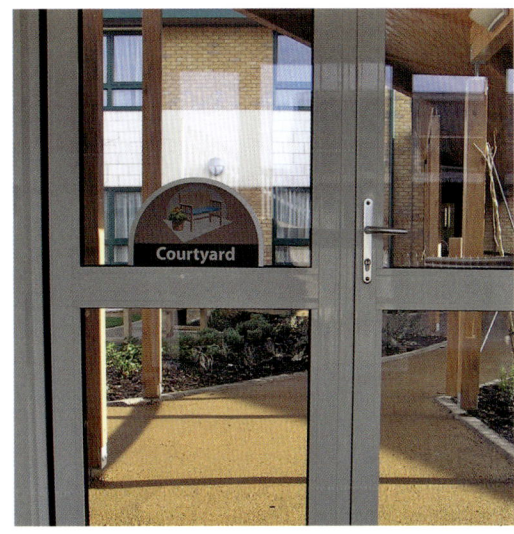

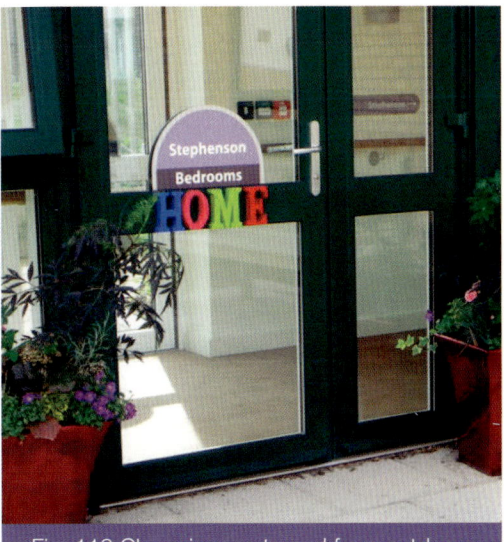

Fig. 113 Clear signage to and from outdoor space

Thresholds

Many people with dementia have visuospatial problems, which mean they have difficulty in processing or interpreting visual information about where objects are in space. For them, any change in colour and contrast between different flooring and/or a too obvious threshold, can look like a step, which can cause hesitation and lead to a possible fall. Thresholds should be level for frail elderly people, many of whom shuffle, walk with a walking aid or are pushed in a wheelchair.

'In-between' space

It can be very helpful to have some sort of 'in-between' transition space linking the inside and outside areas so that people can go out in all weathers and can have somewhere to change. Coat hooks and umbrella stands can be placed in this space along with shoe benches and traditional barometers. This 'in-between' space may take the form of a verandah, lobby or roofed area just beyond the exit doors. The other advantages of spaces such as these are outlined in Chapter 6: Site and climatic considerations.

In summary

Every effort needs to be made to avoid frustration when someone wants to go outside, as frustration raises stress levels and can lead to challenging behaviour, which is upsetting for residents and staff alike.

Key points:

- doors to outside space should be highly visible and easy to use
- doors should be able to be fixed open or at least have a slow door closing mechanism
- glazed walls and doors should allow good visual access for staff as well as residents
- thresholds should be level without abrupt changes in floor colour
- a lobby or other intermediate space (e.g. verandah) is a very useful feature.

4. Layout and design of outside spaces

Clearly different sites will have varying potential for complexity of layout in terms of both building and outside space.

However, there are some general design principles that apply to all arrangements and these are as follows:

- people should be drawn outside by the design and layout, either because they are curious, or because they are attracted by something of interest
- since many people with dementia can recall details from their childhood (but not more recent events), the design should incorporate plants and other elements that might trigger early memories
- seats and tables are essential to encourage people outdoors.

In the same way that outside spaces should draw people out, they also must lead people back inside and paths should take people back to doors that lead into appropriate and recognisable parts of the building. Ideally, there should be only one door by which residents enter and then leave the garden, with a looped path leading from it and back to it. But this is not always straightforward as some outside spaces are shared with several units, so differentiating very strongly the external doors may be important. This can be done with clear signage, objects and colour, as well as using specific plants as 'markers'.

Walking around the outside spaces, providing essential exercise, should be a journey with things to look at and enjoy on the way, with a combination of planting, lawn, and hard surfacing, as well as places to sit and rest in sun and shade. A gate that is easy to open and opens both ways can give a reassuring feeling of freedom to go anywhere.

In terms of more detailed design, the following should be considered, depending on space and layout.

Paved areas

Patios large enough for tables and chairs are really useful for eating and other activities that can be done outside, and these should ideally be immediately adjacent to communal rooms within the building.

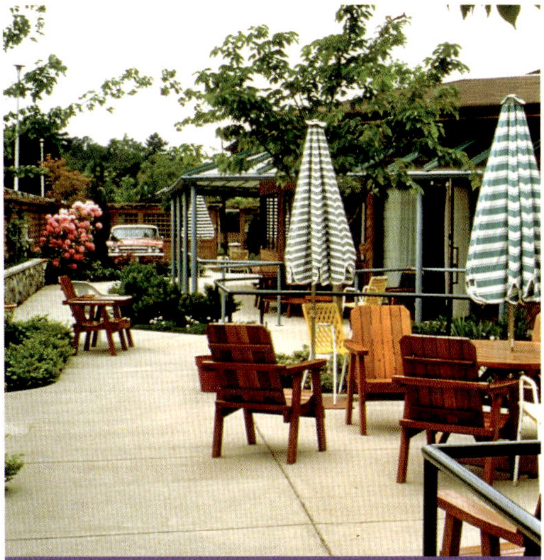

Fig. 114 Tables, chairs and parasols for comfortable outdoor use

Such areas need protection from the elements to ensure maximum usage, for example, the use of parasols, an awning that can be opened out, or a simple roof structure to provide protection from a shower of rain or from strong, direct sun. Guisset-Martinez (2011) describes a hospital garden in Nancy where there is space for meetings to be held outside as well as for a wide variety of other activities.

Noise levels may be increased by large areas of paving. This can be useful in an outside communal space, where gentle background noise may encourage people to venture outside. However, although some paving may be required under bedroom, office or medical room windows for cleaning and maintenance, it should be kept to a minimum for several reasons:

- people could collide with an outward opening window
- the privacy of people in the rooms behind the windows is compromised

- sound and noise can be reflected into the building if the width of paving is sufficient
- water overflow pipes may project near ground level
- it may compromise security in terms of people breaking in.

Paths

Paths should lead somewhere, at the very least around a feature and back again so that there is a journey to be accomplished. Features might include a tree, a sculpture, a summerhouse or simply a route through an arch or pergola to another space. Paths should not lead to dead ends or locked gates – these can exacerbate a sense of frustration and cause confusion in wayfinding.

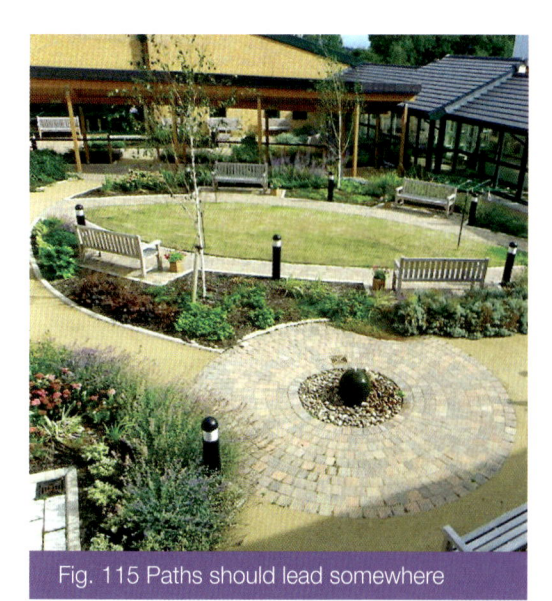

Fig. 115 Paths should lead somewhere

Seating along the paths

Seats should be provided at regular intervals along the paths, so that they can be seen as a destination point for each stretch of pathway. This will help to encourage those who are not so able to walk. Where there is more than one seat, the seats should be laid out to enable people to chat facing each other; seeing the person you are chatting to also helps those whose hearing is not so good.

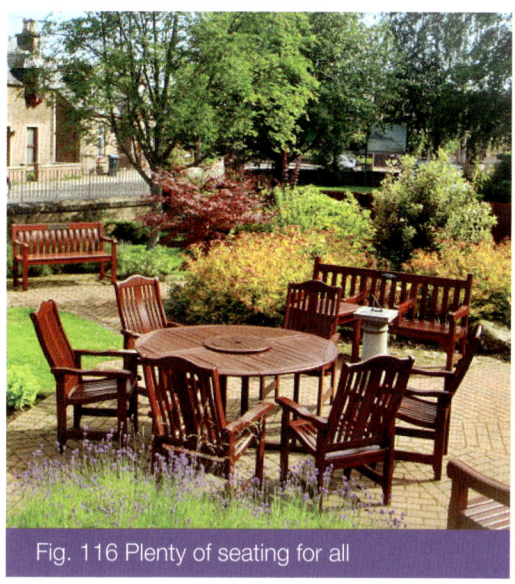

Fig. 116 Plenty of seating for all

Interesting objects

Objects help everyone navigate through their environment by providing 'memory triggers'. Objects, particularly those that have some local affinity, can be very useful; for example, a home with residents who come from a fishing or farming background might have a boat or farm equipment placed in the garden to attract people outdoors. A small, safe water feature can also be an attraction as can a shelter with seating. Case study 3, Werruna, shows how farming objects are used to alert and prompt people to what they might do outside.

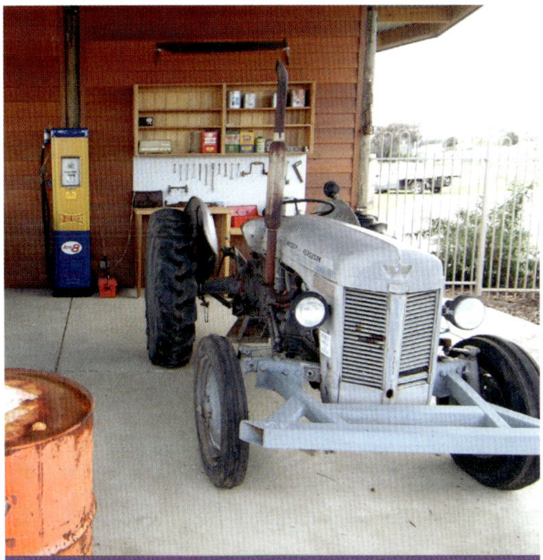

Fig. 117 Tractor, petrol pump and tools in the farm shed at Werruna

Places to go

A destination point, for example a gazebo, greenhouse or chicken coop will encourage people to take exercise.

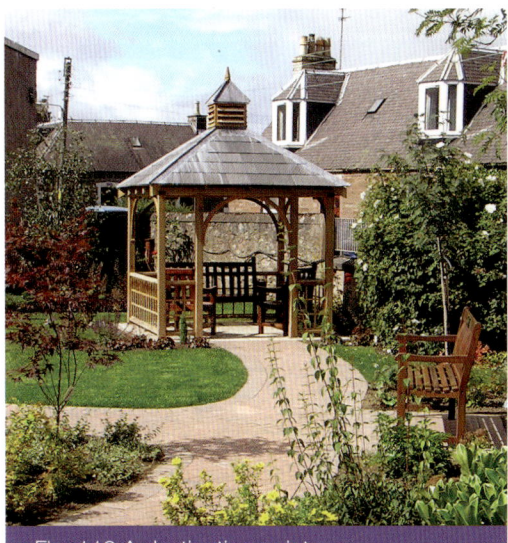

Fig. 118 A destination point

Live animals

Animals will certainly attract people to go outdoors and in this respect chickens, ducks and rabbits are all useful. Case study 3, Werruna, has many different types of animals for the residents to look at, reflecting their agricultural background. Where space is more restricted, bird baths and bird feeders may be appropriate, for example on a balcony or roof terrace.

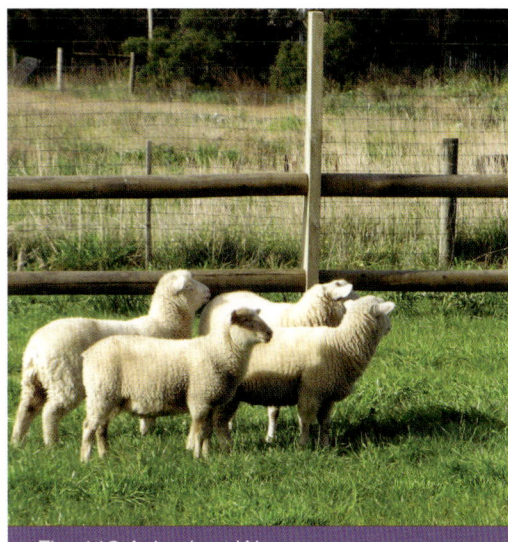

Fig. 119 Animals at Werruna

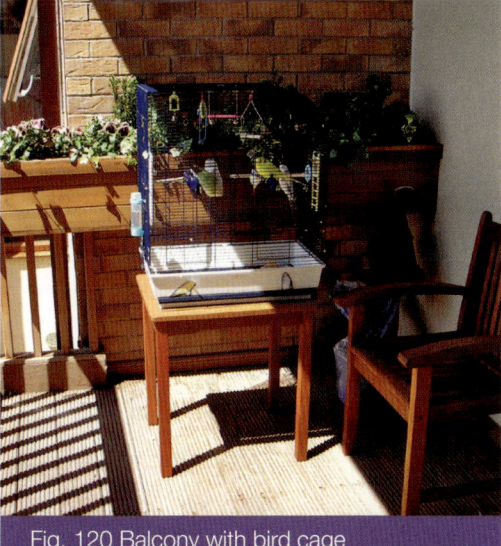

Fig. 120 Balcony with bird cage

Part 3 Chapter 8 Design principles that apply to all outside spaces

147

Places for retreat

Some people really need quiet spaces, somewhere to escape and be private. If there is enough ground, a place to 'retreat' can be really helpful and much appreciated and in this instance, plants with memories attached, perfume, and colour can help to achieve a restful and healing place. However, this place of retreat should be very carefully located and designed so that it has an element of privacy but is still visible to the staff from a well-used interior space.

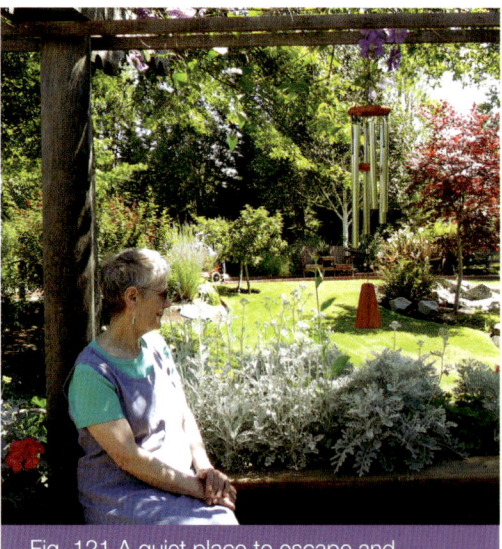

Fig. 121 A quiet place to escape and be private

Shelter

Cohen-Mansfield (2007) noted that one of the main reasons people did not use gardens was because of the weather, e.g. it is too hot, too windy or too sunny; and of course in northern temperate climates, too cold, rainy or windy (see Chapter 6). Outside spaces should be able to be enjoyed in any weather, although clearly every effort needs to be made to maximise shelter from sun, wind or rain and this must be a key consideration in any layout. Shelter needs to be provided, either by the building or by built features such as walls, trellis with planting or densely planted areas.

Shelter should allow people to simply step outside without being exposed and in this respect, the 'in-between' space noted above can be very useful. A shelter in the centre of the garden, such as a gazebo, where people can sit out of the sun, wind or rain can be a good attraction to encourage walking (see Fig. 118).

Key points:

- the outside space should attract people to go outside and make it easy to find their way back again
- a range of types of space, places to go, seating and items of interest will promote activity, exploration and walking
- items of local interest can add to the experience
- a quiet retreat can be much appreciated
- shelter from the elements is essential
- waymarking objects can assist wayfinding
- avoid large areas of paving directly outside bedroom windows, offices or medical rooms, where privacy and security may be compromised.

5. Hard surfaced areas

Hard surfaces such as patios and paths are key features in all outdoor areas. They provide a safe surface to walk about on as well as a directional guide for people with impaired memory and, or impaired vision.

As well as being safe, level, non-slip, and with no trip hazards etc, surfaces need to feel and look safe, so a smooth and non-reflective surface is important. Achieving this is not without problems, in that the surface needs to be non-slip without making it difficult for people who walk with a shuffling gait or who use walking aids to move along more comfortably.

Colour contrast edging can be helpful for people whose eyesight may be impaired.

There is much debate as to whether such edgings should be raised to prevent walking frames with wheels and wheelchairs from running off the edge of a path. On balance, however, raised edges can lead to additional cost in providing drainage and may also cause trip hazards at changes of direction.

Most older people begin to have problems with glare so, if concrete surfacing, slabs or pavers are selected as the pathway material, they should be tinted. A light buff colour will cause fewer problems with reflected sunlight. Asphalt does not create a glare problem, except sometimes when wet, and is more heat retentive than concrete. However, it may not appeal on aesthetic grounds and care needs to be taken to ensure that adjoining patios/ramps do not contrast with the black surface, thereby looking like a change in level.

Another critical issue in selecting materials for paving in areas where people may be using a walking frame or other walking aids is the need to avoid cracks that catch and snag the implements and cause frustration or even a fall. Expansion joints in concrete should not be more than 4 mm wide to be certain to avoid this problem, and joints between paving slabs should be pointed only very slightly recessed. Butt jointing of slabs is not recommended however, since this can cause problems in the long-term with weed growth and differential moisture absorption.

Slopes need to be gradual with highly visible handrails provided to ensure people feel steady and comfortable when moving around. Current Scottish legislation (for example) calls for handrails to be provided for any slope of 1:20 or greater in a ramp access to a building and other countries are likely to have similar regulations.

Encouraging walking is a key role for outside spaces, and as such, outside spaces should feel very easy and safe to navigate and providing handrails may be necessary to achieve this.

This is because we know that a person with dementia may see an undisguised, dark manhole cover as a hole, planting bed or other obstacle and therefore try to avoid walking over it.

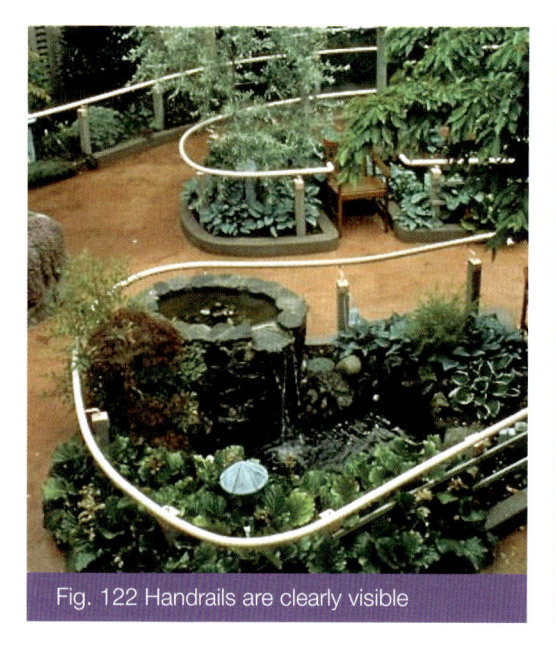

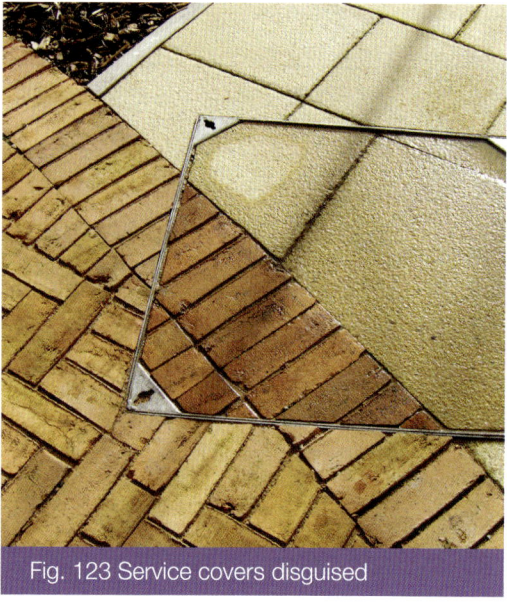

Fig. 122 Handrails are clearly visible

Fig. 123 Service covers disguised

In addition, steps should also be provided as an alternative to the ramp, as people who are physically mobile often find steps easier to use.

Balconies and roof terraces provide different challenges in that a more varied range of flooring materials is available, but the same principles apply.

Again, it is necessary to bear in mind that people with dementia may have visuospatial problems and therefore design should avoid strong changes in colour except for guidance in direction or for use where you want to dissuade people from going. Unavoidable access points to drains and other underground services should ideally be concealed in planting beds. If manhole covers are unavoidable in hard surfaced areas, recessed covers should be used in which the paving pattern can be inset.

Where manhole covers cannot be avoided and a recessed cover has not been used, paths and patios should be designed to allow space for objects such as seats to be placed over them.

Key points:

- use non-slip paving materials but not so rough-textured that they impede movement
- tint paving material to minimise glare problems
- use handrails for slopes, and contrast colour for the actual rail
- use consistent colour unless you want to deter people
- conceal manhole covers using recessed covers.

6. Planting

The actual plants, shrubs and trees used in the outside space will vary hugely with the location of the facility and tastes and culture of the resident groups. Outdoor spaces are frequently focused on having plants that were either popular during the youth of the residents or have an attractive perfume, and clearly both are important. However, it should be borne in mind that for many older people outside spaces were (and still are) functional spaces, rather than spaces just for sitting and admiring the flowers and shrubs. Stephen Judd notes this in Chapter 4 in respect of the Australian backyard.

Such spaces included shared yards, small allotments, areas for functional activities such as clothes drying, storage, chickens, and so on. Some people may have had no private outdoors spaces and would have used municipal parks for exercise and socialising.

Plants can, of course, be a great source of activity, for example, vegetables, fruit and herbs can be grown and harvested, bulbs and annuals can be planted and enjoyed, flowers can be picked and arranged, planting beds can be weeded and it is always useful to have some raised beds for people who struggle to bend or who use a wheelchair.

Plants make excellent landmarks, especially trees. They can attract people and can provide good orientation for finding your way around an outside space. Trees are most effective if they are striking and look similar throughout the year. A silver birch (UK), for example, has striking silver bark throughout the year.

Trees and plants attract birds and wildlife, which can provide endless enjoyment.

Trees can also provide shade from the sun and shelter from wind and rain, so a seat under a big tree is a benefit. In addition, trees are good for people who live above the ground floor to look out into. People on balconies and roof terraces will enjoy watching the branches of a tree, bird life and seeing the seasons change.

General plants attributes for all situations

The following list indicates general attributes of plants that are useful for gardens for people with dementia:

- plants with year-round interest so that there is always something to enjoy; this means plants that announce the seasons (spring flowers, summer flowers, autumn colour), colourful flowers and foliage, evergreen or shapely plants, plants that move in the breeze, plants that look good in the rain (see Case studies 6 and 8)

- plants that might trigger memories by their type and perfume; in the UK these might include plants such as roses, clematis, stocks etc.

- edible plants that relate to food and kitchen gardens, such as fruit trees, herbs and vegetables, which again might trigger early memories

- plants that have a variety of textures in both the foliage and the flowers; in Australia these might include the wattle, grevilleas and eucalypt trees (a group including Eucalyptus, Corymbia and Angophora)

- plants that attract native wildlife and birdlife into the garden

- warm-coloured plants, as ageing eyes can more easily discern colours in the white/yellow/orange/red range than in the blue or lavender ranges

– this is not to preclude plants with blue leaves or flowers, but to make designers aware of this issue

- thorny and/or vigorous plants against fences only where required to deter climbers, otherwise they are best avoided

- trees, small and medium sized, except where there is a park-sized outdoor space. It is important that trees near paths or sitting areas do not have a heavy leaf fall that can cause surfaces to become slippery, or fruit or seeds that might hurt the person sitting underneath (for example, from experience, beech nuts falling can be quite painful!)

- grass/lawn areas that encourage people to walk on it without shoes and sit and smell the freshly-mown grass.

Poisonous plants should be avoided at all costs, because berries, other fruits and leaves may be eaten at some point, plants will be picked and sap may irritate. The Royal Horticultural Society in the UK has excellent guidance on this on their website under 'Potentially harmful garden plants' and there are many other web sites that can be paged to find similar information on appropriate plants in other countries.

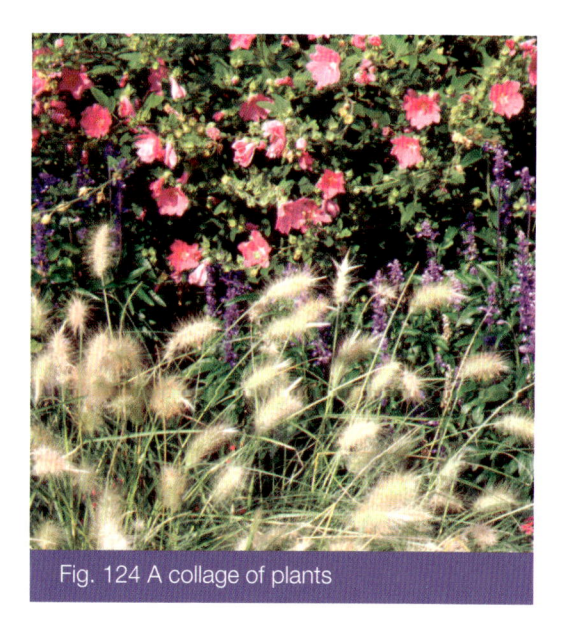

Fig. 124 A collage of plants

Green Roofs

In many countries, and in particular in city environments, green roof design is being positively encouraged (as is shown in Case study 2, Villa Ichikawa, Japan) and has great potential in providing more usable outdoor space. Therefore, the technical design of roof gardens and terraces needs to be taken on board at the outset of a building design. On existing roof gardens or roof terraces, there may be technical constraints on developing planting, but if at all possible, planting beds should be designed into the space and raised to allow for sufficient soil to support a good range of plants. On small roof gardens and terraces, moveable planters may be the only option and these should be carefully chosen to provide a sustainable medium for plants as well as for activity for the users, yet not provide a means for climbing which might endanger the user.

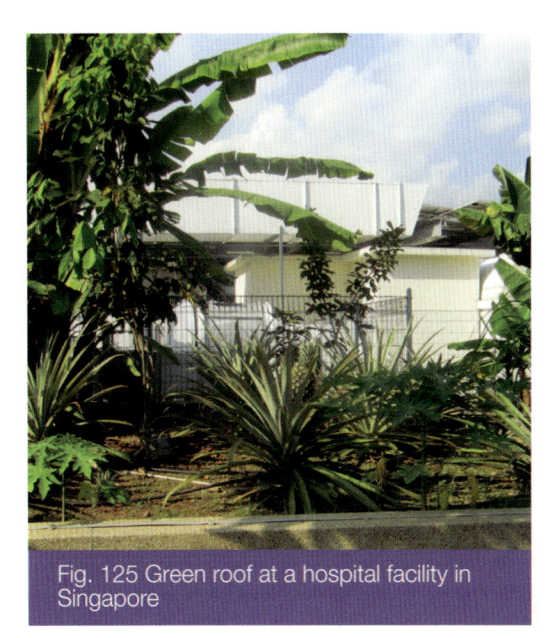

Fig. 125 Green roof at a hospital facility in Singapore

Key points:
- use plants to give year-round interest
- avoid poisonous plants or plants that cause ill effects if eaten or touched
- grow edible plants so they can be harvested and enjoyed
- emphasise flowering plants in the yellow/orange/red colour range
- use trees that make good landmarks
- consider carefully ways of incorporating planting into roof gardens and roof terraces.

7. Features

The potential list of garden features is endless, so here we just give some ideas, many of which have been already been mentioned or are noted in Chapter 9. It is important that the outdoor spaces feel homelike, are appropriate to the culture, and incorporate items that might trigger long-ago memories.

Designers should consider all the potential activities that could take place outdoors (see Chapter 9). At the very least, good seating, tables, a hard surfaced area and planting are always needed. The design should be sufficiently flexible to allow for appropriate outdoor activities that may be developed over a period of time.

Water features

Water is a great attraction but it needs to be made safe. Ponds, in particular, can be hazardous, although they have the enormous additional asset of providing a home for fish and somewhere for birds to get water.

Safety can be maximised by providing a metal mesh over the top which, if well designed can be very attractive; or by incorporating a waist-high grab-rail, fence or wall that will discourage residents from getting into them.

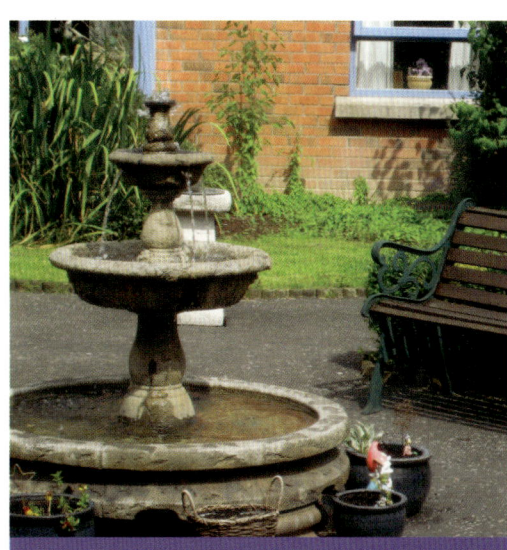

Fig. 126 Water is a great attraction but needs to be made safe

153

Moving water features can be much enjoyed. In hotter countries they are often part of the cultural heritage and encouraged because moving water enhances the microclimate by cooling the air. However, it should be noted that still water (especially in tropical areas) may not be feasible due to potential insect breeding and indeed all water features require careful and dedicated maintenance to ensure their safety.

In selecting a fountain, the resulting sound is important as it is not necessarily always pleasant. Some can sound like wet fabric slapping, some like a constant thumping, some like urination - a good water feature should be soothing to listen to. It is important therefore to assess this before investing. A waist-high 'trickling' fountain can be a pleasant addition since it provides a soothing sound (if there are seats nearby); people can touch the water, yet there is no lying water to tempt people to get into.

The proximity of a toilet should be considered if a moving water feature is planned because it may induce an urge to urinate.

Reminiscence objects

Objects that trigger memories have been mentioned and are generally under-used. They depend on the background of the residents and must be culturally appropriate, as outside spaces and how they are used vary hugely from one culture to another.

Case study 4, Haugmotun, illustrates a development that is not only culturally appropriate, but also incorporates many aspects of country life that the residents will know and understand.

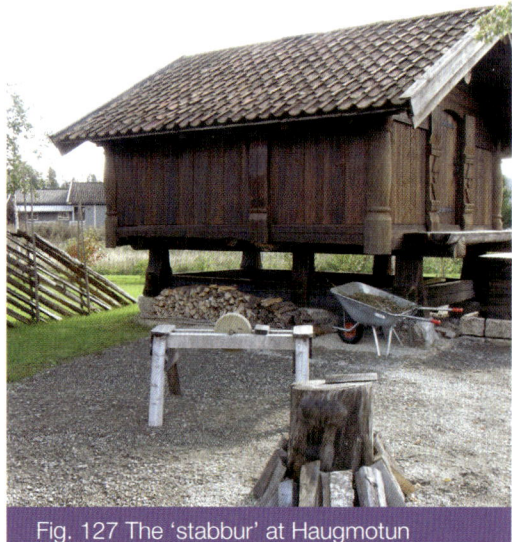

Fig. 127 The 'stabbur' at Haugmotun

In many parts of the world, sheds, greenhouses, chicken coops, washing poles, areas where things can be mended, e.g. a bicycle or car, all provide great 'activity potential' and are discussed further in Chapter 9. Items such as postboxes, phone boxes, bus shelters and so on can also be useful as reminiscence features within the garden, but they need to be incorporated in such a way that the overall 'message' of garden is not compromised. It is important to avoid creating a 'disneyland' atmosphere as this may be thoroughly confusing to the person with dementia.

Eating outside can be hugely enjoyable and it is worth allocating space for a solid and well-made barbeque or even a built-in one.

Features for non-residents

Non-residents include staff, adult visitors and children as well as visiting professionals such as occupational therapists (OTs) and physiotherapists.

Fig. 128 Space for a solid and well-made barbeque or even a built-in one

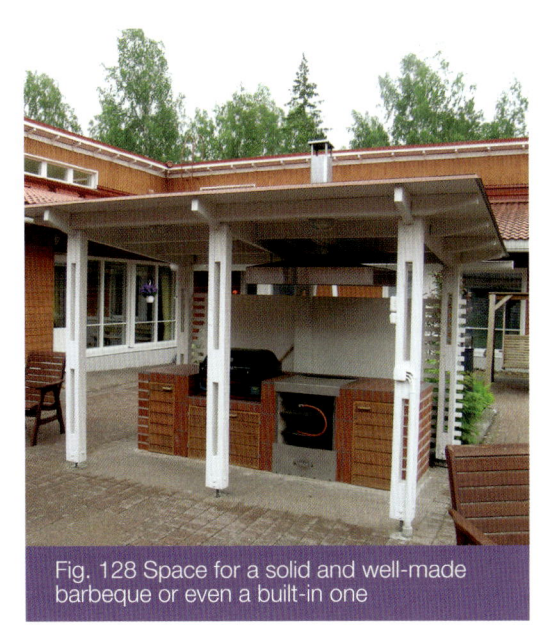

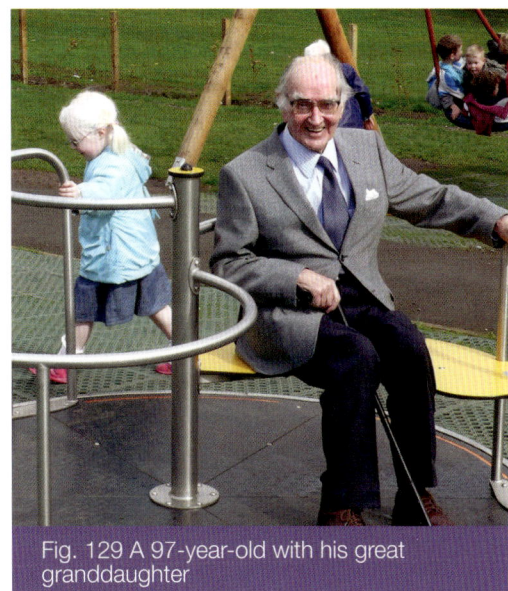

Fig. 129 A 97-year-old with his great granddaughter

Staff will benefit from having their own outside space, if the site allows. They may want to hold outside meetings on good days, have their meals outside or have a well-earned break for a coffee and/or smoke outside. This space would ideally have an alternative door and be visually concealed, for example, by a hedge.

Adult visitors will appreciate space where they can sit with their relative or friend who is a resident, and have things to look at and talk about with them.

Smaller children are likely to appreciate a play area to keep them occupied during visits. They can be very troublesome if they are bored and conversely they can provide enjoyable entertainment if they are playing on things like climbing frames and slides. However care must be taken to ensure that these items are safe for the person with dementia to use as well.

Visiting professionals such as occupational therapists and physiotherapists may like features that maintain activity regimes (see Chapter 9).

Key points:

- tables, chairs and benches should always be provided, taking account of the activities that may happen outside
- designs should include for features that are culturally appropriate, items of reminiscence, that may reflect the past lives of the residents
- water features must have regular maintenance budgeted for
- space for a barbeque or one built in is good for encouraging social contact
- dedicated space for staff to relax outside on their breaks is useful if space allows
- play equipment for young visitors can help with visits and provide enjoyment to all
- features that can help maintain activity regimes are useful.

8. Furniture

Furniture for use in any outside space for older people must be robust, comfortable and stable. This is because older frail people tend to sit down with a lurch due to weak muscles and will usually need to use seat arms to help them get up again. All seating should have backs and sturdy arms projecting just beyond the seat edge so that older people can push themselves up from a seated position.

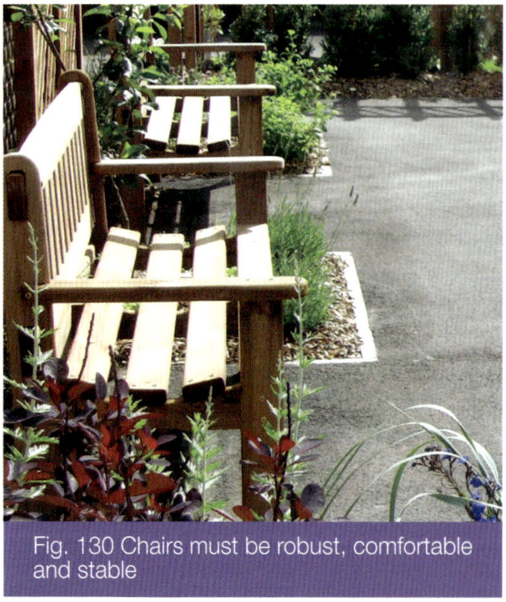

Fig. 130 Chairs must be robust, comfortable and stable

A classic example of good seating is the typical wooden park bench with sturdy back and arms, and such seating can be obtained in a variety of sizes from single seats to benches for six people or more.

It is reassuring for people with dementia if the next seat along a path can be seen from the one being sat upon, and this will encourage walking. Robust wooden benches have the additional merit of being year-round furniture, which can be enjoyed, perhaps with a cushion, in dry weather. Wood is a good material because it is warmer than stone or metal and tends to dry faster after rain or dew.

Other important outdoor furniture includes tables and chairs for activities and eating outside, particularly on a patio just outside the principal access to the garden. Again, this furniture needs to be robust and comfortable. An adjustable and appropriately secured parasol/umbrella above the table can be really helpful so people can sit in shade as the sun moves.

Key points:

- solid, robust benches with arms
- tables that are stable and suitable for wheelchair users
- parasols/umbrella for use in sunny or drizzly weather.

9. Toilets and taps

The proximity of a toilet will give people the confidence to go outside without worrying. Some care homes provide an outside toilet on the basis that this is not only convenient but is what this generation would have had in their younger days.

The toilet door needs to be very clearly identifiable with colour contrast and a sign that is consistent with other toilets in the unit. If a toilet is not near the outside space it needs to be very clearly signed by the door leading in from the garden so that people coming in, in a hurry, can find it easily and quickly. The other advantage of a toilet near to the garden is that it allows people to wash their hands after gardening activities without having to traipse through the building.

An outdoor tap is essential for watering the garden, filling buckets, and washing down the patios. However, it may be necessary to decide whether this is something that is used with supervision only and this will dictate whether it is sited prominently or not.

Key points:

- nearby or easily accessed, well-signed toilet
- nearby outside tap.

10. Maintenance

Good and regular maintenance is essential. So many outside spaces become unusable because they are not properly maintained. Naturally, they should be designed to minimise maintenance but no outside space is ever maintenance-free.

Some residents will really enjoy feeling useful undertaking small garden jobs and the following case study shows how some involvement in maintenance may be beneficial to the resident.

Mr M was a nuisance to the handyman in his care home because he wanted to use the big mechanical mower and he was very insistent having been a gardener himself. He was clearly keen to be helpful. The problem was solved by providing him with his own small, non-mechanical mower, which he could use anytime he wanted.

However, it is not feasible to plan that garden maintenance be achieved as part of activities with residents, as only a small amount of this may result in useful maintenance.

Although some relatives may be willing to help, reliance on volunteer gardeners usually results in patchy work as numbers drop off and many volunteers may not be good gardeners!

A proper maintenance schedule must be drawn up, with specifics as to what has to be done through each season of the year, and implemented with a budget ring-fenced for it. It is a good idea to encourage garden maintenance staff to see their role as an integral part of the care service and to work creatively with residents whenever possible.

The following key points illustrate some of the factors that need to be taken into account when establishing a maintenance budget.

Key points:

- hard surfaces need to be brushed, washed and often treated to get rid of moss and algae; joints may need attention to keep the surface safe to use
- grass needs to be cut regularly and fertilised as required
- planting beds need to be weeded, fertilised and watered as required
- bushes need to be pruned and herbaceous plants divided
- trees may need to be thinned
- there needs to be a budget for planned replacement planting as plants die or become overgrown and unattractive
- water features need to be treated and maintained to keep them healthy
- any animals (e.g. rabbits, chickens etc) need dedicated care.

11. Miscellaneous extra considerations

There are many other considerations in the design of a successful outside space.

Conservatories

Although not strictly an outside space, a conservatory may often form part of or lead to an outside space. Considerations of hard surfaces, furniture and planting are the same. In Case study 1, Clare Cooper Marcus notes that the large conservatory is heavily used in colder weather for horticultural activities.

The design also needs to be carefully considered to avoid a glazed roof casting confusing shadows over the floor.

Verandahs

Similar to conservatories, these areas provide useful intermediate spaces and are perhaps more often found in countries with hotter summers than those in northern Europe. They provide areas for activities as they are open to fresh air, yet provide shade from summer sun. They are also useful for people who do not wish to stray too far from the building, yet like to watch the garden activity.

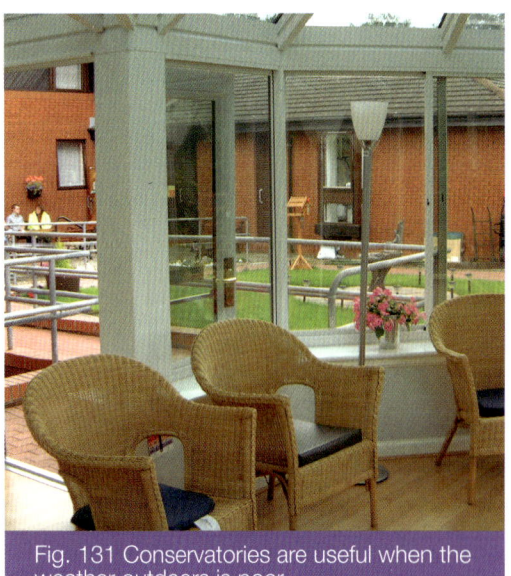

Fig. 131 Conservatories are useful when the weather outdoors is poor

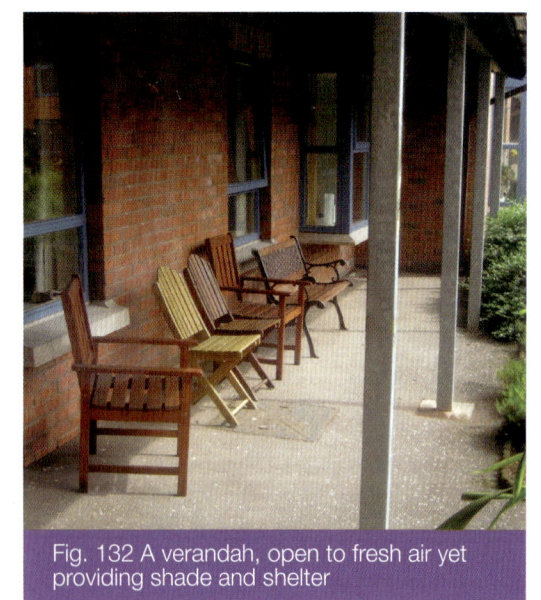

Fig. 132 A verandah, open to fresh air yet providing shade and shelter

A conservatory can provide an area where coats and hats can be stored and people can change their shoes. This can be a very useful space for indoor gardening, potting or horticultural therapy throughout the year. However, temperature and over-bright light can be serious considerations and solar reflective glass and blinds should be incorporated to ensure that these spaces are usable all year round.

Terraces

These are often semi-enclosed, raised areas of hard surfacing immediately adjacent to the building, accessed from communal space. They are particularly useful for social activities and as a possible location for the barbeque.

Case study 4, Haugmuton, notes a much appreciated terrace.

Canvas tents/awnings

Open-sided and wall-fixed type awnings can provide for occasional shelter and allow forward planning for social events in any weather. They are very traditional and appropriate for the generation currently in care homes as most shops had awnings that were opened out to provide shelter and shade from the elements.

Case study 5, Back Porch, notes the use of a canopy and awnings.

A place outside for smokers

Many older people with dementia may have smoked all their lives. Staff too may be smokers. A dedicated place outside which they may use should be considered.

Lighting

Lighting bollards, if used, should not be too low because they can cast confusing shadows unless sited at centres close enough to light the whole pathway. It is important that if the outside space is to be used in the evening the lighting provides a good overall light. This usually requires high-level downlighting either set on posts like traditional street lights or mounted on the building.

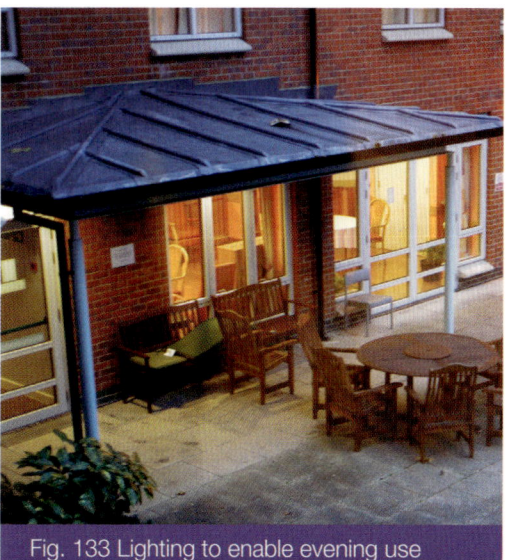

Fig. 133 Lighting to enable evening use

For daytime use, lighting levels immediately inside the building on the way in from the garden should be of a higher intensity to compensate for the change in lighting level from outside to inside and prevent momentary blindness and falls.

Heating

Outdoor heating is rarely provided. There are environmental considerations with this to be taken into account. Nevertheless, outdoor heating could, in more temperate countries, potentially extend considerably the time of usage of outdoor spaces for eating and table-based activities, either into the evenings or beyond the summer months. If provided, heating should be mounted high for safety.

Staff attitudes and training

It is important to involve the management, staff and residents or their relatives in the design and management of the outdoor space. Research at a number of USA sites found that management and training do affect the success of outdoor space in a facility for people with dementia as much as the actual garden design (Grant, 2003). Chapter 11 deals with this in greater detail.

The Living Garden (Clare Cooper Marcus' case study) is successful largely because the designer involved so many significant actors in the process: representatives of patients' families, the centre's staff, and horticultural therapists from a nearby botanical garden.

Key points:

- intermediate spaces, e.g. verandahs or conservatories, are useful for encouraging outdoor activity and providing activity space in poor weather
- awnings can provide for occasional shelter and allow forward planning for social events in any weather
- a place for smokers should be included
- lighting and heating can enable outdoor activity later in the day
- inclusive design by everyone who is to be involved usually results in success.

References

Berentsen, V.D., Grefsrød, E.-E., & Eek, A. (2008). Gardens for people with dementia: Design and use. Tønsberg, Norway: Aldring og helse.

Cohen-Mansfield, J. (2007). Outdoor wandering parks for persons with dementia. In S. Rodiek & B. Schwarz (Eds.). *Outdoor environments for people with dementia*. New York, NY: Haworth Press.

Grant, C. (2003). *Factors influencing the use of outdoor space by residents with dementia in long-term care facilities.* (PhD thesis). Atlanta, GA: Georgia Institute of Technology. Department of Architecture.

Guisset-Martinez, M. J. (2011). *Regaining identity: New synergies for a different approach to Alzheimer's*. Paris: Fondation Médéric Alzheimer.

Kearney, A. R., & Winterbottom, D. (2005). Nearby nature and long-term care facility residents: Benefits and design recommendations. In S. Rodiek & B. Schwarz (Eds.). *The role of the outdoors in residential environments for aging.* New York, NY: Haworth Press.

Marshall, M. (2010). *Designing balconies, roof terraces and roof gardens for people with dementia*. Stirling: Dementia Services Development Centre.

Namazi, K. H., & Johnson, B. D. (1992). Pertinent autonomy for residents with dementias: Modification of the physical environment to enhance independence. *American Journal of Alzheimer's Disease and Other Dementias, 7*(1),10–15.

Pollock, R. (2003). *Designing interiors for people with dementia*. Stirling: Dementia Services Development Centre.

Rodiek, S. (2009). *Environmental influence on outdoor usage in facilities for the elderly*. Bethesda, MD: National Institute on Aging.

Zeisel, J. (2011). *I'm still here: Creating a better life for a loved one living with dementia*. London: Piatkus.

Case Study 6
Sydenham Court

Sally Visick and Clifford McClenaghan

Sydenham Court is a purpose-designed two-storey housing development providing care for people with dementia. It comprises 25 flats situated around a central courtyard, which measures 27 metres by 22.5 metres.

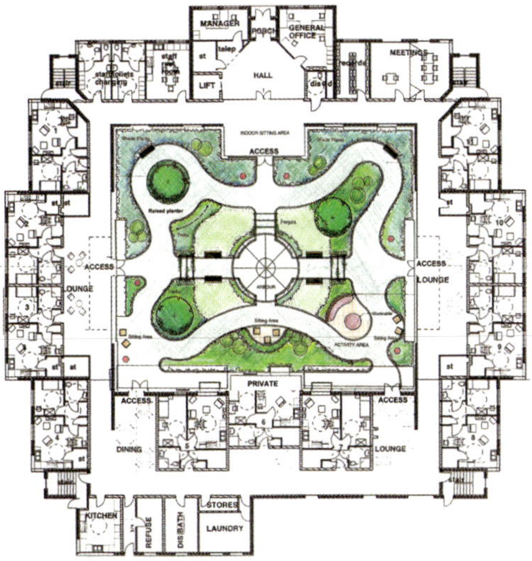

Fig. 134 Plan of courtyard (refer to appendix 1 on page 219 for enlarged version)

Fig. 135 The courtyard, accessible from corridors and lounges

The courtyard is accessible from corridors and lounges on all four sides, offering an unsupervised but visible, safe and secure environment.

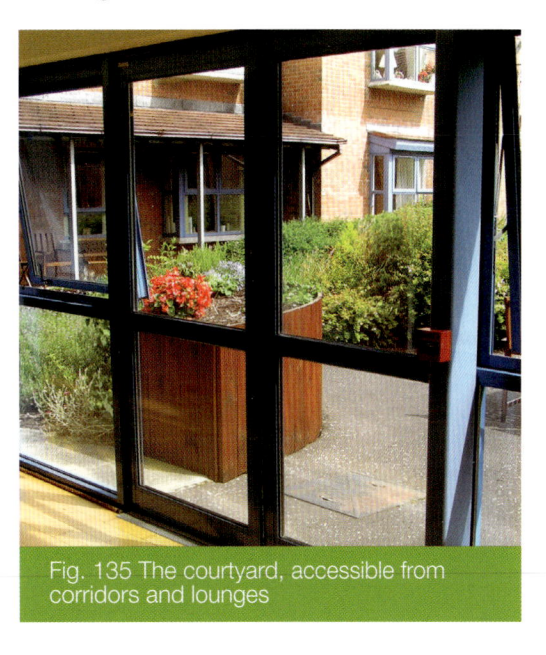

In late 1999, when our clients (the South and East Belfast Health Trust in partnership with Clanmil Housing Association) briefed us, they provided clear guidelines on the landscape design of Sydenham Court. In addition, they gave us a number of reference materials, notably a paper by Annie Pollock, *Landscaping for Dementia Patients* (undated); a handout prepared for a one-day conference at Stirling Royal Infirmary in September 1997 entitled *Garden Design for People with Dementia*; and brief extracts from research by Norman (*Severe dementia – The provision of long-stay care*, Centre for Policy on Ageing, London, 1987) and Cohen and Weisman (*Holding on to Home*, Johns Hopkins University Press, 1991), on the topics of environmental stimulation without stress and ample and safe space for indoor and outdoor wandering.

Conversations with the architect, Clifford McClenaghan, who was already well advanced with the design of the building, were an invaluable part of the process.

Notes for a client presentation in January 2000 highlight key features of the proposed sketch design – continuous circulation, spatial subdivision, symmetry and asymmetry, restful areas and activity areas and resting points on route. Concerning planting, these notes suggest that the main structure be provided but that there should be opportunities for the tenants to contribute and they highlight the importance of fragrance, texture, sun/shade, seasonal effect and the use of evergreen species. Possible trees are white-barked birch, crab apple, rowan, cherry and pear – all small species that offer a variety of interest at different seasons of the year via form, flower, fruit, foliage or bark effects.

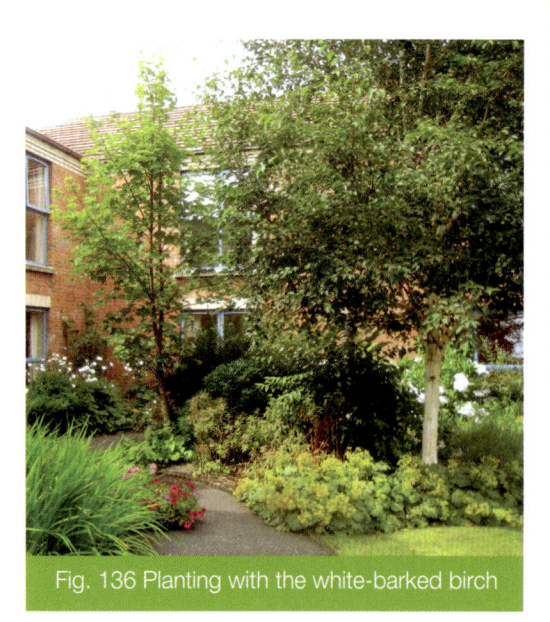

Fig. 136 Planting with the white-barked birch

Looking back over more than a decade, what stands out in the memory is that Sydenham Court was a trail-blazer in terms of supported independent living for people with dementia.

The landscape, particularly of the internal courtyard, was seen as an active contributor to residents' wellbeing, part of a safe and restful environment, where potentially confusing stimuli were minimised and opportunities for agreeable interaction with the outdoors were maximised. There were certainly budgetary constraints which meant that the full concept as designed was not completed at the time in every detail, but there was no doubting the commitment to an 'active' landscape.

The overall site was restricted and not without its difficulties, occupying a position on a relatively steep slope looking north-north-west across Belfast Harbour to the Antrim Hills. Once car parking, circulation and incidental requirements such as bin storage and oil tanks, were catered for, the remainder of the space outside the building was largely planted to screen or provide privacy from adjacent sites and to create a 'green' outlook for the tenants.

On the south-east elevation there was just enough room for a few private garden spaces serving ground floor apartments.

Fig. 137 Private garden spaces serving ground floor apartments

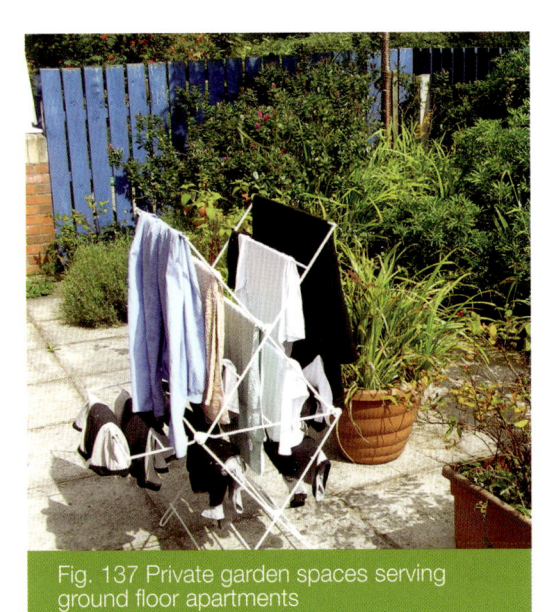

Although small, these gardens are a practical and valuable addition to the living space.

The main focus of the design scheme was the courtyard at the heart of the building, accessible from all four sides of the ground floor and visible from the upper storey. The space was symmetrical about its NNW/SSE axis, but the off-centre positioning of the doors on the east and west sides created the opportunity to have a balanced rather than a symmetrical composition for all four quadrants.

One of the key considerations for the layout, informed by background research, was the need to provide a continuous circulation route so that residents were never confronted with a dead end. To this end, the design evolved, with a central area wrapped in a gently sinuous outer path, creating a butterfly-shaped plan form. Alternative routes were introduced by aligning paths across the courtyard with three of the access doors, offering a degree of variety as well as creating a central space. Each one of the four 'wing' sections was slightly different in plan form from the others. We planned two of the sections, diagonally opposite each other, as activity areas with a raised planter in one and a working area with a raised bench in the other. The other two sections were intended to be more tranquil with the emphasis on the stimulus of the planting. More contrasts came from the varying aspects, with sunny and shady sides, lighter and darker areas and the resulting variety in plant selection.

The plan provided for quite strong spatial subdivision with planted pergolas acting as gateways to the central space, which in turn was to be enclosed with an arbour. The importance of providing well-distributed resting points was recognised with provision for fixed benches throughout as well as spaces for occasional seating. The plan also included 'signposts' – simple visual prompts to remind people of the location of an exit. The notes for the January 2000 presentation suggested that these signposts could be sculptural pieces or bird feeders or wind chimes or distinctive plants and my annotations suggest that the idea of wind chimes and bird feeders were particularly welcomed at the time. The planting plan did include strategically placed 'landmark' plants – a pair of camellias framing the main central door on the south side, a Japanese maple beside the east door, a white-barked birch close to the west door.

Hard surfaces within the courtyard were all paved in asphalt and there was considerable discussion at the time about the best way to treat the edges – how to strike the difficult balance between having enough of a raised edge to direct water to gullies effectively while not creating trip hazards. The budget did not extend to a continuous drainage system that would have allowed the level between hard and soft surfaces to remain flush and eventually it was decided, in consultation with the client, to lift grassed and planted areas by 50 mm and edge them with a timber trim.

The planting plan for the courtyard, with a roster of more than 100 species, was much more intense, diversified and gardenesque than the average institutional project. In the scheme as drawn, three specimen trees provide the tall structure – Himalayan birch (Betula jacquemontii), rowan (Sorbus 'Sheerwater Seedling') and flowering pear (Pyrus 'Chanticleer'). Himalayan birch is hard to beat in elegance of form, lightness of branch structure, ethereal winter presence and the almost edible quality of the fresh green spring foliage. Pyrus 'Chanticleer' produces startling white blossoms on bare twigs against rather dull, dark bark colouring and is a striking harbinger of spring, while rowans reliably produce a treble hit of flower, fruit and autumn foliage even before taking into consideration their attraction to garden birds. Specimen shrubs, strategically distributed throughout the space, were selected for interesting foliage and form (Acer palmatum dissectum), seasonal impact (Magnolia stellata, Camellia and Rhododendron), fragrance (Hamamelis, Choisya and Philadelphus) or plain old-fashioned familiarity (Hydrangea).

On the SSW-facing, sunny side of the courtyard, larger shrubs (Buddleia, Philadelphus and Choisya) were anchored at lower level by sun-loving evergreens (Hebes, Cistus, and prostrate Ceanothus). They, in turn, were interspersed with an array of hardy perennials, which included familiar garden favourites (Lychnis, red-hot pokers, asters, columbines and heathers). Lavender fringed the informal sitting area to provide fragrance and pleasantly tactile foliage, and culinary herbs were concentrated within the adjacent and equally sunny 'wing' section to the east. Wind was never a real issue, as the site is not particularly exposed.

On the shadier side of the courtyard the emphasis was on variety of form, leaf texture and colour. At low level, old-fashioned staples (London pride) rub shoulders with Hostas, Bergenia and Heuchera, while higher up Skimmia, Viburnum davidii, Philadelphus coronarius 'Aureus' and bamboo were chosen for contributions that don't depend on flower. Box hedging defined and enclosed the central circle with clematis and jasmine and wisteria selected for the pergolas and arbour.

In the event budgetary constraints meant that the design was not implemented in its entirety – the pergolas, arbour, and raised bed - workbench and seating were all omitted at the time, although seating and several smaller raised beds were introduced through subsequent fundraising. The positioning of the trees and specimen shrubs, combined with the plan form, achieved some degree of spatial articulation, but this was very much weaker than would otherwise have been the case.

Reports elsewhere suggest that the courtyard has come to play a central role in the lives of its residents in many different ways and that it has successfully embraced minor evolutions and additions to its fabric, including a garden shed and a water feature. The latter addition is interesting: design guidance when we were developing the scheme suggested that water features were not particularly suitable for this type of facility. But in the end a landscape scheme of this kind is only a starting point.

It is for its owners, in the truest sense of the word, to make it their own and this they have done.

This outdoor space gives residents freedom to explore, to sit in the sunshine or garden in a relaxed atmosphere. Although the housing association maintains the garden, the residents have formed a gardening club and spend time looking after the plants and growing vegetables such as beetroot, peas, lettuce and also rhubarb and herbs.

The gardening club has a 'dig it/eat it' programme and prepare vegetables for main meals. All this activity promotes feelings of self-worth and provides useful, meaningful occupation, with almost 90% of residents taking part.

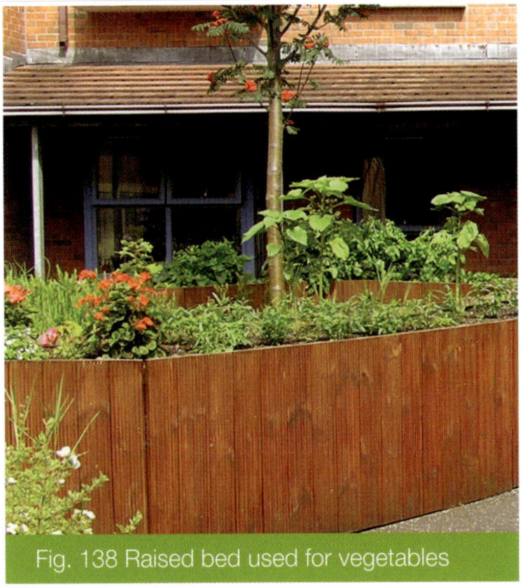

Fig. 138 Raised bed used for vegetables

The tables and chairs and covered sitting areas provide the opportunity to take the sun and relax or shelter and contemplate the birds, which come to bathe in the water feature.

On a good summer's evening, barbeques are held and music is provided for all to enjoy. Relatives also organise summer fetes, coffee mornings and the nearby country Streamvale Farm has been known to bring farm animals along for the interest of the residents and especially for the residents' grandchildren.

The staff have noted that if the courtyard was not available, it would be impossible to allow people outside into the busy, densely-populated area surrounding the scheme, with the result that anxiety levels would go up and sleeping patterns would be disturbed.

Although there is no outside toilet, there is access to facilities nearby. There have been no toilet problems.

The tenant's forum planned the water feature, which is central to this outdoor haven in an otherwise busy and noisy urban environment.

Mrs McC, an energetic resident, describes the garden as always accessible, with doors always open and staff always on hand should they be needed. She enjoys the opportunity to get outside, to walk on the level paths and sit in a safe and interesting space. She is a keen gardener and loves the ability to potter about in the garden shed or tend to the vegetables in the easy, reachable raised beds. She always feels happy in the garden and can't imagine what it would be like without it.

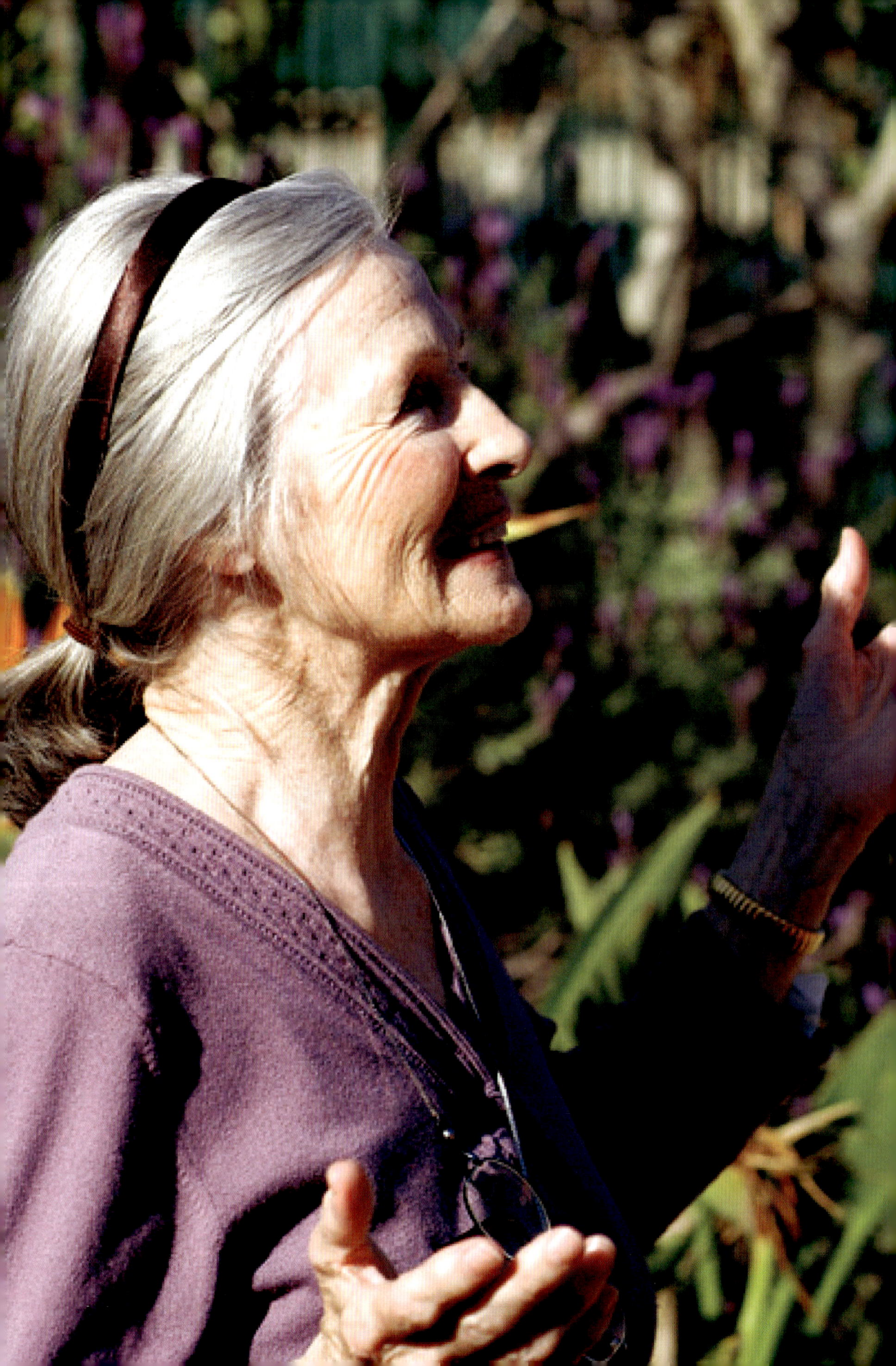

PART 4 USING THE OUTDOORS

Chapter 9
Activities and outside space
Teresia Hazen and Maria McManus

Designers and staff as well really do have to understand the activities that might take place in an outside space in order to plan and design for them, as these activities will impact not only on the garden design but also the building and how the two relate to each other.

Meaningful activities are recognised as a critical component of good quality dementia care (National Institute for Health and Clinical Excellence, 2008; College of Occupational Therapists (COT), 2008). Getting outside and being outside are central to health and wellbeing, and it is important, therefore, to include the opportunity to do activities – to engage the person and to add pleasure and quality to the day by encouraging people to go outside and to stay out.

Activity is a critical means by which we as human beings express ourselves and interact with the world around us and as such, activities are essential to human existence, health and wellbeing (COT, 2007). Lack of activity and lack of pleasure in activity are associated with higher rates of mortality or depression, reduction in social functioning, physical wellbeing, increased isolation and loss of quality of life (Mozley, Sutcliffe, Bagley, Cordingley, Challis, Huxley & Burns, 2004; Alessi, Yoon, Schnelle, Al-Samarrai & Cruise, 1999).

There are many types of activity. Some are about restoring and reinforcing long-held skills, abilities and knowledge; some provide multi-sensory stimulation; if you include sitting, watching and reflecting (which may be all that very impaired people with dementia can manage), then we are thinking of activities that are interesting for people to watch as well as areas within the garden for calmness and quiet. Finally, we need to consider activities at night because this can be a time of great stress for many people with dementia.

There are also activities that we would describe as normal, everyday outdoor activities that people will have undertaken in their own outdoor spaces all their lives. These may include hanging out or taking in the washing, shaking the dusters outside, emptying the compostable waste bin, sweeping the garden path, cleaning the garden furniture and repairing or repainting exterior wooden items (e.g. the hen coop, rabbit hutch, trellis, planters), putting out food on the bird table, having a cup of coffee, tea and/or having a cigarette and so on. It is important not to forget these everyday tasks as many people will get great pleasure from them.

Many of these may be included in the more specific headings summarised below:

1. Activities that encourage social interaction
2. Activities that enable a person to achieve their creative potential and self-expression
3. Activities that assist physical health, activity and exercise

4. Activities that engage the brain
5. Activities that restore and reinforce long-held skills, abilities and knowledge
6. Activities that provide multi-sensory stimulation
7. Activities that are less physical such as sitting, watching, reflecting
8. Lastly, outdoor activities that can be undertaken in the evening when the light is fading.

This chapter relates closely to Chapter 2 on the benefits of being outside and Chapter 11 on how staff can encourage people to go outside. This chapter will look at ways in which each of the activities noted above can be achieved outside. Of course many, if not most, activities have several purposes and advantages but some sort of order is needed to assist readers who are planning activities outside. It is assumed that staff will work with relatives and friends as well as the residents to ensure that the activities are appropriate for each individual. This will not only reinforce resident/staff relationships, but ensure that staff have a sound knowledge of a person's past and preferences that they then make central to a person's care plan (see Chapter 11).

In parallel with this, it is vital to remember that whilst getting outside and being outside are central to health and wellbeing, people don't necessarily go outside just because the weather is good and the space is attractive. They go outside because:

- it is easy to go out and they feel safe
- there is something to do outside or something to look at
- the environment is welcoming and appropriately designed for a range of activities, including being on your own
- the design provides a microclimate that is comfortable to be in.

Quotes from Marthe Raske's study of an enabling garden (2010) are inserted throughout the text.

1. Activities that enhance social interaction

It is essential that the activities which a care facility provides have meaning for the person and that those activities are also viewed as the means by which people with dementia are encouraged and supported to engage with each other, with their environment, with care staff and with their families. In this way, activities become a vehicle for much that is life-affirming and therefore central to quality of life. The relationship between the carer and the person with dementia lies at the heart of this work. As such, activity becomes a way to 'be together' in the moment and to enjoy pleasure, fun, satisfaction and a sense of achievement.

We exist in a social world and in general humans are happier when not alone. Our experience of the social world directly contributes to our sense of wellbeing and emotions such as satisfaction, belonging, pleasure or, conversely, ill-being, anxiety, fear and oppression (Kelly, 2007). 'At the coalface, the quality of the lives of people with dementia are dominated by the individual interactions experienced, day by day, minute by minute.' (Hughes & Baldwin, 2006, p.12)

The following describes some of the activities that promote social interaction:

Table-based activities

Eating outside can be really pleasurable when the weather permits. Sometimes this can relate to produce from the garden. We all enjoy jam, apple tarts and fruit pies and fresh fruit picked and eaten such as strawberries and raspberries. Barbeques can provide a welcome change of menu with lovely smells and finger food. Picnics can make ordinary lunch more interesting, with sandwiches wrapped in greaseproof paper as they used to be and tea and coffee from a flask.

Games such as cards, chess, draughts and jigsaws can all be played outside.

The daily newspaper can be read and its crosswords attempted over a cup of tea or coffee.

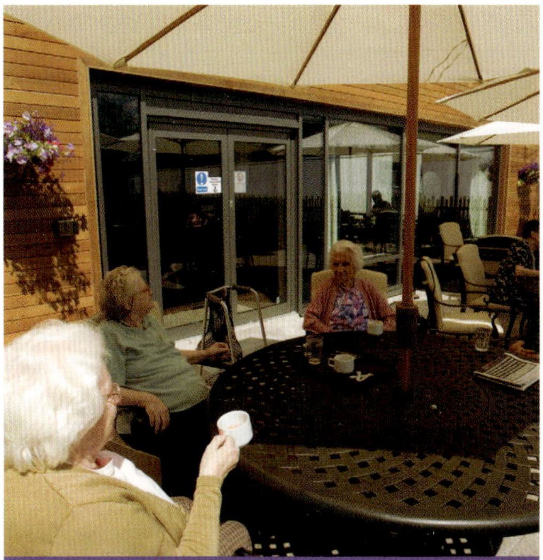

Fig. 139 A cup of coffee outdoors with friends

Painting (mentioned below) and craftwork such as patchwork or knitting is often easier outside where there is very good light and is an activity often enjoyed with a group of others. When our hands are busy, conversation is often easier. Reading poetry together can be hugely enjoyable especially if the poems are familiar from schooldays in the 1940s and 1950s. Many of the poems are about outside – weather, forests, flowers etc.

Activities men, in particular, will enjoy

A motorbike engine or upturned bicycle will provide small groups with welcome activity, as will a parked car that has disabled locks and engine. Many men can happily wash a car or lean into the engine and reminisce. This may also appeal to some women for whom cars and bicycles were important and perhaps those who were ATS[12] girls in the Second World War.

For Australian men, mowing the lawn was a weekend ritual and nothing can replace the sense of satisfaction of seeing the lawn tidy and neat whilst enjoying a cold beer on the back verandah.

An example of a car in a garden for people with dementia is illustrated in Chapter 3 (see Fig 15), and a Sunday drive was a ritual for many men and their families.

Caring for animals

Caring for animals will be a familiar activity for many older people. During the war, many families had chickens and rabbits. Residents can gain a lot of pleasure from feeding hens and rabbits, and helping to clean their accommodation, as Garuth Chalfont explains in his description of Charnley Fold in Case study 7.

Encouraging birds into the garden, without the responsibility of ownership or effort to tend to them, can also give pleasure. Seeing and hearing birds can be therapeutic or can provide familiar sounds that many people find calming.

---

[12] The Women's Auxiliary Territorial Service was officially launched on 9 September, 1938.

Growing plants

Many older people will have grown their own flowers and vegetables in gardens, allotments or on the land if they have been farmers. This can be a very social activity with lots of conversation about what to plant, working through seed catalogues, planting seeds and cuttings, transferring to raised beds, pots or flower/vegetable plots and then weeding, cutting, harvesting.

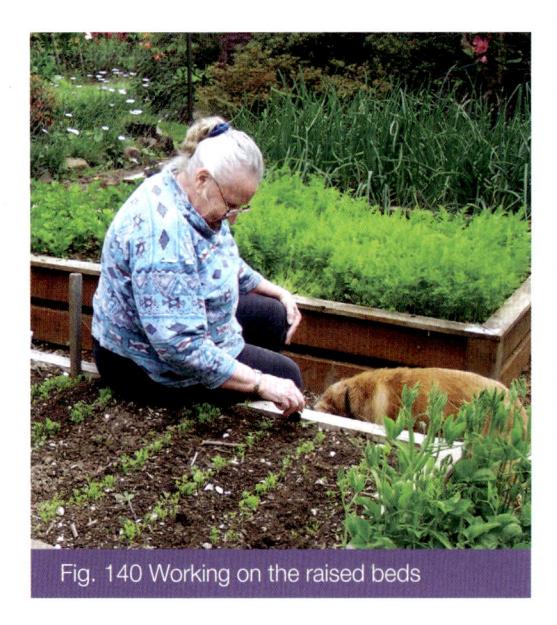

Fig. 140 Working on the raised beds

Some people prefer to work on their own, with their own project, rather than on a collective project with others. There will still be plenty to talk about and comment on. In Yuji Okubo's Case study 2, the residents enjoyed growing and harvesting on a rooftop garden.

"If you had a garden, what would you want in it?… thinking that we would plant flowers and herbs. But, the residents wanted vegetables."

"The residents get a big kick out of cooking and eating produce out of their own garden." (Raske, 2010)

Fun

Most activities can provide fun but there is particular hilarity in some games, such as croquet, bowls and putting, for those who are participating and for those who are watching.

2. Activities achieving creative potential and self-expression

Residents who are not attracted to horticulture and gardening may be engaged through other related activities. For example, people who love art may enjoy painting and stenciling pots, using the fruit and flowers for still life studies, or painting shells, stones, leaves, pictures of the birds and so on.

A joint project to create a mosaic might be an enjoyable group activity.

Many artists may prefer work in a conservatory, covered external space or outside because the light is better and often the outside world provides more interesting subjects to paint or draw, providing inspiration, light and perspective.

Fig. 141 Using flowers for a still-life study

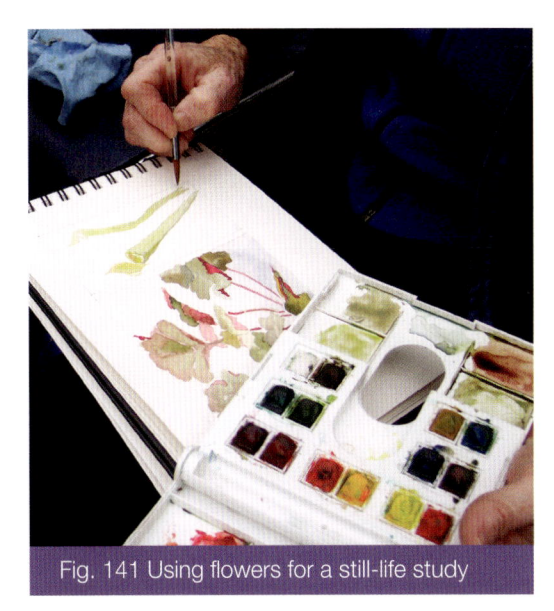

3. Activities that assist with physical health, activity and exercise

Scientists have found that staying physically active and exercising regularly can help prevent or delay many diseases and disabilities, and in some cases, exercise is an effective treatment for many chronic conditions. This is discussed in more detail in Chapter 2.

What is the difference between physical activity and exercise? For the purposes of this book, we define **'physical activity'** as activities that get your body moving such as gardening, walking the dog and sweeping the patio and **'exercise'** as a form of physical activity that is specifically planned, structured, and repetitive such as weight training, tai chi, or an aerobics class. Including both in the activity plan will provide older adults with health benefits that can help them feel better and enjoy life more.

Including 'exercise' in what is perceived as social activity may enable therapy to be undertaken without the resident even being aware! And this is beneficial to those who are nervous of exercise or who enjoy inactivity.

"When he is outside and it's nice, he reverts to walking, less shuffling his feet; and when he pulls weeds he is physically more active."

"We bring therapy patients out here for balance and gait training. It takes a little pressure off of doing therapy." (Raske, 2010)

Normal ageing involves a general decline in the functioning of all the body's systems and the emergence of chronic conditions in people with dementia is no different. The caregiver must have an understanding of the individual's stage in the ageing process and their chronic health issues as well as their dementia in order to develop an effective activity program.

Generally, older adults who are inactive lose ground in four areas that are important for staying healthy and independent. These are endurance, strength, balance and stretching, and flexibility. Research suggests that seniors can maintain, or at least partially restore, these four areas through exercise and physical activity, and that doing so improves fitness. Spending at least 30 minutes in moderate activity, such as a brisk walk or raking leaves, on all or most days of the week has remarkable health benefits for older adults (Agency for Healthcare Research and Quality (AHRQ), 2002).

The outdoor setting is ideal for this and can be a key to improved health and wellbeing for all older people and particularly those in a care setting. Well-designed garden environments can provide for socialization, activity programs, independent activities, exercise, active gardening space and opportunity for therapy sessions.

Everyone can benefit from using or working outdoors but seniors can get particular benefits from gardening because it:

- is an enjoyable form of exercise and a part of the leisure history of many older adults
- increases levels of physical activity and maintains mobility and flexibility
- encourages use of all motor skills including walking, reaching and bending
- improves endurance and strength
- reduces stress levels and promotes relaxation
- provides stimulation and interest in nature and the outdoors
- improves wellbeing as a result of social interaction
- stimulates the senses.

We now look at the specific areas that are important is retaining good health:

Endurance

Endurance activities help increase breathing and heart rate. In the garden, these might include:

- pushing grandchildren on the swings
- sweeping the paths
- working in the garden
- mowing the lawn
- raking leaves
- walking for increased periods of time over the weeks and months
- walking two or three times each day; the walking path in the garden could be measured so that the seniors walking or their caregiver could count the laps and keep a chart to record daily laps and progress;

a sign such as 'Garden Walk' could be placed at the start and end of the walking circuit.

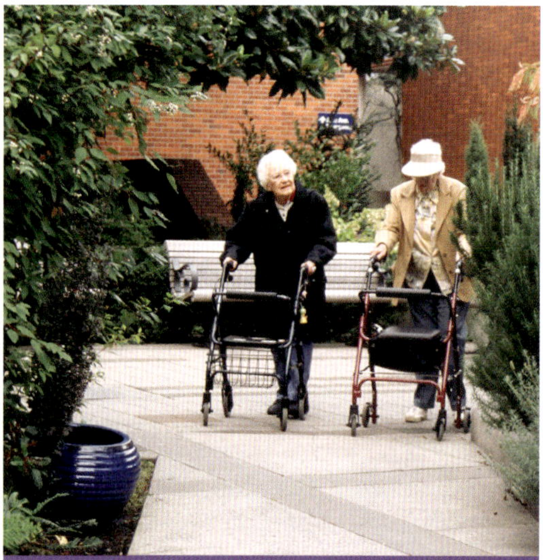

Fig. 142 Walking two or three times a day

Strength

These are activities that strengthen muscles, help maintain muscle strength and improve balance. Activity ideas include:

- carrying baskets of fruits and vegetables
- wheeling a cart or barrow with supplies
- lifting small bags of potting mix, compost and mulch in the garden
- stacking pots
- washing pots.

Balance

These are activities that can help improve a person's ability to control and maintain body position, whether they are moving or still. Good balance is important to help prevent falls and avoid the disability that may result from falling.

Activities that will help this are:

- walking on an uneven sidewalk without falling
- reaching to pick green beans from the bean teepee
- reaching to clip sweet peas from a wall trellis
- moving from a sitting position to a standing position on the edge of a raised bed or seating wall.

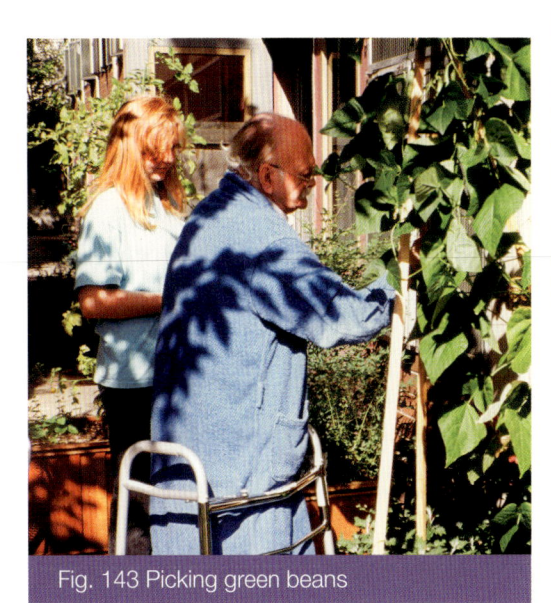

- looking over your shoulder and in all directions to see and greet friends in the garden.

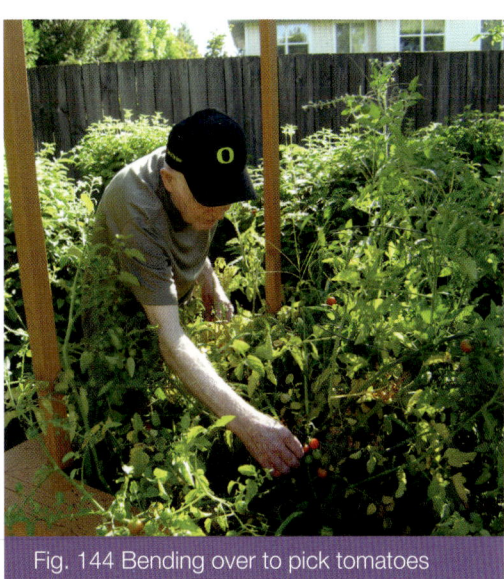

Fig. 144 Bending over to pick tomatoes

A range of motion is developed and maintained by:

- reaching to feel or pick a daisy from a tall container
- passing a watering container to a friend
- reaching up to pick a green bean from the trellis.

Fig. 143 Picking green beans

Stretching and flexibility

Stretching and flexibility activities help older adults remain limber and to retain a range of movement and include:

- bending over to the raised bed to pick tomatoes
- reaching for a tool on the shelf in the garden shed or an apple in the tree
- emptying a small bag of planting mix into a large container
- pulling a sweater off over one's head when getting too warm with gardening work

Fine and gross motor skills are supported by:

- deadheading (pinching off dead blooms) of marigolds, geraniums and other flowers
- collecting rose flowers and pulling them apart to make sachet materials. Perhaps also stripping lavender from stems and adding them to the mix, then placing all of these in the middle of a handkerchief or fabric and tying with a ribbon.

4. Activities that engage the brain

There are plenty of things in the garden that can engage the brain, for example wildlife including birds, squirrels, bats and insects; seasonal plants; the changing weather and daylight conditions.

Identification charts of common garden wildlife could be kept nearby and a bird table installed and maintained with food and water to encourage visits by birds. With a digital camera this can be recorded and subsequently discussed, written about or painted. Seasonal counts of the birds and bats could be undertaken and the internet used to link to conservation organisations and websites and to find out what to expect from the seasons and reinforce the stimulus for art and writing projects. Other links could be made to television programmes such as (in the UK) the BBC's *Springwatch* and *Autumnwatch* as well as having magazines and books related to the subject readily available in the activity room as a resource for creative activities.

Currently (2011) in the UK, Bupa are working with the Royal Society for the Protection of Birds (RSPB) and piloting the creation of care home grounds that will attract wildlife and encourage meaningful activities relating to this, for example, ponds, hedgehog hotels (as they called them) building bird boxes, having the right plant life in the garden etc. People are involved in all aspects from the gardening/woodwork to painting and drawing. This has had a hugely positive outcome, especially for those with dementia, and now it is being rolled out across the UK. RSPB train the staff, who get a certificate. All staff are involved, from maintenance staff to nursing staff and even the chef!

Familiar hobbies are often easier in the garden. Mrs P, for example, is an elderly lady who lives in Edinburgh in a sheltered housing complex. She sits outside whenever the weather permits, as there the bright light helps her to read the paper and do her crosswords, and undoubtedly this will also help her to sleep well too! (see Chapter 3)

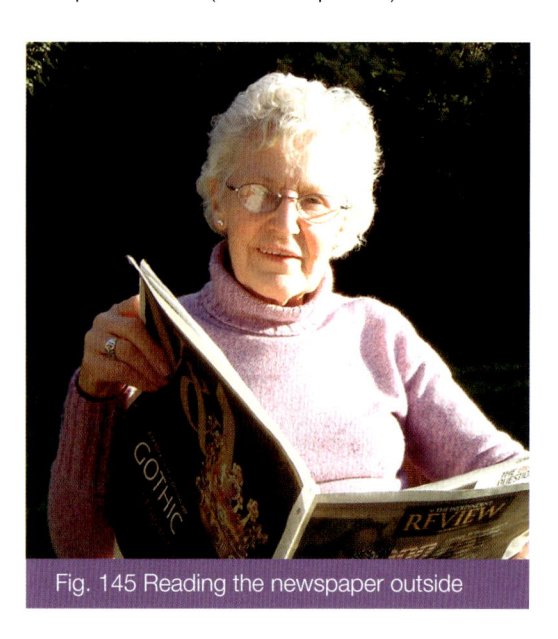

Fig. 145 Reading the newspaper outside

5. Activities that restore and reinforce long-held skills

The person with dementia may well know much about growing fruit and vegetables and flowers, or have had a life-long interest in birds and wildlife. In this way, being outside and maintaining those interests and reinforcing known skills and abilities are an important aspect of reinforcing the sense of self as well as promoting orientation to time and to the seasons.

"He can't concentrate on anything for very long. So television is not effective for him because he can't follow the story line. He doesn't read stories or books. These are activities

he did before but he's not able to continue them because of the progression of the dementia. But gardening is something he can still do and enjoy very much."
(Raske, 2010)

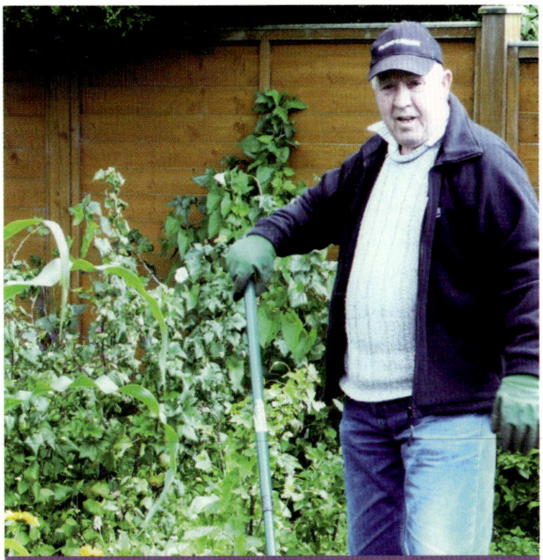

Fig. 146 Enjoying a visit to the garden

Reminiscence arises from almost all outside activities especially if those activities have been tailored to past habits and memories.

6. Activities that provide multi-sensory stimulation

Sensory stimulation needs to be addressed on a daily basis and year-round to support all five sensory realms. This work can help to compensate for sensory changes and losses, to maintain function and to provide a high level of resident engagement in meaningful activities. The garden and its produce can help with this, as described as follows:

Visual stimulation
- observing the garden from the view out of the window to the garden
- comparing the size of two different types of fruit or vegetable at harvest
- observing the night sky
- watching the birds in the bird feeder/birdbath.

Tactile stimulation
- handling the potatoes at harvest; talking about the texture, weight and size in the hand
- feeling the herbs, for example, rosemary, sage and thyme. How are they different and alike?
- having a footbath as described in the Japanese Case study 2
- feeling the cool change in the air, driving away the heat of the day
- gathering flowers for a bouquet, feeling the different textures, placing them in a vase.

Gustatory stimulation
- gathering apples and having an apple tasting event
- picking strawberries from the raised bed; washing, hulling and preparing a favourite dish
- picking blueberries or cherry tomatoes; washing them and eating them fresh from the garden
- cooking lunch on the barbeque.

Auditory stimulation
- watching and listening for birds on the morning walk
- watching a hummingbird and listening for its sounds
- how do the different grasses sound in the wind?

Olfactory stimulation

- looking at, feeling, and smelling the herbs, for example, rosemary, sage. How are they different? How do they smell and feel? Which do you prefer?
- talking about afternoon smells on the afternoon walk; are they different from morning smells?
- talking about the smell of freshly cut grass
- smelling the sausages and onions cooking on the barbeque
- noticing the smell of rain in the air, or perhaps the coming thunderstorm.

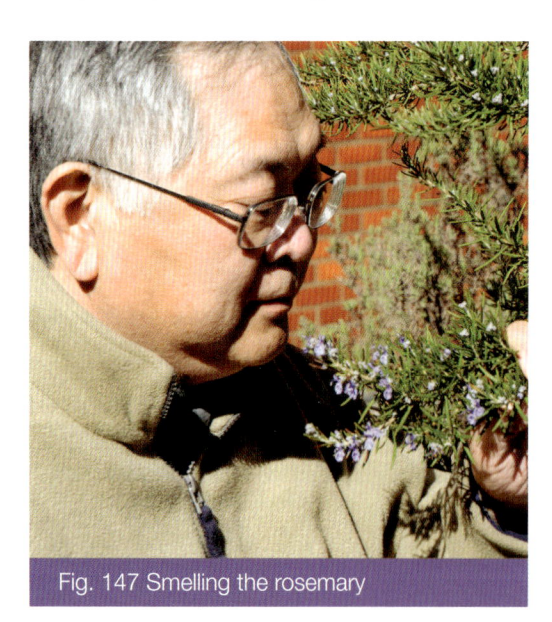

Fig. 147 Smelling the rosemary

Obviously, the many sensory garden attributes and activities will have to be tailored to the climate – what you can do in a hot summer in southern Europe, America, Asia or Australia, the flowers that can grow, and the birds you might see, will not be the same in the cool and often wet regions of the UK and northern Europe. However, picking and tasting brambles, picking and smelling lavender and putting it in with your clothes or under your pillow to help you sleep, and listening to the gentle sound of rain falling are just as important in stimulating the senses.

7. Activities that are less physical

For people who want or need to sit, some will find that watching the wind in the trees or the sun on flowerbeds is enough, whereas others will want to watch things that are moving.

An aviary or chicken run can provide hours of pleasure. For others, watching visiting children can be very engaging and in this respect, you could consider including play equipment for children. By doing this, when family members come to visit, it becomes a much more pleasurable event for the children and families alike, thus reinforcing family bonds and helping to sustain relationships as well as providing something to watch. Children may also be engaged in the many outdoor activities, and intergenerational work is positive and helpful. Many older people with dementia seem to relate more easily with the young.

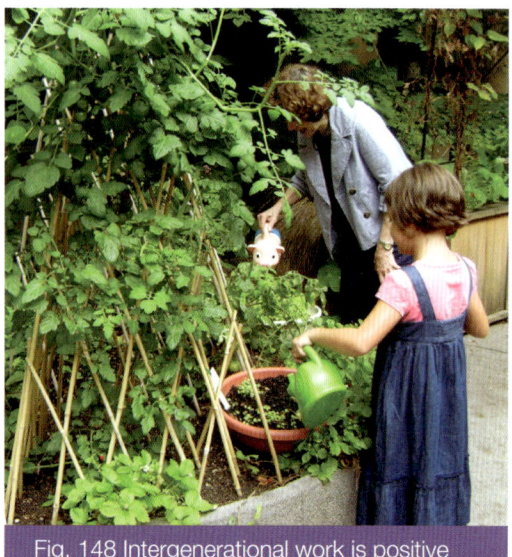

Fig. 148 Intergenerational work is positive and helpful

Some people really like watching a water feature but for others this activity will just result in anxiety about the location of the toilet. If a garden is well used and full of activity, there will be plenty to watch and choices to make.

Watching the sunrise and sunset can bring great pleasure and again reinforces the sense of time, or rising and going to bed.

8. Outdoor activities in the evening

Many cultures (in particular in parts of the world with very hot summers) regularly use the cool of the evening to take a walk with family or friends – in Spanish they have a word for this: 'Paseo' – a slow and leisurely walk, often at night when the air is cool. There is no reason why people with dementia shouldn't also enjoy the outdoors at night, taking gentle exercise, listening to the night sounds, looking at the stars and so on – this is discussed in more detail in Chapter 10.

> *Key points*
> - activity is vital to a meaningful life, involving and encouraging:
>   - social interaction
>   - creativity
>   - physical exercise and therapy
>   - restoration of skills and multi sensory stimulation
>   - opportunities for self reflection.

References

Agency for Healthcare Research and Quality. (2002). *Physical activity and older Americans: Benefits and strategies.* Retrieved from http://www.ahrq.gov/ppip/activity.htm

Alessi, C., Yoon, E., Schnelle, L., Al-Samarrai, N.R., & Cruise, P.A. (1999). A randomized trial of a combined physical activity and environmental intervention in nursing home residents: Do sleep and agitation improve? *Journal of the American Geriatrics Society, 47,* 784-791.

Alzheimer's Society. (2007). *Dementia UK: The full report.* Retrieved from http://www.alzheimers.org.uk/site/scripts/documents_info.php?documentID=342

Alzheimer's Society. (2007). *Home from home: A report highlighting opportunities for improving the standards of dementia care in care homes.* Retrieved from http://www.alzheimers.org.uk/site/scripts/download_info.php?fileID=270

Ashton-Schaffer, C., & Constant, A. (2005). Why do older adults garden? *Activities, Adaptations & Aging, 30*(2).

Brawley, E. (2004). Gardens of memories. *Alzheimer's Care Quarterly, 5* (2), 154-164.

Chapman, N., Hazen, T., & Noell-Waggoner, E. (2005). Encouraging development and use of gardens by caregivers of people with dementia. *Alzheimer's Care Quarterly, 6*(4), 349-356.

Marcus, C.C., & Barnes, M. (Eds.) (1999). *Healing gardens: Therapeutic benefits and design recommendations.* New York, NY: Wiley.

College of Occupational Therapists. (2007) *Activity provision: Benchmarking good practice in care homes.* Retrieved from http://www.cot.co.uk/sites/default/files/publications/public/Activity_Provision_2010.pdf

Hughes, J.C., & Baldwin, C. (2006). *Ethical issues in dementia care: Making difficult decisions.* London: Jessica Kingsley.

Kelly, F. (2007). *Well-being and expressions of self in dementia: Interactions in long-term wards and creative sessions.* (PhD thesis) Retrieved from https://dspace.stir.ac.uk/handle/1893/207 https://dspace.stir.ac.uk/handle/1893/207

Mozley, C., Sutcliffe, C., Bagley, H., Cordingley, L., Challis, D., Huxley P., & Burns, A. (2004). *Towards quality care: Outcomes for older people in care homes.* Aldershot: Ashgate.

National Institute for Health and Clinical Excellence. (2008). *Occupational therapy Interventions and physical activity interventions to promote the mental wellbeing of older people in primary care and residential care.* Retrieved from http://www.nice.org.uk/nicemedia/pdf/PH16Guidance.pdf

Rodiek, S. & Schwarz, B. (Eds.) (2007). *Outdoor environments for people with dementia.* New York, NY: Haworth Press.

Raske, M. (2010). Nursing home quality of life: Study of an enabling garden. *Journal of Gerontological Social Work, 53*(4), 336-351.

Simpson, S. & Straus, M. (Eds.) (1999). *Horticulture as therapy: Principles and practice.* New York, NY: Food Products Press.

Therapeutic Landscapes Network. Retrieved from http://healinglandscapes.org

Wells, S. (Ed.) (1997). *Horticultural therapy and the older adult population* Binghampton, NY: Haworth Press.

Case Study 7
Charnley Fold

Garuth Chalfont

Introduction

Charnley Fold is a 'one stop shop' for older people's mental health services, resources and treatment, located in Central Lancashire and operating since 2008. The NHS, Lancashire County Council, Age Concern and Alzheimer's Society cooperated in providing a health and wellbeing centre and support facility, including an enhanced day care service supporting older people with complex mental health needs, including dementia, to maintain their independence. The site is on the outskirts of Bamber Bridge, south of Preston, set back from the main road by a row of houses, and surrounded by a small farm holding and an industrial site. Chalfont Design consulted on the renovation of the site (formerly a care home) and designed the outdoors for therapeutic and rehabilitative purposes. They continue to provide staff training to maximise use of the landscape, and to guide future garden development.

A staff team operates the day centre five days a week, serving a total of 60 participants, each attending for one to four days a week over a 12 week session. This allows time to assess their needs, set goals, assign them to appropriate groups and review progress. A typical session of the gardening group on a Monday afternoon might involve strolling around the garden, identifying tasks that need to be done, feeding the birds, watering plants in the greenhouse and outdoor pots, transplanting seedlings to larger pots and trimming back dead wood on lavender plants. The group has also been involved with caring for the four chickens which live in an octagonal, wooden, aviary-type chicken coop.

Design philosophy

The design approach embeds the philosophy of care into the physical setting, ensuring that the landscape, the building and the staff work together to achieve wellbeing for the service users. The philosophy of care enables each individual to freely access, engage with, enjoy and benefit from the environment. The aims of the design are, briefly, to:

- facilitate rehabilitation and therapeutic opportunities through connection to nature
- enable service users to regain and maintain skills and abilities
- maximise staff's ability to provide an enhanced service
- improve happiness and wellbeing through an interesting, year-round outdoor experience.

This includes familiar domestic activities such as pottering in the garden, feeding the birds, planting, pulling weeds and watering tomatoes in the greenhouse, or simply sitting and watching others or taking a walk.

Beyond caring for the person, occupying their time and providing sensory stimulation, service users are enabled to maintain and develop relationships, to be creative and pursue emerging interests, to use the gardens, nature and the outdoors as tools for communication, and to experience personal freedom through an open-door policy of direct, easy, safe and year-round access to outdoors.

Physical layout and design elements

Charnley Fold occupies approximately 7000 square metres on a relatively level site, about a third of which is green space and planted areas.

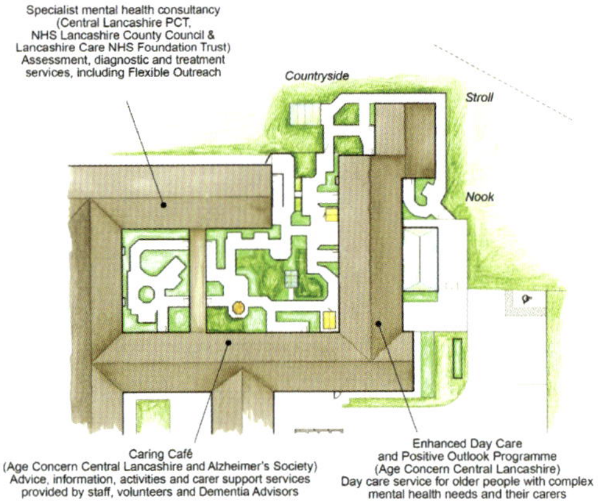

Fig. 149 Building and courtyards (refer to appendix 1 on page 220 for enlarged version)

About 540 square metres are designed for intensive therapeutic and rehabilitative uses. Specific design elements and structures are used to support the design philosophy. For instance, interior spaces were opened up during renovation to maximise daylight, natural ventilation and views out. Spaces outdoors are designed and furnished to support a range of activities – active and passive, domestic and wild, solitary and group, productive and recreational. This requires trellises, a greenhouse, sheds, raised beds, pergolas, arches, water features, chairs, benches, work tables and arbour seats (built and/or installed by a local joiner).

Paths and activity areas are tightly integrated. There are multiple circulation loops connecting the indoors and the gardens, encouraging people to look out onto and to visit the outdoors.

Participants can independently access the garden areas through numerous doors.

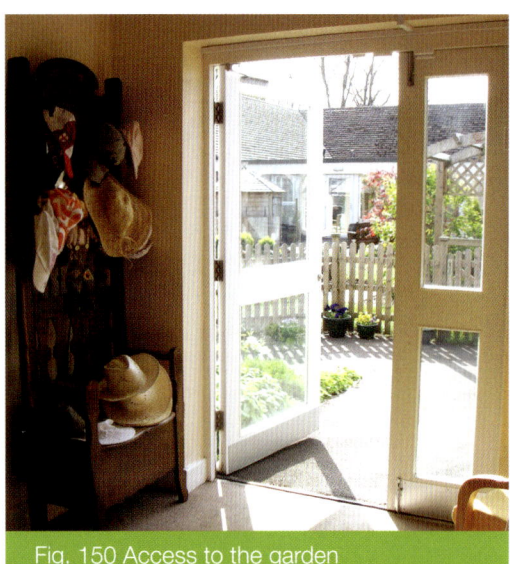

Fig. 150 Access to the garden

The paths are smooth tarmac with one large patio area laid with paving slabs.

Spatial archetypes

One innovation at Charnley Fold is the creation of *7 Meaningful Spaces*, which are based on archetypes of normal, familiar outdoor places. Archetypal spaces are culturally relevant, they resonate with meaning and they prompt behaviour. A place that is recognisable and familiar, with multi-sensory cues, will help a person know what to do there. Such places encourage people to take ownership and to participate in ways that feel right for them, whether it is sweeping, digging in the soil, feeding the chickens or simply watching. Examples at Charnley Fold include *The Pocket Park, The Back Garden* and *The Yard*.

The *Back Garden* contains the greenhouse and is edged with a picket fence; a gate is located at each end of a small patch of grass. There is a 1.2 metre-long bench in the corner with red peonies and a miniature almond tree blooming nearby.

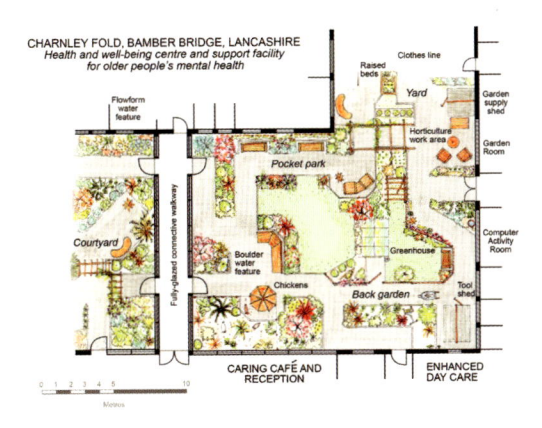

Fig. 151 Garden layout (refer to appendix 1 on page 221 for enlarged version)

The benches are separated by a dwarf apple tree surrounded by lavender, looking onto a small, square lawn with flower borders and with a boulder fountain located nearby.

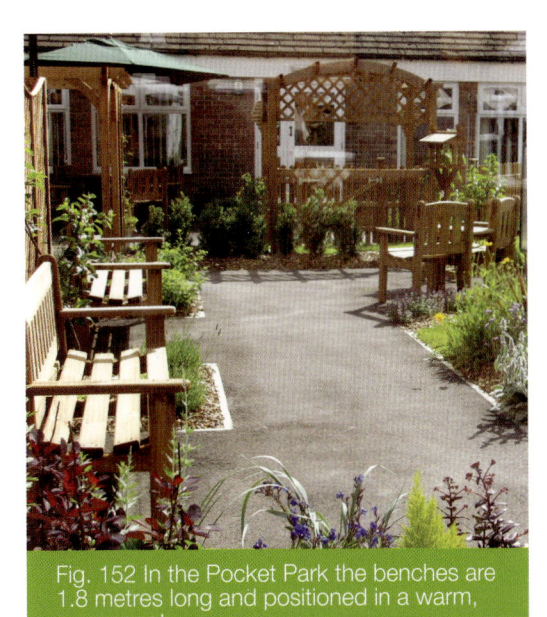

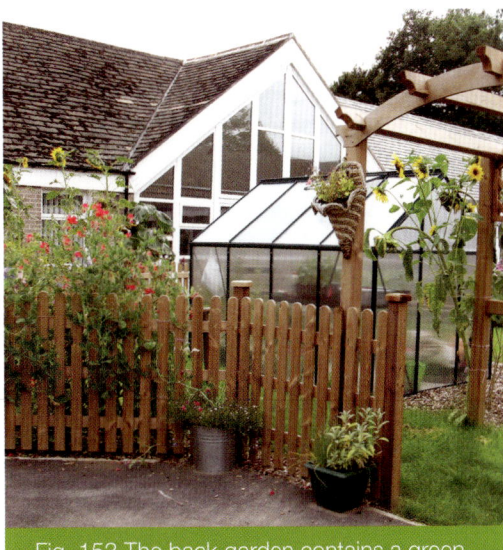

Fig. 153 The back garden contains a greenhouse and is edged with a picket fence

A garden gnome stands beside the greenhouse, which overflows with plants at various stages of growth. Outside the fence is the larger of two sheds, with its garden supplies and equipment neatly organised and labelled, so all gloves and tools can be returned to their rightful places.

Fig. 152 In the Pocket Park the benches are 1.8 metres long and positioned in a warm, sunny spot

Fig. 154 In The Yard you will find raised beds, a compost bin and clothes drying on the line

Coat stands laden with hats and coats can be found near the doors. A doll's pram is located just inside the door where it prompts people to take it out for a stroll around the garden. Such familiar items encourage independent use of the spaces by triggering memories of how tools and equipment are used, and by giving clues about what can be done.

Changes, surprises and lessons learned

- ask for enough outdoor taps and electric points to anticipate future needs

- there are two water features – a boulder fountain and a flowform. Both can be seen from indoors and attract attention and comment. I have since used water features that come as a single unit, needing no assembly and requiring minimal installation, just an electric socket nearby. Stand it on the ground or attach it to a wall, then add water and turn it on. There are pros and cons to both. But in terms of the costs, maintenance, repairs and downtime, the fewer workmen involved, the less time it takes to sort out problems and the more likely that it will be running on any given day. Self-contained units are less problematic and just as effective in providing the look, feel and sound of water that brings such pleasure

- provide edge space such as a porch and a covered walkway. For budgetary reasons this was not included in the building works. So now a door is to be added to an activity room to make it into a garden room, with double doors to the outside. A clear roof is to be constructed on the existing pergola, thus giving immediate edge space outside the room

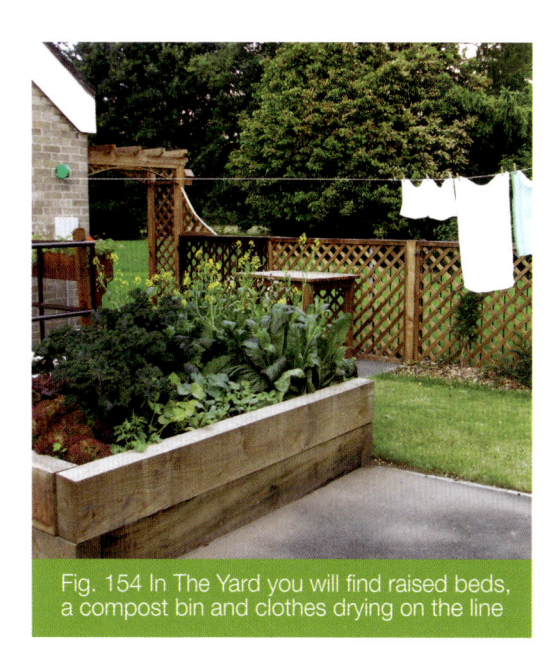

A hops vine scrambles over the pergola and a restored, blue mangle draws constant comment. Around the corner from the clothes line, a thrush has built her nest atop an arch adjacent to the wall, where she produced four eggs that hatched this spring.

Such spaces flow easily from one to the next and provide incentive for conversation and involvement, drawing a person in and through the garden, stopping at points of interest along the way.

Enabling space

Just as an archetype prompts behaviour, a space can enable activity simply by its physical design. Paths afford walking on and gates invite opening and closing. A line of pots filled with soil, or a wheelbarrow of plant material beside the compost pile, all say something is happening, people are about and work is underway. Props such as a sweeping brush, trowel, watering can or badminton rackets are set out in appropriate places around the garden, prior to participants arriving each day.

- as the greenhouse was well planted and much used, the need for more cultivation space became evident, especially space where a number of people could comfortably participate. A polytunnel was suggested in a focus group and funds were raised. Surprisingly, staff voted for the whole floor to be paved, with staging added along each side. So there is no ground level planting area as one would expect. It was certainly cheaper than a wooden structure or a greenhouse, and it will be ideal for small group activities and will extend thermal comfort during early spring and late fall

- the staff team has suggested that no view of cars should be allowed from interior activity rooms as it would impact negatively upon concentration levels of service users during a session. This is a day centre and people will be expecting to leave, so watching cars arrive will be a distraction. I do, however, advocate a view to the outside world in a residential care environment, particularly from the garden

- chickens have been a great addition although we did not plan them from the start. Luckily, the perfect spot for the coop and run was available, right in front of the café/reception area window. I would recommend that you plan for animals of some sort (chickens, bees, rabbits, etc) in the design stage, so an appropriate amount and type of space is set aside.

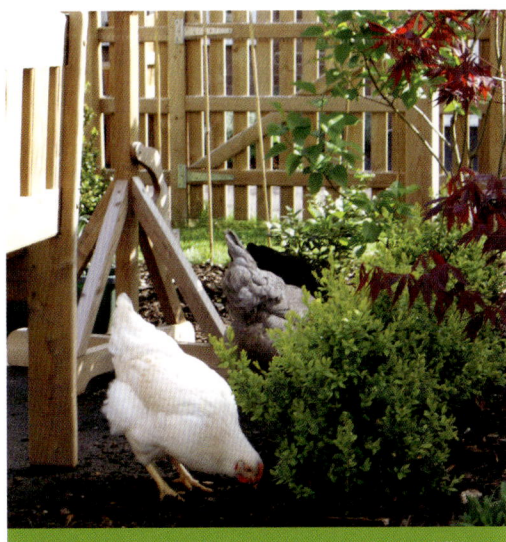

Fig. 155 Chickens have been a great addition

Evaluation

The enhanced day care service and use of the gardens were evaluated after one year. From that evaluation came some key points contributing to the success of the garden. Quotes are from service users and staff.

- **garden is mood altering:** "A person can walk off a temper… sit down, look around… temper's gone. Sweeping up can also be therapeutic. He's not brushed in months and he's back into it… second time in two days."

- **everyone has some outside time every day because the doors are always open:** "They have the freedom to come out; they're not stuck inside."

- **the garden has many walking routes through and around it which are being used:** "There's a purpose to walking outside but it's their purpose."

- **plants with a sensory quality such as lamb's ear are the thin end of the wedge:** "If they touch that and enjoy it, then I can introduce them to other plants."

- **produce is an essential part of the plan:** "Plants are being grown to sell, or fruits grown to jar and sell."

- **chickens are a magnet, an instant draw:** "Chickens bring them out… to sit and look at something… some continually walk but will stop there and look at the chickens. Everybody can see them from wherever… using benches to sit and watch them… eye-catching… talking point. Chickens require daily attention… so people look at the garden as well, it gets them out."

- **each group does something about the garden or in the garden:** "It's very unusual not to see someone in the garden. Even people who watch from the lounge window have been seeing a bird pulling a piece of string from the fence or a fat robin."

- **being in the garden is the key to engagement:** "People who don't like gardening like to just have a walk around, do two or three things in the gardening group, just join in… don't realise they're gardening."

- **offer spaces for gardening, games or craft:** "They can do whatever they want – independence is promoted."

- **create the garden and cater the service to suit a wide range of interests:** "More of the outdoors is used… I'm seeing it coming together. The garden doubles the size of the service. Very unusual not to see someone in the garden. Hardly anyone takes a nap here."

Further reading

Chalfont, G. (2011). Charnley Fold: A practice model of environmental design for enhanced dementia day care. Social Care and *Neurodisability*, 2(2), 71-79.

Chalfont, G. (2009). *Charnley Fold. Enhanced day care (EDC) garden: One year assessment report.* Retrieved from http://www.chalfontdesign.com/files/media/Charnley_Fold_Gardens%20Report_May_2009.pdf

Chapter 10
Using outside space at night
Colm Cunningham

Using outside space at night is not routinely considered in the planning and delivery of aged care facilities for older people and people with dementia. The design of the built environment has many functions, one of which is to provide the residents of that place with pleasurable spaces to use. People living in aged care have lived lives that included going outside at night. They will have spent time outside watching the sun go down, enjoying drinks with friends, having a cigarette or having a warm drink before settling for the night. The experience of having a quick cup of tea or coffee at the back door before heading off to an early morning job is also a common and relaxing experience older people in aged care will have done to prepare for the day ahead.

The attention now being given on enhancing support for older people at night, including the important work of Kerr and Wilkinson (2011), has demonstrated the need for a major shift in the approaches to care at night. One critical issue that has been highlighted through this work is the need to consider that going 'back to bed' may not always be what the person needs. Some people do not sleep well at night. Staff need to be provided with skills, techniques and resources to facilitate choices for older people and people with dementia at night. If a person with dementia becomes anxious at night, the use of the outside space may be a valuable and therapeutic tool.

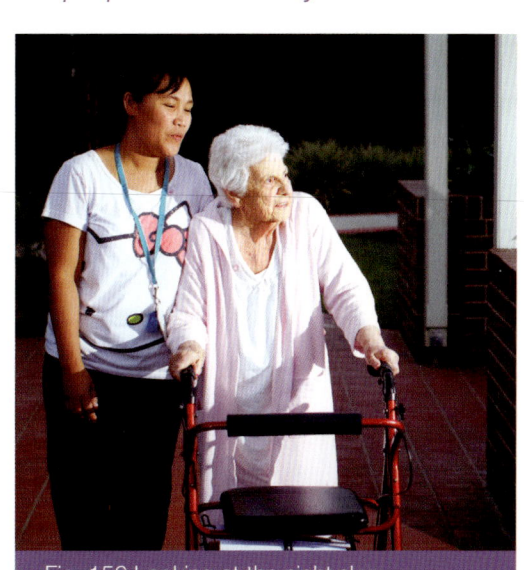

Fig. 156 Looking at the night sky

While it may be thought that the warmer climate in the southern hemisphere makes going out at night safer because people will not be at risk from cold or bad weather, there is nothing to stop an older person sitting outside with the right clothes and coat. Planning for these situations is important, for example in Scotland in June the sun may not set until 11pm, so ensuring that the routine of the day and staff planning allows for people to go outside later is important. With the introduction of outside heaters this is increasingly possible.

The outside space does not disappear as we enter into night-time. It therefore should offer the older person and staff something to engage with. Having things that are interesting to look out on at night and are eye catching is an easy starting point. This requires that the design of the space and lighting allows for this space to be viewed.

Fig. 157 Night view of bowling green

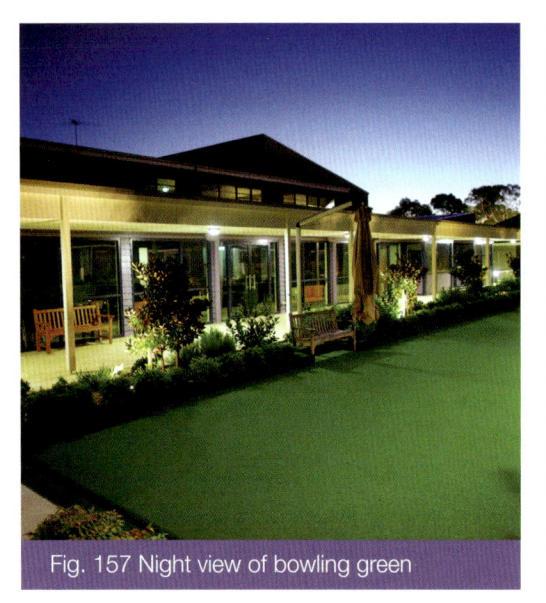

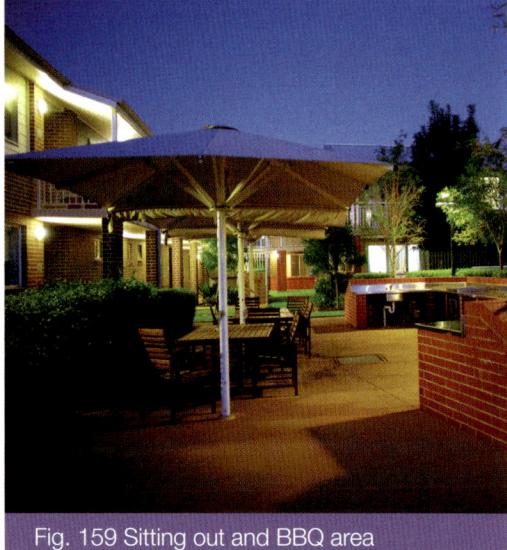

Fig. 159 Sitting out and BBQ area

Changes of the space with the seasons can also maintain people's interest, for example a feature of pumpkins in October, or even better, actually seeing them grow in the garden.

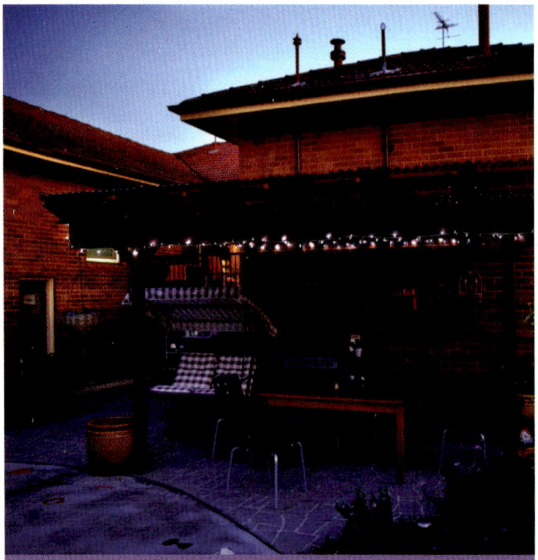

Fig. 158 Lighting allows for this space to be viewed

When it comes to the idea of letting someone go out at night, there are many perceived barriers to this happening. The early part of the night-time is when all staff are engaged in reports from day to night shift. The routine is also focused on getting people who want to go to sleep settled for bed. There may, therefore, be a concern of risk to unobserved residents of such things as falls or chills due to the cold. If the space has been designed to ensure that access is easy, for example lighting which avoids pools of light and dark spots and that there are safe areas for people to sit, then an assessment relating to risk should be based on the individual and not a global ban on access to outside.

The areas for sitting do need to be considered though, as they may be a problem if placed next to a room where someone is trying to sleep.

Activities outside should also be thought of, to allow for a positive use of the space, for example sitting with a member of staff reading the paper, or playing cards or board games, as these can just as easily happen at night.

Fig. 160 Chatting over a magazine and getting some night air

Fig. 161 Ready now to relax before going to bed

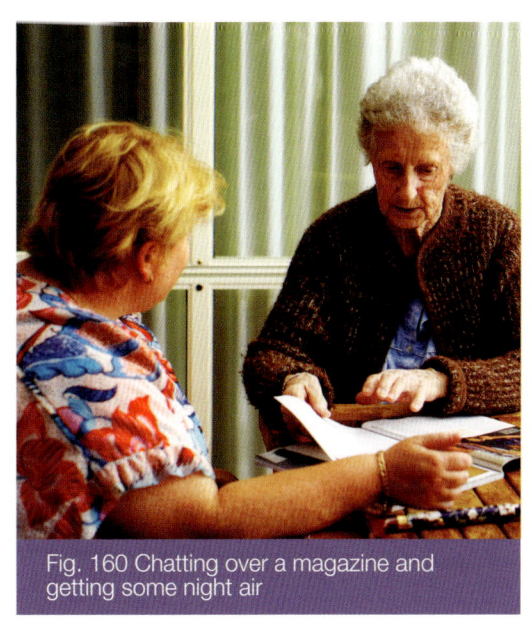

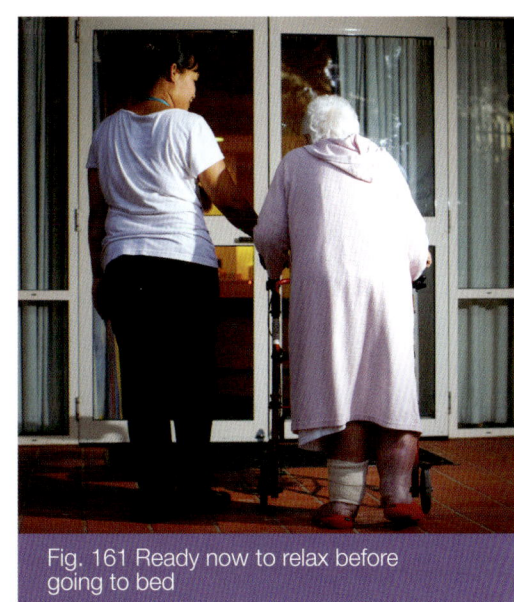

For staff working in a care home or hospital, long shifts and, in particular, night shifts can be stressful. The use of outdoor space at night for these people should also be considered.

One nurse working in an intensive care ward notes how night-staff frequently use the 'trimtrack' outside at night in their breaks – or immediately after a shift – as this not only relaxes them but removes some of the stress of the working environment.

Case studies

Krisi

Outside space at night may also provide comfort and support. Krisi had lived in Pine lodge for six months and had dementia. At night she wanted to go outside. It was discovered that Krisi wanted to pray and she wanted to pray outside under the tree. A member of care staff would go out with Krisi and kneel with her under the tree. Krisi would then say her prayers and it was found that then Krisi would be ready for a cup of tea and to relax before going to bed.

If Krisi could not go out, the risk was that she would become anxious and unsettled. Having a safe outside space and staff willing to use this for her benefit was really important to her care and formed part of her night-time care plan.

Joy

Joy was a very active 85-year-old woman who had lived on the land all her life until she was admitted to a city psychiatric hospital following the onset of dementia. Joy was a very determined and organised kind of woman prior to the onset of dementia and this personality type came through strongly in every aspect of Joy's life. Her lack of insight and need to be constantly working and organising everyone often caused Joy to be at risk of harm from the other residents who did not tolerate her behaviour and would place her at risk of injury.

Joy was transferred to a small, specialised unit for people with dementia who displayed behaviours of concern. Despite the best intentions of the team and her family, Joy became very overstimulated by the environment in which she lived and early on in her admission Joy was able to remain awake, singing and talking loudly for 48 hours non-stop, day and night. Interventions in place were not successful in reducing the agitation so the team implemented the 'hands off' approach to try and calm her after ensuring that her problems were not caused by physical or medical symptoms. Maintaining her safety and reducing the likelihood of injury or damage to property became the team's aims of care.

Managing Joy during the night-time period was especially challenging as she had the capacity to disturb other residents because of the constant noise and rattling of their door handles. The team, including her family, decided that if Joy wanted to go into the garden area at night that this would be helpful as she had been noted by many to be happier and more settled in this area during daylight hours. The garden was flat, secure and safe and staff had good visual access to provide supervision without needing to be at her side constantly. There were low lights that enabled Joy to see the plants and she happily gardened and talked while she worked. The garden contained small trees, annual plants in raised garden beds and bulbs. Joy pruned plants manually, weeded and generally enjoyed herself. Because it was winter and very cold, staff dressed Joy in warm clothing and ensured she did not become cold.

The availability of a safe, secure area that met the needs of the resident is an example of a supportive environment that is able to reduce the level of disability of a person with high care needs. The staff ability to manipulate the environment to assist the resident to calm in her own time and in her own way was effective and the resident did eventually settle and have reduced severity and frequency of episodes of overstimulated behaviour.

While this intervention was only needed short-term and is an extreme example of behaviour management (meeting the needs of a person with dementia) an outside area is an essential feature of a unit caring for this population, even during the night.

Henry

Henry was a man in a low-care, dementia-specific facility who paced continuously as part of his normal lifestyle. Prior to admission Henry had a set pattern of walking for miles around his neighbourhood. This behaviour continued after admission where he paced through the living area and went into the garden and returned to the living area by a second door. Henry did this pacing day and night and would have been very agitated if his obsessive repetition had been disrupted. He lived very happily in this cottage until his condition deteriorated suddenly and he died.

The team was very happy that Henry was able to continue a practice that helped his feeling of wellbeing.

Key points

- use of outdoor space at night-time is beneficial for staff and residents alike
- by good design, outdoor spaces can be safe at night-time – but sitting areas should not be near bedrooms where their use might disturb people sleeping
- use of outdoor space at night may satisfy personal and/or cultural traditions and thereby limit agitation in the person with dementia.

Reference

Kerr, D., & Wilkinson, H. (2011). *Providing good care at night for older people: Practical approaches for use in nursing and care homes.* London: Jessica Kingsley.

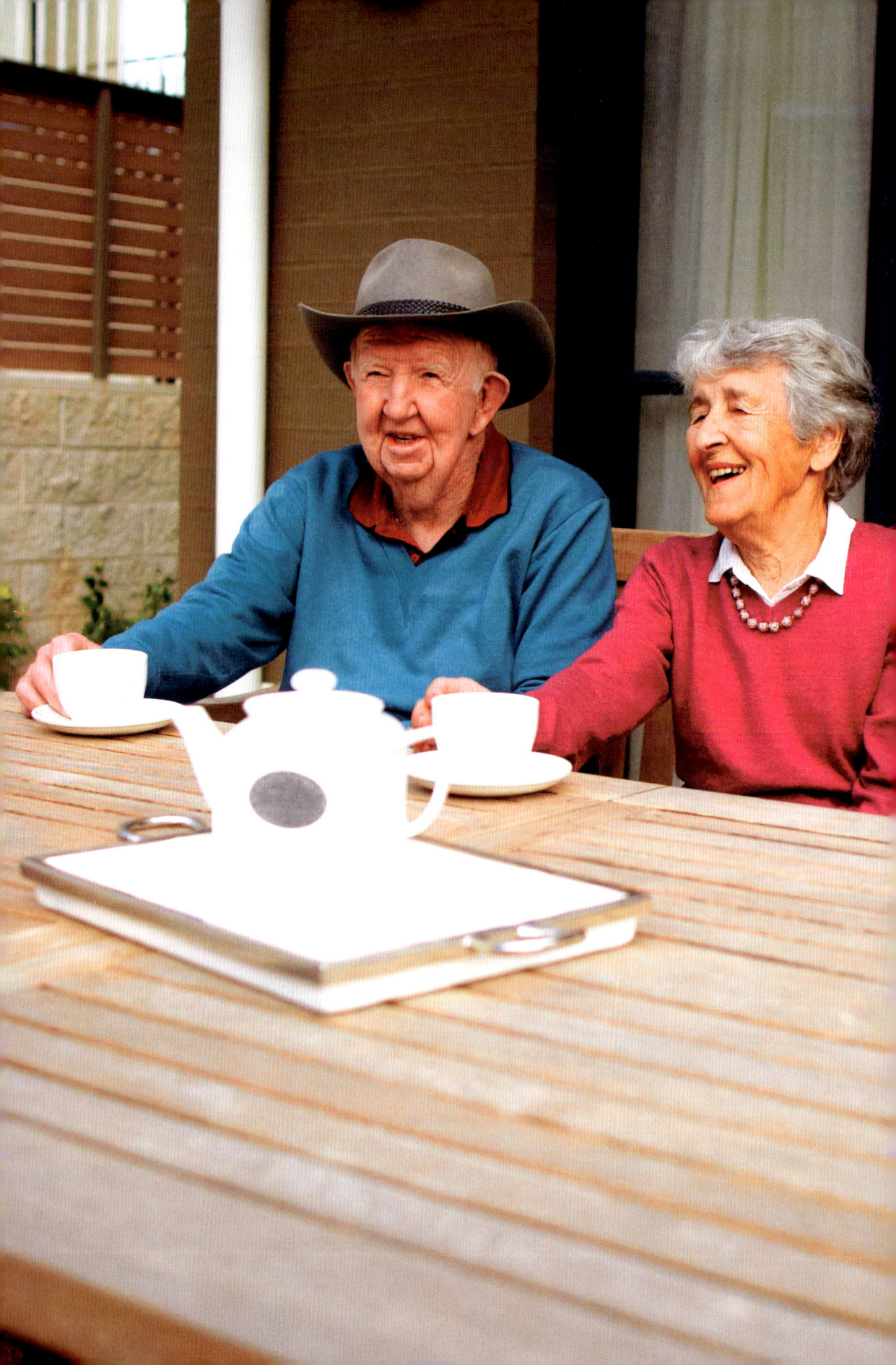

Chapter 11
How relatives, friends and staff can facilitate being outside

Edith Macintosh

This chapter offers some helpful suggestions and guidance to enable people with dementia to enjoy the benefits of being outside. Many are practical, common sense ideas, which are simple to do and relate directly to supporting an individual's wishes. There will be some overlap with this chapter and Chapter 9 on activities, particularly in relation to those activities usually done inside which could be taken outside.

The benefits of going outside at any time of day are many and not just for the person with dementia. A person's sense of wellbeing, experienced from enjoying the outside, will have a positive impact on relatives, friends and staff.

If going outside meets the needs of the person with dementia, it will improve their overall quality of life, giving a sense of physical, mental, emotional and spiritual wellbeing.

1. Organisational policy and practice

People with dementia do not always have the physical ability to go outside, the communication skills to make their choices easily known or the ability to initiate an activity. Relatives, friends and staff therefore have a responsibility to enable and support individuals to go outside.

In busy and demanding care settings, making time to do this can be seen as a challenge and is often related to the numbers of staff. However, in many care settings where this is done there is anecdotal evidence that clearly shows that investing in this way of working reduces demands on staff in the long term. If staff make the time to build relationships with individuals, really get to know their story along with their likes and dislikes, they are then able to support them to live a fulfilling life, which will include taking part in activities outside and enjoying the outdoors.

All staff in a care setting must be supported, empowered and given permission to develop an enabling approach in partnership with individuals rather than simply carry out tasks. This way of working adopts an approach that is 'doing with' rather than 'doing to' when supporting someone in daily activities. Giving an individual the right amount of support in relation to his or her own abilities is very empowering, particularly for someone living with dementia.

This may mean a significant change in culture and practice. To achieve this approach there must be commitment to the following:

- person-centred care
- an understanding of the value of going outside
- leadership by example, particularly by senior staff, so that other care staff understand the importance of this.

Staff and others will then be encouraged to create a positive, activity-orientated culture, which includes the use of outside areas.

It may be helpful to develop or revise a 'mission statement' for the organisation, which has an emphasis on enabling individuals to go outside.

A mission statement is a formal, short, written statement of the purpose of a company or organisation, which guides the actions of that organisation:

- it should spell out its overall goal to provide a sense of direction and guide decision making
- it provides a framework or context within which the company or organisation's strategies/policies are formulated (Haschak, 1998)
- it can be added to publicity materials such as information packs, recruitment packs, brochures and advertisements and clearly displayed in the care setting itself.

To do this well, staff, friends, relatives and the local community should be included in developing the mission statement. This can be done in a variety of ways including one to one conversations, meetings with relatives and friends, resident meetings, questionnaires and so on. There are many books and websites available for advice on how to develop a mission statement, for example, Mission Statement Builder, available from <http://www.franklincovey.com/msb>.

It is important to note however, that a mission statement will only be effective if there is active influence and the objective to encourage it to happen. Also, the mission statement and philosophy have to match the physical environment, for example, no locked doors to outside areas if the mission statement and philosophy recognise the importance of outdoor spaces for the wellbeing of a person.

Case study

The mission statement said that every effort would be made to maintain links between the resident and his/her family. The outside space provided an important way of achieving this with an area specifically for families to use with seats, a table and a climbing frame for small children. Another point on the mission statement, which translated into practice outside, was the statement: "We aim to provide opportunities for our residents to continue activities and hobbies which they have enjoyed".

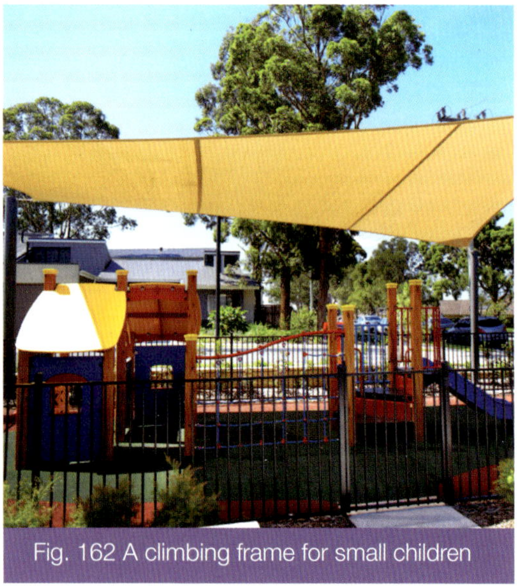

Fig. 162 A climbing frame for small children

A specific organisational policy on enabling individuals to go outside is an excellent way of embedding the key message about the importance of this in the overall running of the care setting, giving clear guidance on how to do this well. This can then be included in induction processes and can be made available for residents, family and friends.

The policy gives a powerful message about the vision and values of an organisation and empowers staff and others to embrace these on a day-today basis, thus creating positive belief in the value of the outdoors (Rodiek & Schwarz, 2007).

Key points
- embed the use of outside spaces in an organisational policy to create positive belief in the value of outdoors
- develop an enabling approach to care – 'do with' rather than 'do for'
- develop/revise a mission statement that includes the use of outside spaces.

2. The person at the centre

We are all unique individuals with unique likes, dislikes, hopes, dreams and ambitions. If these are fulfilled, individuals can live a life that has meaning and purpose. We all require being needed and valued and feel that we can contribute to society in some way, and this is no less so for individuals with dementia.

The outdoors can provide the ideal place for this to happen.

In order to support individuals to go outside we need to discover what they enjoy doing outside that can be done regularly or on a daily basis. To do this, it is essential that appropriate relationships are built and staff and others really get to know the individual. This requires spending time with them, listening and talking, looking at pictures or items which may be of personal value or interest, hearing from relatives and friends and getting to know the individual's life story which should include past, present and future.

Many individuals may have a preference as to what time of day they like to go out. This may be, for example, first thing in the morning for an early morning walk or later, after they have had lunch. Having that information included and shared provides staff and others with an opportunity to support the individual's preferences and more successfully enable them to go outside. This activity of getting to know life stories can also be done outside!

Recording all the information is essential so that everyone involved in an individual's daily life can be aware of what they enjoy doing and what can be done outside. This is often called a 'life history'. This life history document must be a 'living document', which is reviewed and updated regularly (every six weeks if possible) as people's likes and dislikes can change. This should be kept with the care plan and/or with the individual if appropriate, so that staff, family and friends can read it and support the individual in the most appropriate way through this knowledge.

A variety of life themes may become apparent when the life history is gathered that will give more opportunity to consider how individuals can be enabled and encouraged, through activities they enjoy, to go outside. These themes may include:

- hobbies e.g. gardening, walking, fishing, putting a bet on the horses
- employment e.g. postman, farmer, builder
- everyday chores e.g. hanging out the washing, sweeping the leaves
- clubs e.g. bowling, bird watching, hiking
- family and friends e.g. taking grandchildren out, going shopping

- food and drink e.g. lunch with friends, going to the pub, having a picnic.

Drawing on past experience and engaging individuals in what they have previously enjoyed will facilitate going outside. Most people's 'typical day', if living in their own home, would have included activities outside, and it is important to support people to continue to enjoy their 'typical day' if living in a care setting.

If an individual had a hobby or they carried out a particular role in life that they could continue to do in some way in a care setting, this should also be facilitated.

Some examples of how this has been achieved in some care-home settings

- a care home purchased a hen house and hens as one of the residents was a farmer and loved being outside. He now takes care of the hens. One of the ladies likes to put an apron on with large pockets and gathers the eggs each day using the apron pockets

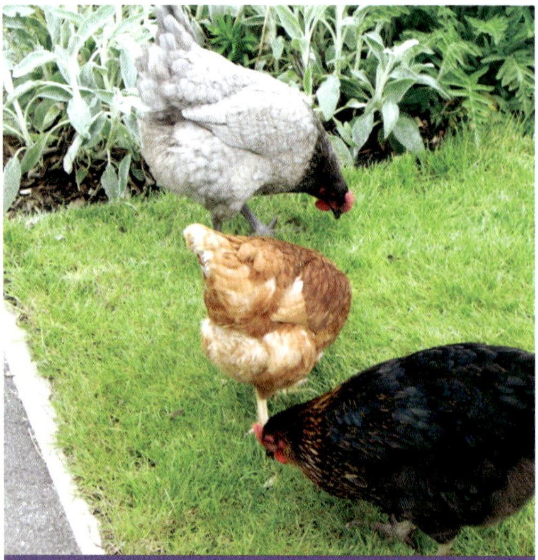

- at one care home it was discovered, after staff researched a gentleman's background, that the reason this particular gentleman became restless each day at 3pm was because he had always gone out at that time on his tractor in the fields where he farmed. As a result of this, a solution was found for his restlessness, and subsequently each day this gentleman had the opportunity to go out with the gardener on his ride on tractor to cut the grass

- some care homes have a washing line and particular residents enjoy hanging out their washing regularly

- some care homes have bird feeders at bedroom windows where it is known the resident enjoys bird watching and this then encourages people to venture outside to see the birds

- some care homes have dogs and residents walk the dog. This is done with a staff member if need be

- in one care home the manager owns a horse and arrives at work on it. The residents have the opportunity to feed it and spend time with the horse

- when a lady who enjoyed the outdoors all her life and going out in all weathers was required to live in a care home, one was chosen which had large gardens and water nearby. This care home always enables residents to get out into the gardens and further afield. This particular lady had a nominated carer who ensured she got outside each day. The smile on her face when her husband visited showed him just how much she had enjoyed it

Fig. 163 Caring for the chickens can give great pleasure

- the water at the care home was a small lake and this lady was able to enjoy the sun shimmering on it and the birds around it
- a gentleman who liked to place bets when living in his own home is supported by the care home staff where he lives to have daily visits to the bookmaker if he wishes
- many care homes encourage residents to be involved in planting vegetables in the garden, which they then look after and harvest when the time is right. The residents then get involved in preparing and cooking the vegetables for the meals in the care home.

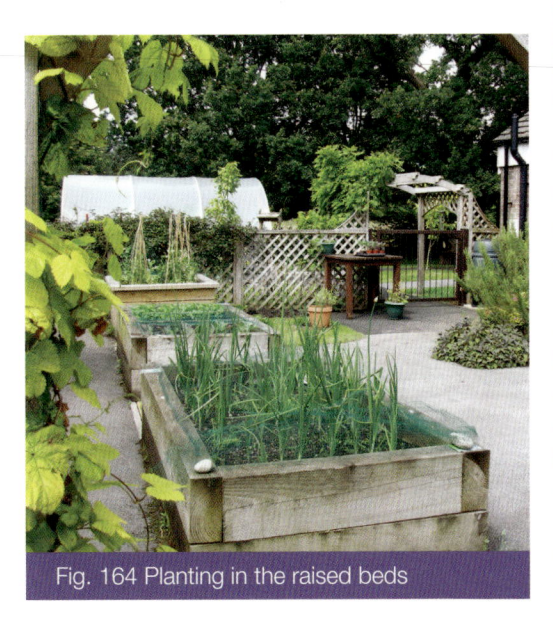

Fig. 164 Planting in the raised beds

As well as drawing on people's past experiences, staff may also need to use their own initiative and make suggestions about possible activities outside in the garden or the community in general.

There may be something that has always been a particular ambition for someone, which although very simple, they may never have had the opportunity to do, for example learning to bowl, looking after a pet, going swimming and so on. It may be possible for staff to help this person fulfil that ambition.

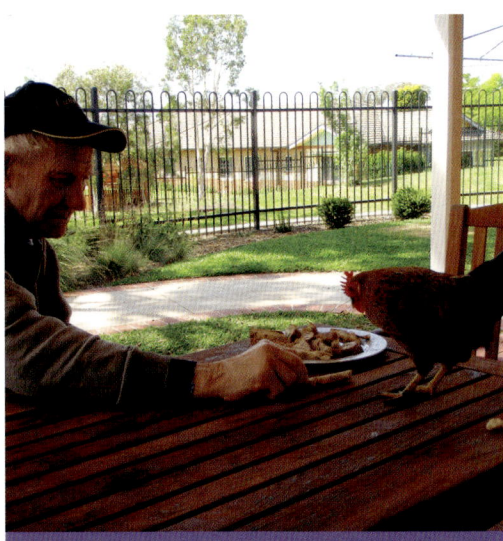

Fig. 165 Enjoying the company of a pet

Engaging in certain activities outside or in the community can raise the issue of risk. It is important to think carefully about risk in the context of a risk/benefit assessment and to be aware that risk-averse practices can breach a person's human rights. When caring for someone else, there is a natural desire to try to reduce risk as much as possible. However, this may mean missing out on benefits and restricting someone's freedom (Nuffield Council on Bioethics, 2009). It is suggested therefore that staff should:

- look at the risk and the benefits and make a judgement based on balance to encourage positive risk-taking
- recognise the long-term benefits as these may outweigh the risk

- incorporate this process into risk/benefit assessment policies and procedures, taking into account the interests of the individual with dementia and also close family and friends who may be the most risk averse.

If the activity is going to give someone pleasure and improve their wellbeing significantly, giving them a greater quality of life, then this may outweigh any identified risks. Risks can be modified to an extent, which still allows people the freedom to contribute to society in their own way.

An example of balancing risk with benefit

If someone enjoys sweeping leaves outside but is unsteady on their feet, there may be concerns about this individual falling and injuring themselves. If there is a benefit to this person being able to do this activity in terms of their pleasure and quality of life, this risk should be managed to support this person to sweep the leaves.

For example, it could be arranged that this activity is done when a friend visits, or a staff member has time to accompany the individual, or if there is a risk of falling that it is analysed and managed in a way that identifies when the person may be less unsteady. If they are less unsteady at a certain time of day then that would be the best time to do the activity. It may help to ask these questions when considering going outside to do an activity:

- Does the individual want to go outside?
- Is this a beneficial activity for the individual?
- Is the individual, with staff if required, physically able to go outside and carry out the activity?
- Are there any special requirements that need to be met (e.g. clothing, medication, footwear, walking frame, wheelchair, sunscreen etc)?

Managers should seek to challenge those actions that would disturb the balance between the value of an activity, risk and safety. Organisational guidance should always reflect positive risk-taking.

Key points
- get to know people well
- gather life histories and keep histories alive
- use past experiences to support going outside
- suggest new ideas and be an active influence
- employ positive risk-taking.

3. Care planning

A care plan is an agreement between an individual and a care-giver about how they wish to be supported, day to day, in every area of life. Everyone should have an individualised care plan which reflects the strengths and also the needs of the individual. Activity and going outside should be integral to this.

A care plan must be reviewed and updated regularly in partnership with the individual. It is helpful if friends and relatives are included in the care planning process. It is then clear to all what an individual's strengths, needs and preferences are and this can then be reinforced by everyone. A care plan also helps to deal with any issues that arise relating to risk/benefits, and access to records does not become an issue if all the key people are included in the care planning process.

As part of the care planning process it is important to note the following within the care plan:

- when the individual may like to go outside
- what they like to do
- what they may need to support them, for example hat, coat, walking frame and so on.

It would be beneficial to also note any relevant clinical information, for example claustrophobia and agoraphobia. It can be very helpful to have a resumé sheet or booklet which can be kept in an individual's room or with them, which shows, at a glance, likes, dislikes and preferences for a typical day.

If an individual gets frustrated at times and perhaps displays behaviour that challenges others, having the opportunity to go outside to see the birds, smell the lavender or get fresh air can help to relieve these tensions.

This should be reflected in a care plan and communicated to staff, friends and relatives so that everyone can embrace this strategy.

Individuals may consider having an Advanced Directive, which can state clearly at an early stage what their wishes are in relation to day-to-day activity, and if so this should be included in the care plan. An Advanced Directive gives instructions by an individual specifying what actions should be taken for their health and wellbeing in the event they are no longer able to make decisions due to illness or incapacity, and appoints someone to make decisions on their behalf. Many really thrive on being outside and it would be detrimental to their physical and psychological wellbeing for them not to continue to have the opportunity to go outside.

Key points

- a care plan should include the use of outside spaces
- develop a care plan in partnership with all key people
- Advanced Directives may be a consideration.

4. Education and Training

Access to education and training is essential for all staff. This is required to ensure that staff have the opportunity to gain the knowledge and skills to provide the care that meets the needs of the individuals they are caring for on a daily basis. This can be formal or informal and range from general awareness to more in-depth training on various aspects of care. It should include, at a minimum, awareness on why going outside is important for health.

Training can be available online, through training organisations or provided locally by health and social care professionals or others. Valuable learning can also take place through visiting other care settings and shadowing other staff.

Staff must have dementia training appropriate to the skill level required. The Scottish educational framework for health and social care for those living with dementia, *'Promoting excellence: a framework for health and social services staff working with people with dementia, families and carers'*, can help identify the level of training required and signpost people to the most appropriate training.

All staff in a care setting, no matter what their role, should have awareness training in dementia care and in the need for people to be outside some of the time.

It would be helpful for staff to gain an understanding of what activity is and how to facilitate the use of outside space. In the UK, the National Association for Providers of Activities for Older People (NAPA) provides training that would be appropriate. Also, organisations such as the Royal Society for Protection of Birds (RSPB) will provide advice to care homes on creating an outside environment that will attract bird and animal life.

The Dementia Services Development Centre at the University of Stirling has a variety of training materials and courses that would be suitable. An example of an appropriate training course would be 'Meaningful activities with people with dementia'.

Having a good awareness and being convinced of the physical, mental, emotional and spiritual benefits of going outside should increase the priority that individuals give to making it happen!

Benefits such as increased mobility, improved function, fewer behavioural issues, improved appetite, better communication and so on, have been reported – benefits which not only impact on an individual's life but may also affect the lives of relatives, friends and staff, improving their job satisfaction (see Chapter 2).

For all new staff, appropriate training should be included in the formal induction package. Training should be updated annually and recorded on a database so that it can be easily monitored through performance development reviews and appraisals.

Support should be given where necessary to access training through the most appropriate medium.

Ongoing coaching and mentoring is very supportive and empowering for staff. It would be helpful to link training with local specialists such as Occupational Therapists or Physiotherapists who can offer advice and help in this way. They will also be able to explain how outside spaces can support their therapeutic programmes.

To ensure, as far as possible, that the appropriate training takes place and all staff know they are required to complete it, a training and education policy should be made available, detailing expectations.

Key points

- education and training for the appropriate skills set is essential
- a monitoring system should be in place to ensure all staff receive appropriate training which is updated regularly
- include clear expectations of training in a training policy
- find out who your local specialists are, who can advise and support the care home.

5. Essential equipment

Essential equipment for going outside should be easily accessible and available for all to facilitate and enable people to go outside. This should take into account that they may wish to go outside at night as well as during the day and also all year round, even in the snow or rain.

This equipment may include the following:

- clothing for all weathers – hats, scarves, coats, waterproofs, warm gloves, gardening gloves, footwear for wet and dry weather
- mobility aids – stick, walking frame, wheeled walking frame, wheelchairs
- equipment for a sunny day – sun cream, sun brolleys, sun hats, sunglasses.

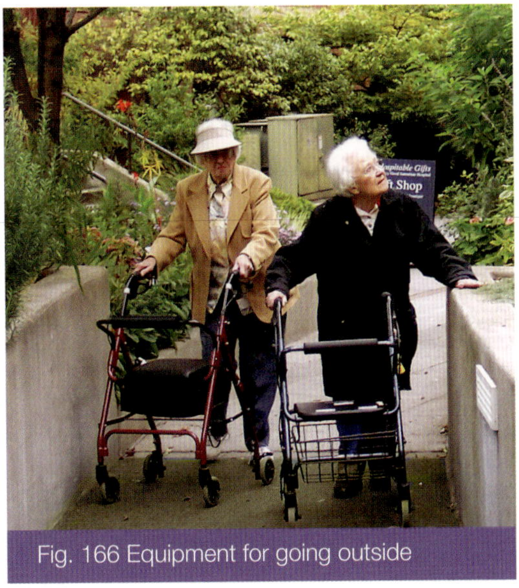

Fig. 166 Equipment for going outside

6. Staff use of outside space

The use of outside space for staff has been mentioned several times in this book. For example, in Yuji Okubo's contribution, he mentions that they use the outside space for breaks. The fact that outside space provides a place for staff to calm down, get fresh air, take exercise and meet in a convivial place should not be underestimated as a way of benefitting the whole community.

Happy and relaxed staff means happier and more relaxed people with dementia.

References:

Berentsen, V.D., Grefsrød, E.-E., & Eek, A. (2008). Gardens for people with dementia: Design and use. Tønsberg, Norway: Aldring og helse.

Brooker, D. (2007). *Person-centred dementia care: Making services better.* London: Jessica Kingsley.

Haschak, P.G. (1998). *Corporate statements: The official missions, goals, principles and philosophies of over 900 companies.* Jefferson, NC: McFarland.

National Association for Providers of Activities for Older People. (2010). *Activity at the heart of care: A guide for managers.* London: NAPA.

Nuffield Council on Bioethics. (2009). *Dementia: Ethical issues.* Retrieved from http://www.nuffieldbioethics.org/dementia

Rodiek, S., & Schwarz, B. (Eds.) (2007). *Outdoor environments for people with dementia.* New York, NY: Haworth Press.

Samuels, T. (2010). The dynamics of occupation and social engagement. *OT News,* April, 28.

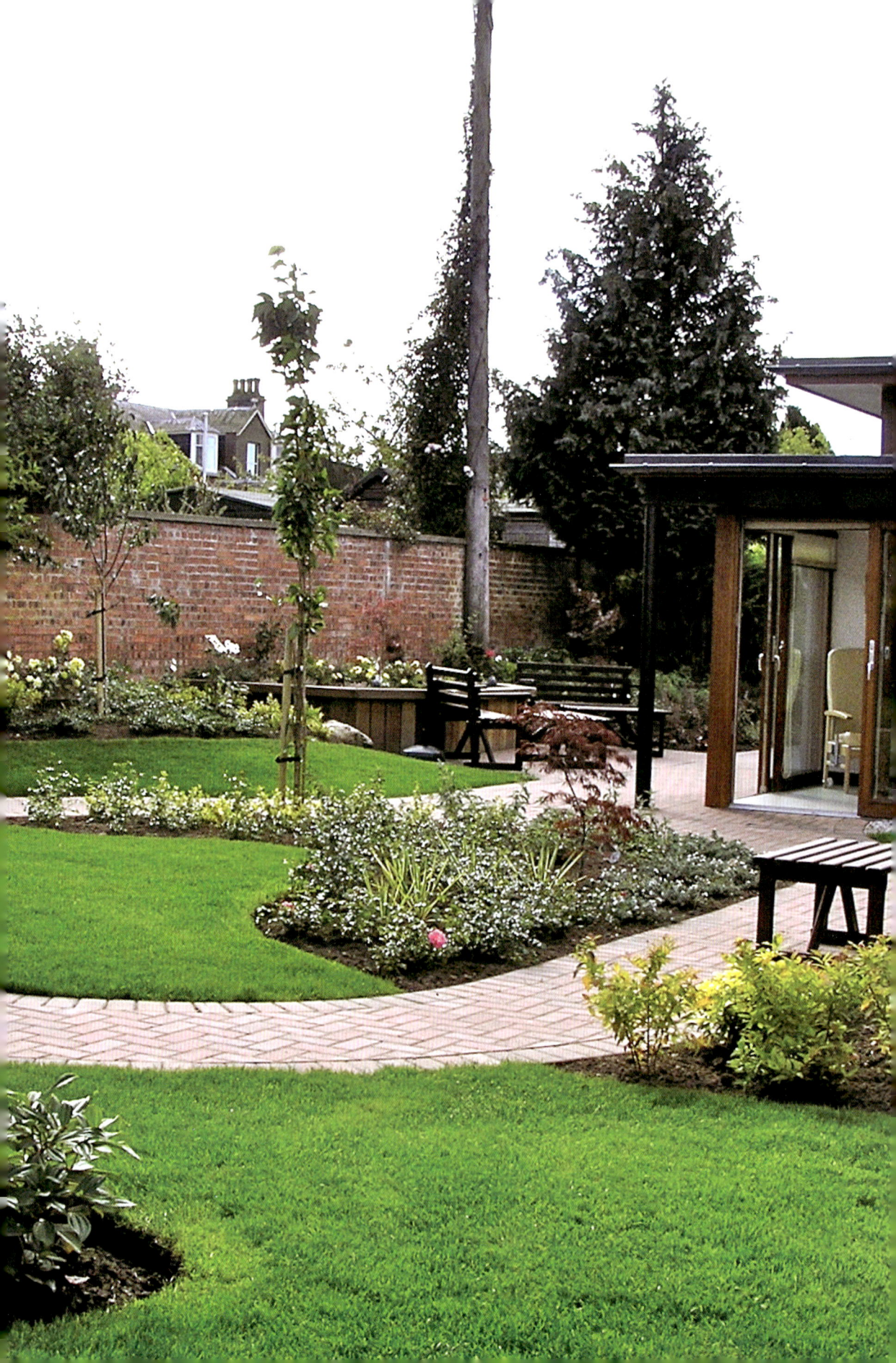

Case Study 8
Blairgowrie Community Hospital

Annie Pollock

Friends of the hospital and staff raised 50% of funding for work to improve the GP unit and the Dementia ward (the Strathmore unit) at Blairgowrie Community Hospital. NHS Tayside matched this funding and in 2005, decided to commission the work, which comprised the provision of two sunrooms for each of the units and garden areas associated with each.

The GP unit garden

This area was at the front of the hospital and was accessed from the nearest ward by a corridor and long, unattractive ramp.

The area was not secure and contained an unmaintained summerhouse in poor condition.

The intention was to make this into a garden that could be used by people in palliative care, people with dementia, the frail elderly, and those in wheelchairs or with mobility issues. The use of this garden would always be supervised.

Fig. 168 During construction

Fig. 169 GP unit garden, complete

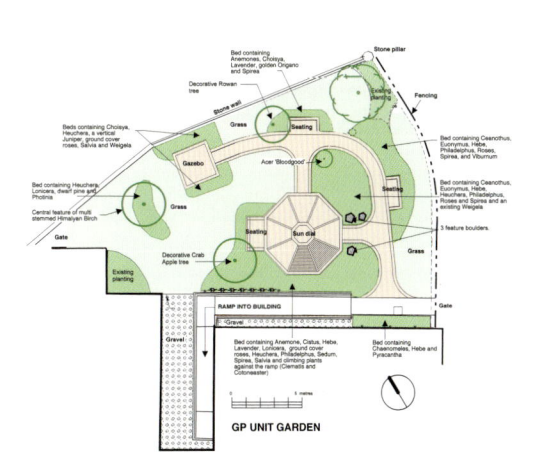

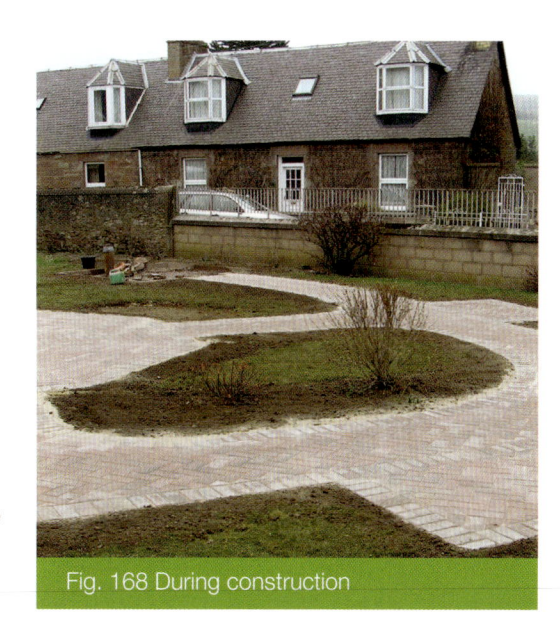

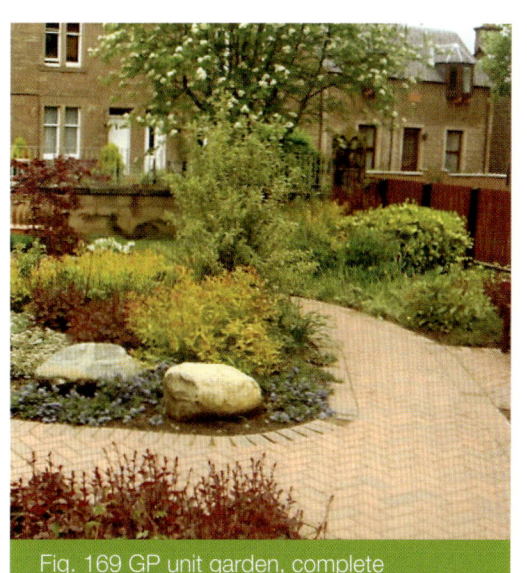

Fig. 167 Plan of GP unit garden (refer to appendix 1 on page 222 for enlarged version)

Fig. 170 Staff using the gazebo

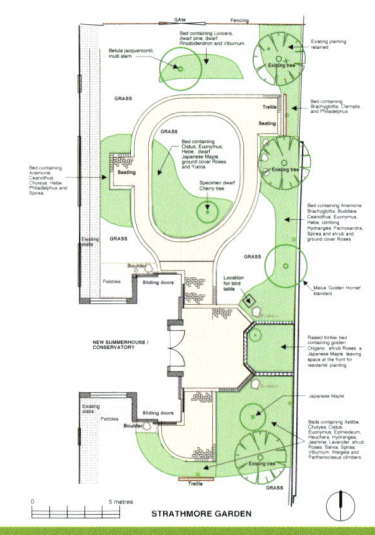

Fig. 171 Plan of Strathmore unit garden (refer to appendix 1 on page 223 for enlarged version)

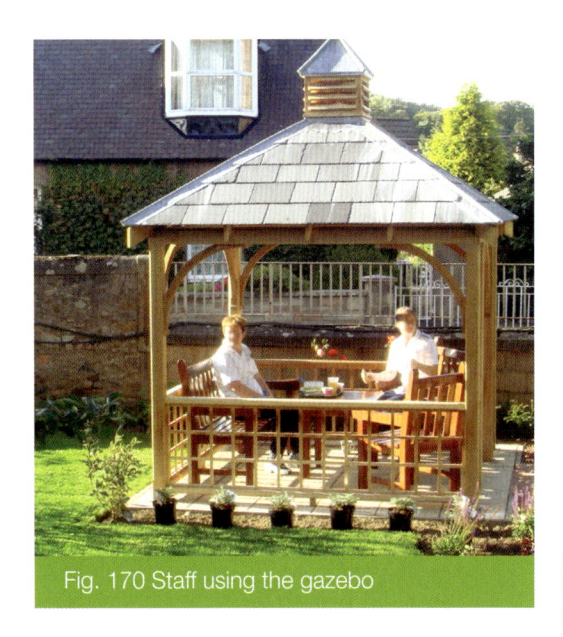

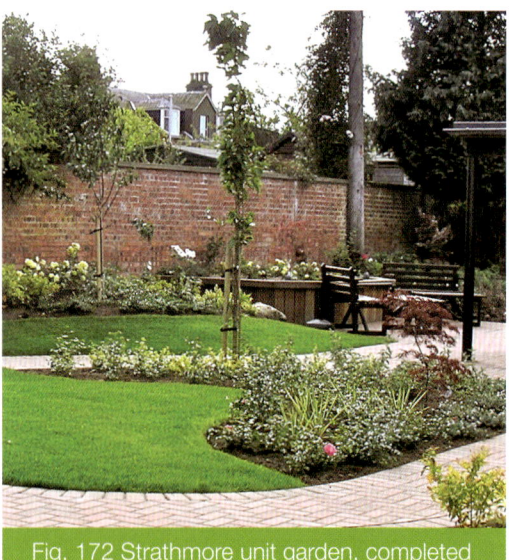

Garden furniture and plants are often gifted in memory of someone who has passed away and many carers still come back to sit in the garden even after their loved one has died.

The Strathmore unit garden

This garden area led out from a dementia ward and allowed patients access to the garden.

It contained a summerhouse that had been gifted but the entrance to it was not barrier-free. There was little else to encourage exercise or enjoyment.

The proposals included for a conservatory (architect designed) and a garden designed for use by people with dementia

The garden served people with dementia for a short time only, since it was closed recently following changes to the service in the area. Currently, it is used by staff only, although is possible that the GP unit will move into the wards, providing easier access for the patients to the garden.

Fig. 172 Strathmore unit garden, completed

Staff have commented as follows:

"The gardens definitely enhanced the patients' quality of life whilst in the Strathmore unit. It allowed them to go into the garden area rather than wandering aimlessly up and down the main corridor. I would like to say that it reduced agitation and therefore a reduction in medication given to patients. It certainly was utilised as a first attempt to reduce agitation and distract patients.

Visitors also enjoyed having time in the garden when they visited their loved ones. One patient enjoyed sitting in the sunroom watching the activity in the garden, whether that be birds or the gardeners attending to the garden.

The garden area also gave staff an opportunity to take five minutes in the middle of a hectic shift. It had a nice calming effect."

One patient, a man in his late 50s who had worked all his life outdoors, was in palliative care in the GP unit. Because he was unable to leave his bed, he could not access the garden via the ramp (which was not wide enough for a bed). So staff wheeled him through the hospital into the Strathmore garden, which he loved, noting: "All I want is to feel the sun and rain on my face…" He died shortly afterwards, but his time in the garden undoubtedly made his last days easier.

Plants

The plants in both gardens were chosen to maximise year-round interest and to include old-fashioned plants that people might recognise from the past as well as plants that were colourful and perfumed

The list included Clematis, Chaenomeles, Choisya, decorative grasses, rock roses and shrub roses, Euonymus, Hebe, Heuchera, Salvia (sage), Sedum, Spirea, Viburnum, Vinca, Weigela, and several small trees – Japanese maple, Himalayan birch, golden crab apple, a small flowering cherry and a decorative rowan.

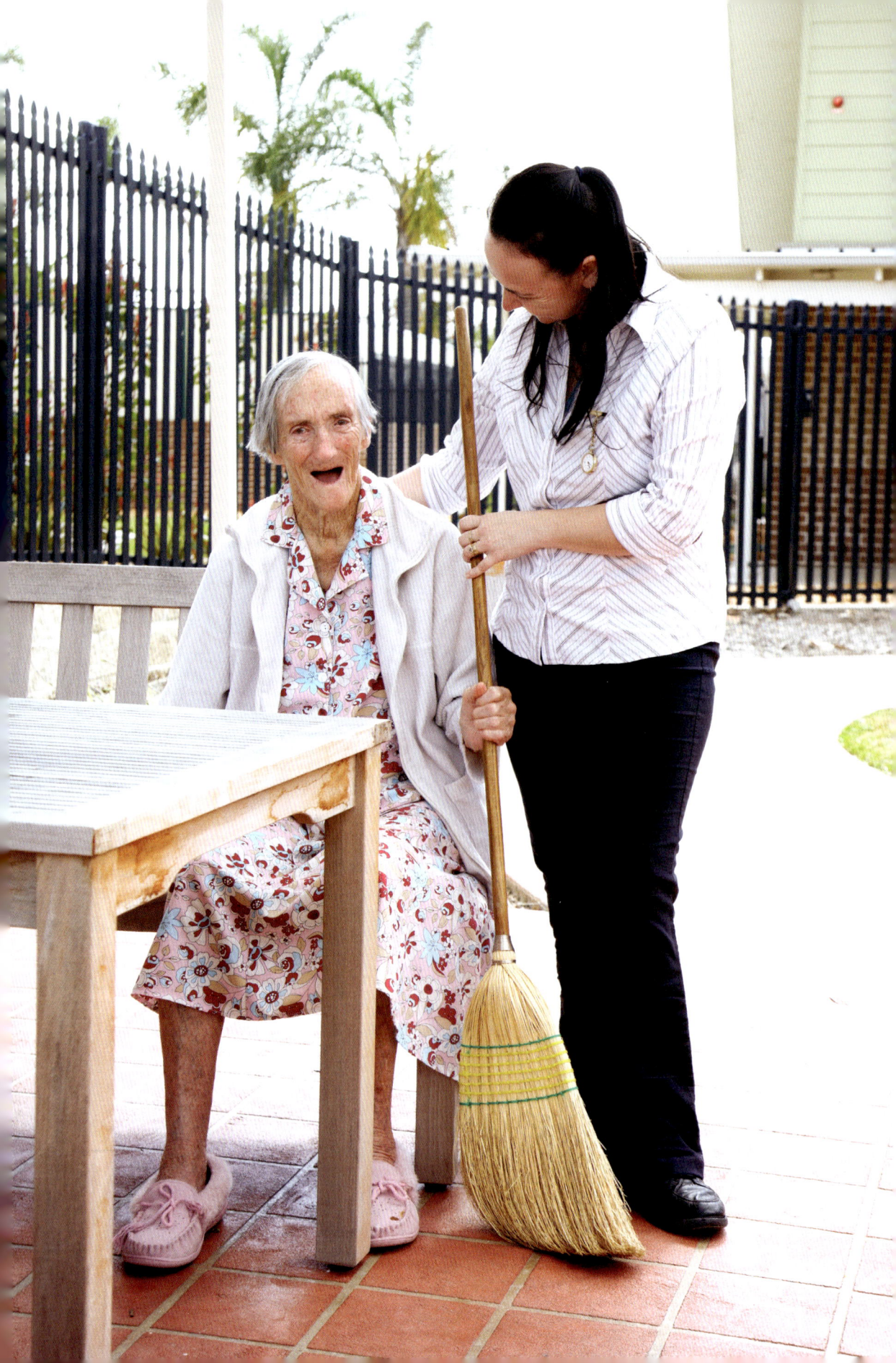

PART 5
CONCLUDING REFLECTIONS

Annie Pollock and Mary Marshall

We have learned an enormous amount from editing this book and writing our chapters. Our contributors and consultants are widely respected experts and they have been very generous with their expertise in their key chapters and every time we have asked for their advice and help. We have also learned a lot from our reading, most notably the remarkable books of research papers collected by Rodiek and Schwarz (2006 and 2007) and P J Littlefair's books on site planning and daylight/sunlight. These books have all been tremendously useful and we commend them to you as references.

Our book is very different; it is a book for people in practice who need to be able to argue the case for outside space and to know how to design it well.

We have realised that the more we know, the more we appreciate that this is a continuing journey of learning. New issues are emerging, new outside spaces being designed and new books being written all the time. Every country has different cultural expectations of outdoor space and different climatic issues to deal with.

This new knowledge does not contradict existing approaches but develops and enhances them, making outside spaces more effective for a wider group of people. We see this book as a station on the journey where a lot of lines have converged, but this is absolutely not the end of the line. The convergence of different aspects of design is the reason this book is different. There are other books specifically about the outdoors for people with dementia: gardens (Chalfont, 2008) and town and city neighbourhoods (Burton & Mitchell, 2006). But in looking at all outside spaces in terms of ethics and rights, technical and design aspects, activities and staffing issues, we think we have produced a book of wide appeal and usefulness.

It has been a book that has grown well beyond its original conception. We started it thinking the book would be about gardens and courtyards for people with dementia, following Annie's attendance at the inspirational Chicago Botanic Garden's course on 'Healthcare Garden Design' in 2009, which is held annually with presentations from key North American designers and researchers. We are members of an excellent design team at the Dementia Services Development Centre at the University of Stirling, so we had a good pool of expertise with which to start. Annie had written a short design guide in 2001, *Designing Gardens for People with Dementia*, and then Mary wrote her book *Balconies, Roof Terraces* and *Roof Gardens for People with Dementia* in 2010. We realised that we had to talk about all outside spaces.

We have known Elizabeth Burton and Lynne Mitchell for a long time and it seemed sensible to include their useful expertise. Because we are so indignant about the restrictions on the liberty of people with dementia who do not get outside, we asked Donny Lyons to contribute, and so it went on and the book now also embraces activities and care home practice. The book has also taken on an increasingly international flavour which started with our case studies and then extended to include our Australian colleagues, Stephen Judd and Kirsty Bennett.

The fact that the book has ended up with an Australian publisher only reinforces our attempt to ensure an international relevance.

In spite of this being a book that is broad enough in content to include climate, human rights and activities to support guidance on design, we are well aware that there are gaps. We are most aware of the gap in cultural diversity. We hope we have helped people to think about this issue and that our case studies, as well as some of our chapters, provide really useful emphasis on cultural differences. However, we would have liked chapters or case examples that drew on experience from the Middle East especially. This is clearly a topic to be addressed by another book, perhaps with a collection of detailed case studies from all over the world.

The reason for all this history is to explain why we feel our horizons have grown along with the book and how pleased we are with the combination (and we hope integration) of a very wide range of aspects of design.

It might be worth reiterating our reasons for feeling so strongly about optimal outside spaces for people with dementia. We are very well aware (and we hope the book makes a strong case) of the crucial importance of the outdoors for mental and physical health. Neither of us can imagine a future when we cannot go outside and we know this is just as strong a feeling for most people with dementia. In some ways it is extraordinary and rather depressing that we need to make the case for people with dementia going outside since they have the same needs and inclinations as the rest of us – they are us! However, as we assembled our arguments and read widely, we felt we could make a strong, pragmatic case for encouraging people with dementia to go outside: happy, fit people with dementia and less-stressed staff do not cost as much. We do recognise that some people will need medication and that going outside is not a cure-all, but it is life-enhancing in every sense. Care homes are not prisons where people are punished; they should be havens where you live out the last few months and years of your life as well and as happily as possible.

The same applies to our towns and cities; enabling people with dementia to go out and about with more confidence can only be a good thing, and this understanding should take its place beside all the other pressures to make our towns and cities fully accessible to people with a range of disabilities. This underlines one of our key beliefs, which is that 'dementia-friendly' is friendly for everyone. Getting outside with ease, dignity and safety is the right of every citizen, and what works in a design sense for people with dementia actually works for us all very effectively.

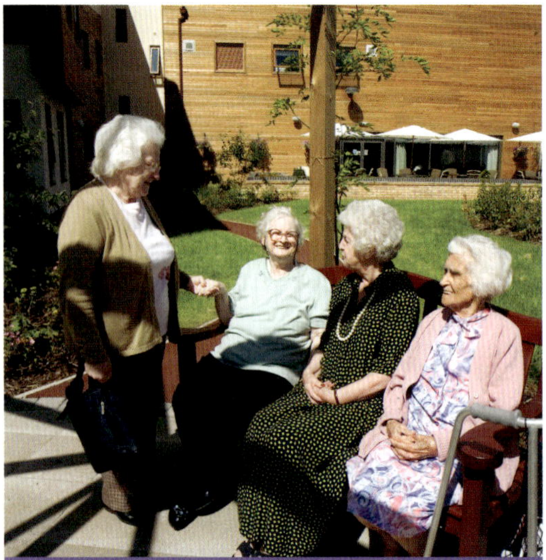

Fig. 173 Getting outside with ease, dignity and safety is the right of every citizen

So we started with a passion and a determination to produce a book to help and in many ways we have been hugely encouraged by the process. We have learned about some exceptionally good practice and we have met and worked with committed and highly knowledgeable people. The task now is to continue the efforts of many others in making sure that when buildings are planned for people with dementia, outside space is not an afterthought. Too often the outside space is simply leftover and unsuitable land with no budget to make the best of it. Outside space must be considered at the outset, as we have said in our chapter on site and climate considerations. Light into the building and access to a good, usable outside space are considerations that should be made when the building is at its footprint stage. Too often the consideration is how to get as many bedrooms on the site as possible. This may be a false economy in the future as people will be increasingly expecting access to good, adjacent outside space for themselves and their relatives. More people may specify this in their advance directives. Balconies, roof terraces and roof gardens are increasingly expected in buildings with more than one floor, even in colder northern latitudes, and in these instances, if well designed, they may actually contribute to the building's insulation in the colder months. In many really crowded cities like Tokyo, Singapore and Hong Kong, there are now policies about greening roofs, as Yuji Okubo explains in his case study.

Another aspect of care, which is achieving greater prominence, is the need for more activities. Relatives are becoming increasingly vocal about the lack of activities and are choosing places that seem to have a buzz of activities. The better homes now routinely employ a person to plan and instigate activities. We are more and more aware in research about the importance of activity for people with dementia and the negative consequences of boredom.

Outside spaces provide huge potential for activities, often ones that are familiar and simple. The outdoors can provide straightforward breaks in routine, which invigorate both residents and staff. Messy activities can be easier outdoors. People who struggle to eat can respond to a change of location and atmosphere.

Of course, outside spaces mean different things to different people. For some people, being outside was part of their job and the focus of their leisure time, like the father-in-law of one of our carers in Chapter 1, who languishes on the third floor of a hospital having spent his life as a policeman and a gardener. Our hearts go out to people like this and we very much intend this book to make it less likely to happen in the future.

We include here a diagram that summarises the various factors that influence the use of outdoor space for people with dementia. This was adapted from the 'Garden-Use Model' prepared by Charlotte F. Grant and Jean D Wineman (Rodiek & Schwarz, 2007).

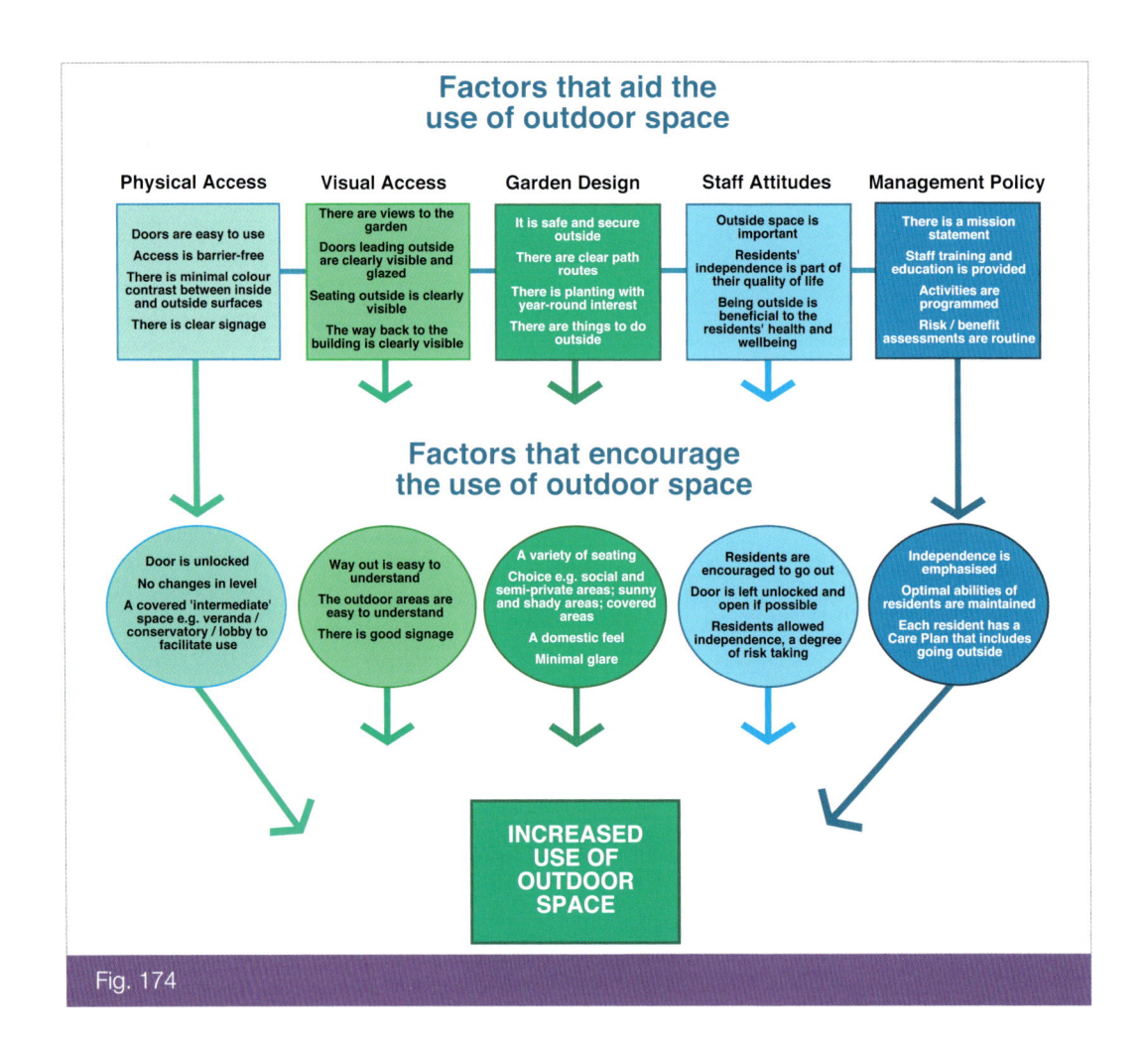

Factors that aid the use of outdoor space

Physical Access
- Doors are easy to use
- Access is barrier-free
- There is minimal colour contrast between inside and outside surfaces
- There is clear signage

Visual Access
- There are views to the garden
- Doors leading outside are clearly visible and glazed
- Seating outside is clearly visible
- The way back to the building is clearly visible

Garden Design
- It is safe and secure outside
- There are clear path routes
- There is planting with year-round interest
- There are things to do outside

Staff Attitudes
- Outside space is important
- Residents' independence is part of their quality of life
- Being outside is beneficial to the residents' health and wellbeing

Management Policy
- There is a mission statement
- Staff training and education is provided
- Activities are programmed
- Risk / benefit assessments are routine

Factors that encourage the use of outdoor space

- Door is unlocked
- No changes in level
- A covered 'intermediate' space e.g. veranda / conservatory / lobby to facilitate use

- Way out is easy to understand
- The outdoor areas are easy to understand
- There is good signage

- A variety of seating
- Choice e.g. social and semi-private areas; sunny and shady areas; covered areas
- A domestic feel
- Minimal glare

- Residents are encouraged to go out
- Door is left unlocked and open if possible
- Residents allowed independence, a degree of risk taking

- Independence is emphasised
- Optimal abilities of residents are maintained
- Each resident has a Care Plan that includes going outside

INCREASED USE OF OUTDOOR SPACE

Fig. 174

It should not be possible to design any space these days without having people with dementia in mind. For example, in the UK, over half the patients in acute hospitals are over 65, and a substantial proportion have dementia. They have a particularly neglected need for outside space, even if only to see it from the window. Most people with dementia are not in special buildings for older people, they are at home and walking around our towns and cities with the rest of us; they need to be able to do this in comfort and safety.

It is our fervent hope that this book covers the key issues for people planning, commissioning, designing and adapting outside spaces for people with dementia. We hope too that it provides enough evidence to make the case for easy access to good outside space an imperative for health and wellbeing.

References

Burton, E., & Mitchell, L. (2006). *Inclusive urban design: Streets for life.* Oxford: Architectural Press.

Chalfont, G. (2008). *Design for nature in dementia care.* London: Jessica Kingsley.

Littlefair, P.J. (2011). *Site layout planning for daylight and sunlight : A guide to good practice.* Watford: IHS BRE Press.

Rodiek, S., & Schwarz, B. (Eds.) (2006). *The role of the outdoors in residential environments for aging.* New York, NY: Haworth Press.

Rodiek S., & Schwarz, B. (Eds.) (2007). *Outdoor environments for people with dementia.* New York, NY: Haworth Press.

Appendix - graphs and plans

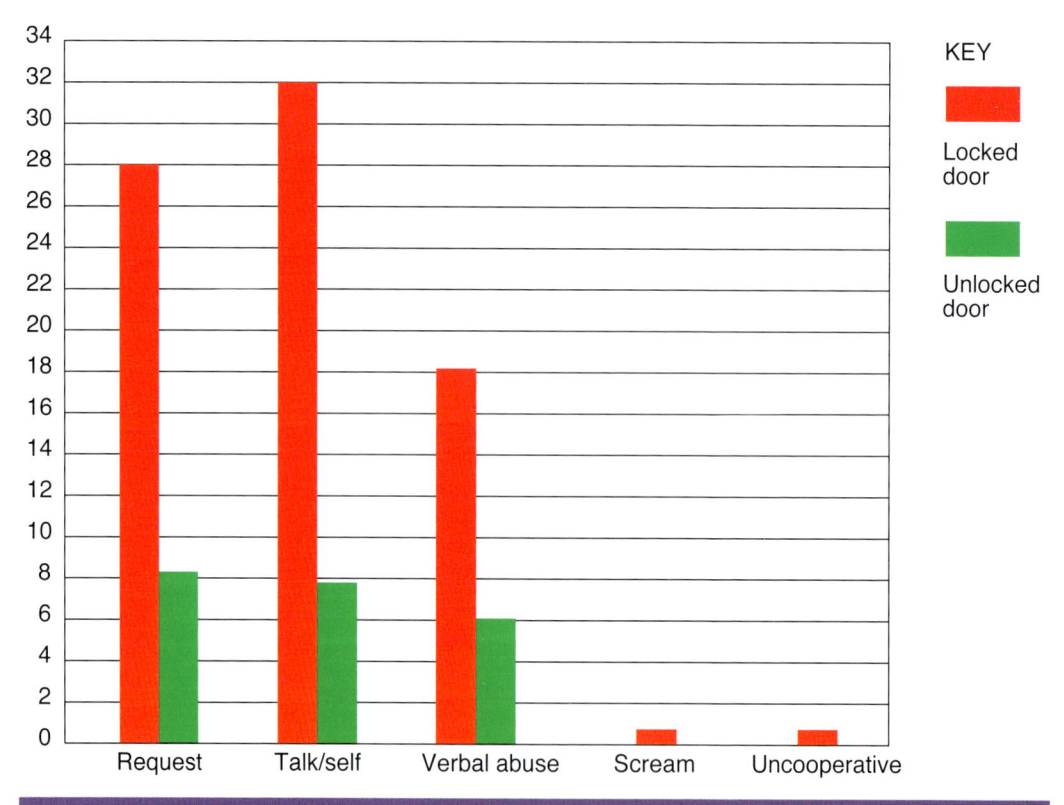

Fig. 8 Verbal responses to a locked and unlocked door

Fig. 11 The garden layout (north is to the top)

Appendix - graphs and plans

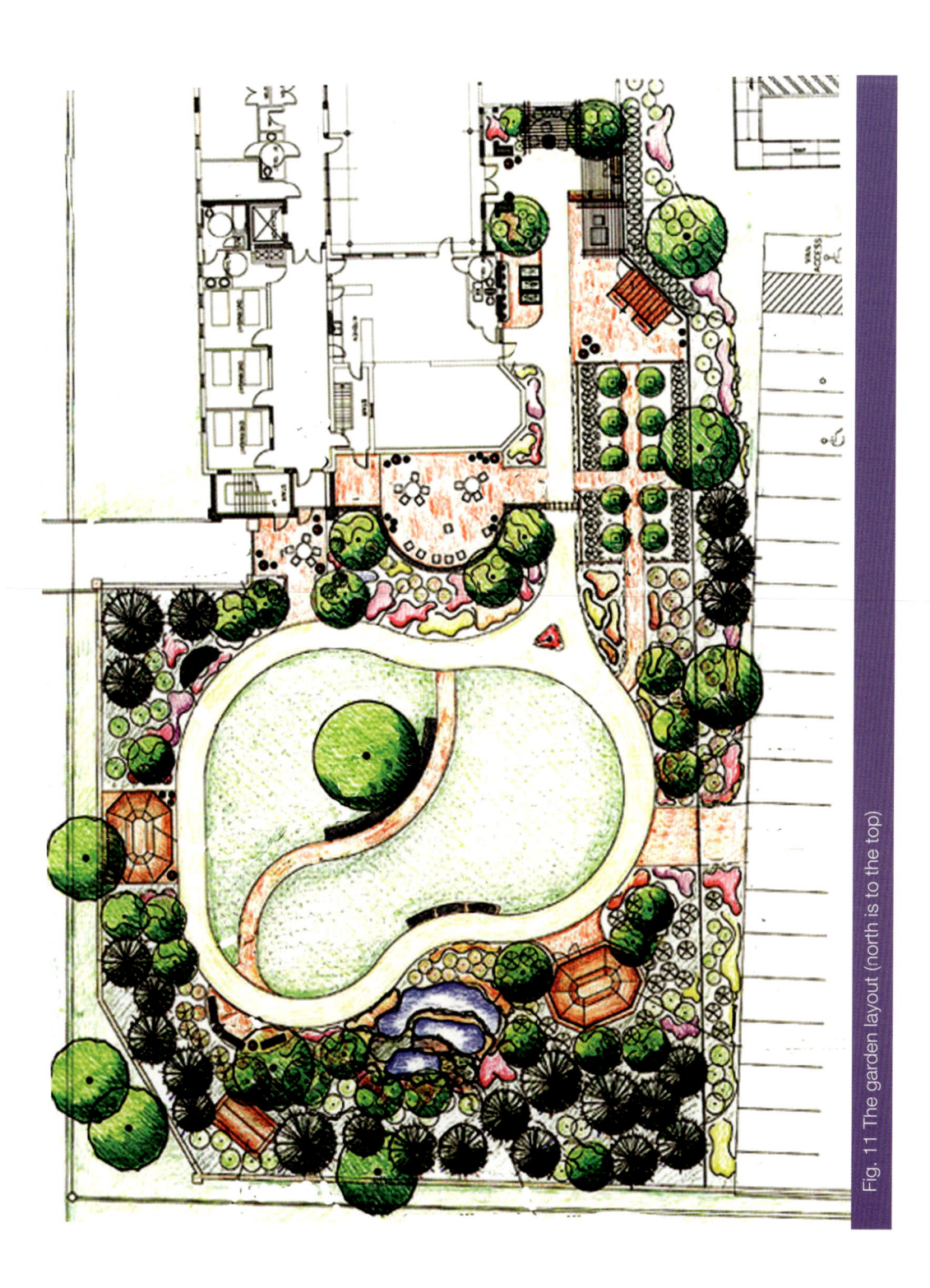

211

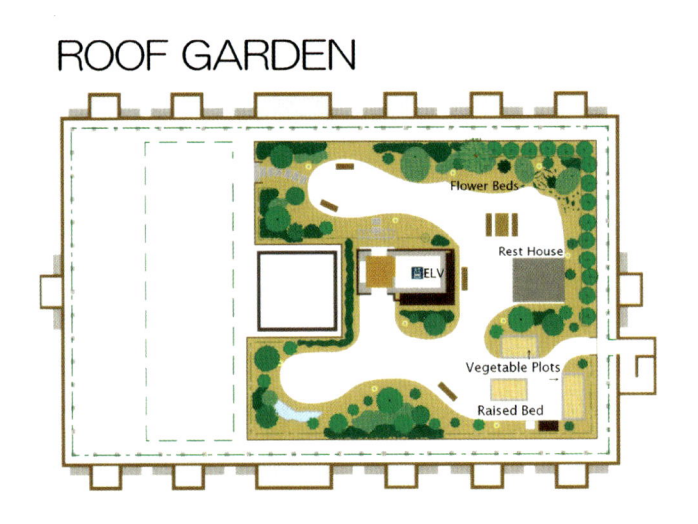

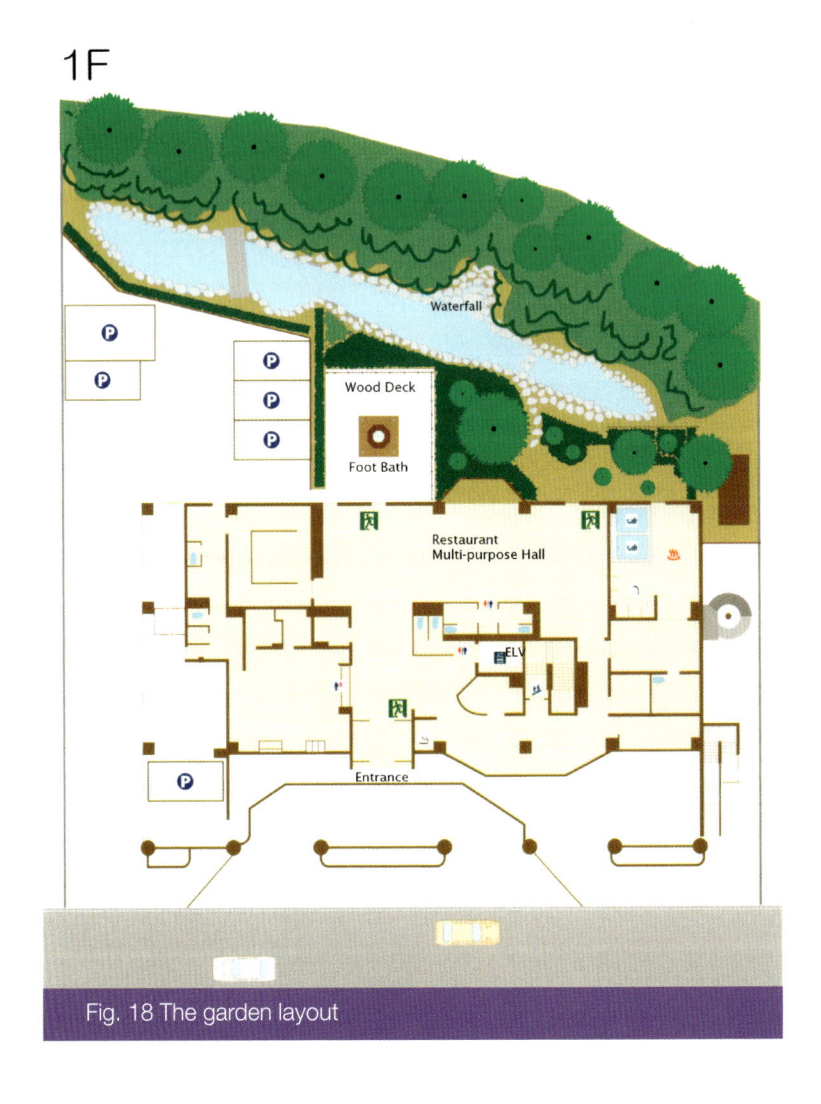

Fig. 18 The garden layout

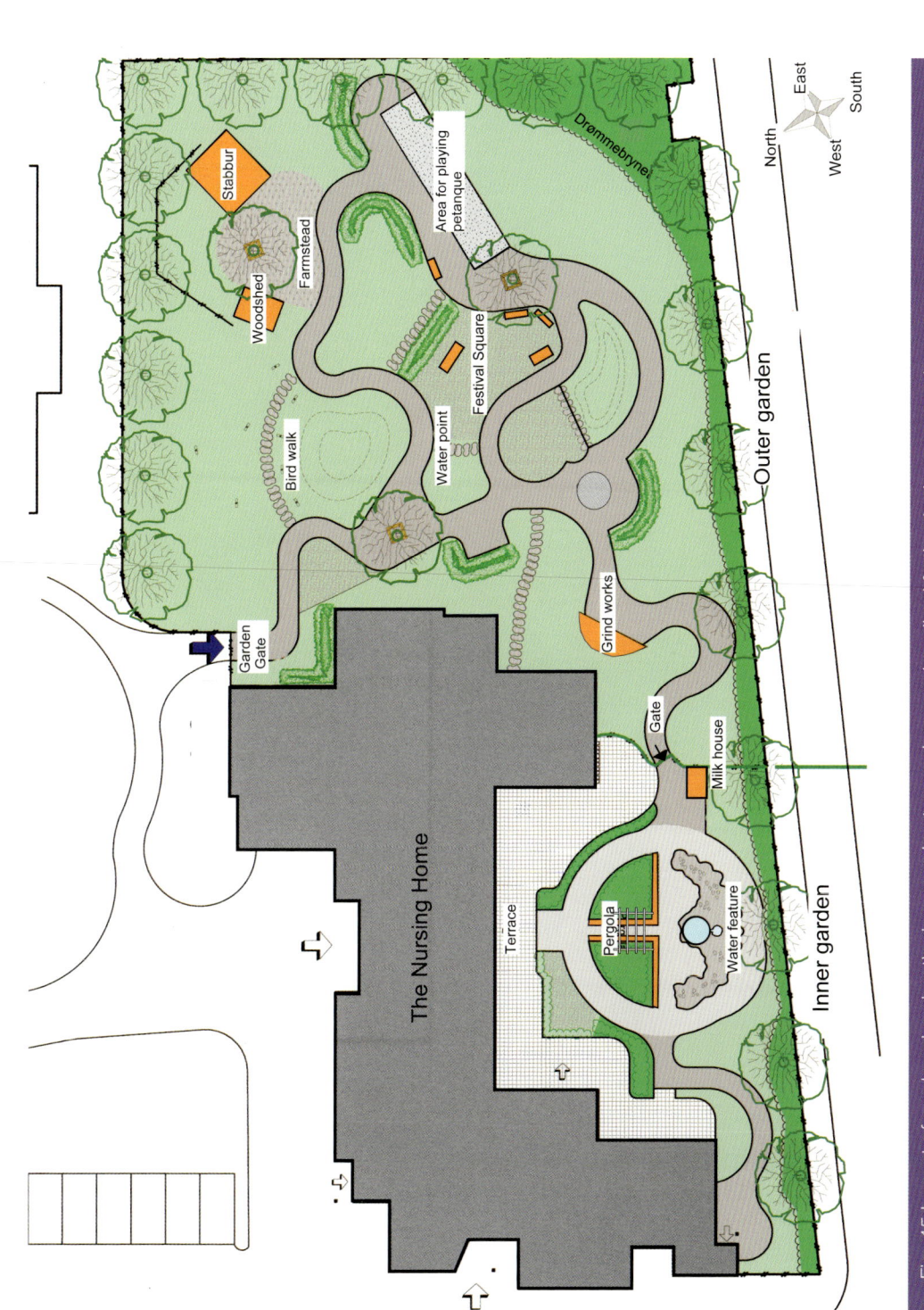

Fig. 45 Layout of garden showing the inner and outer gardens as described further in the case study

Appendix - graphs and plans

213

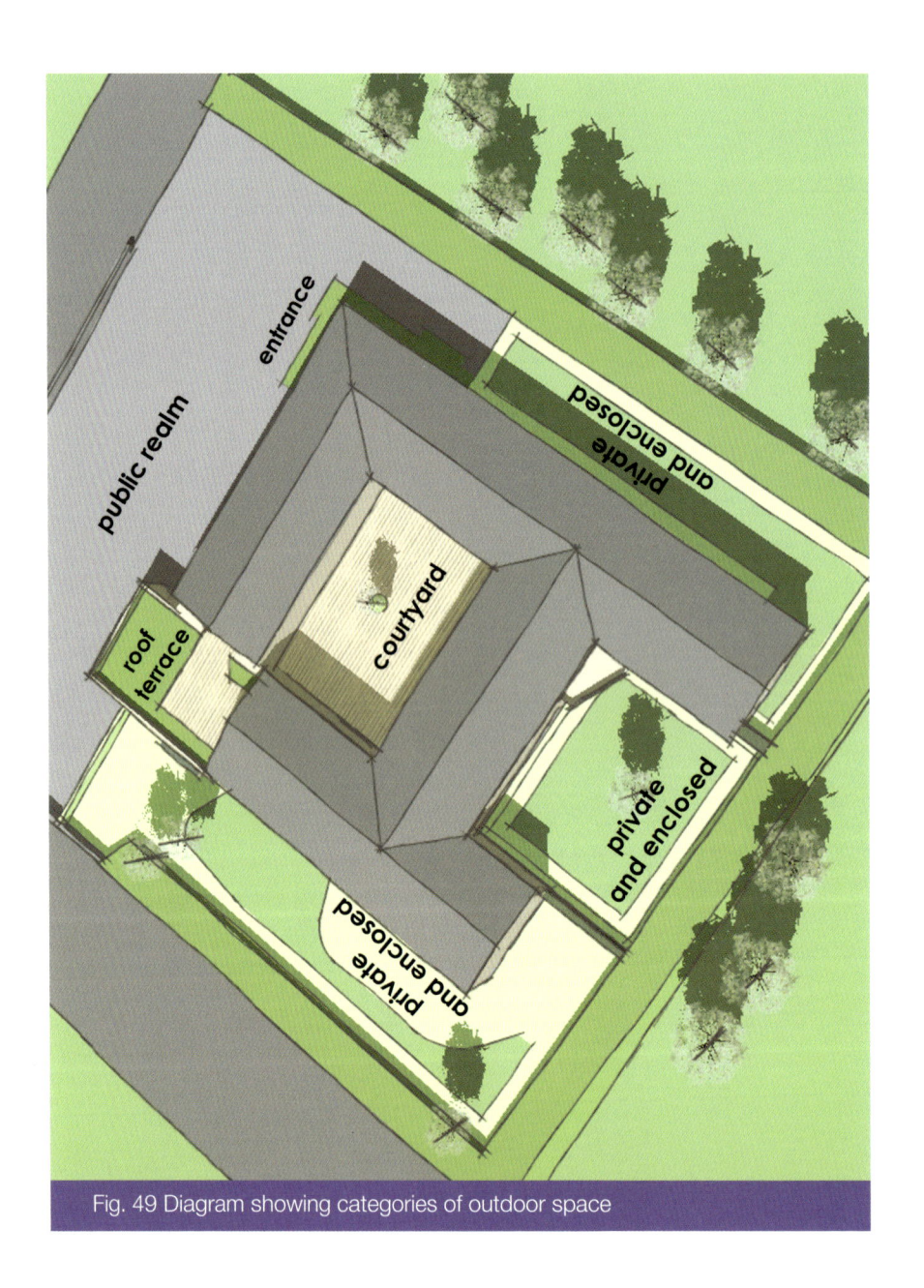

Fig. 49 Diagram showing categories of outdoor space

MARCH JUNE

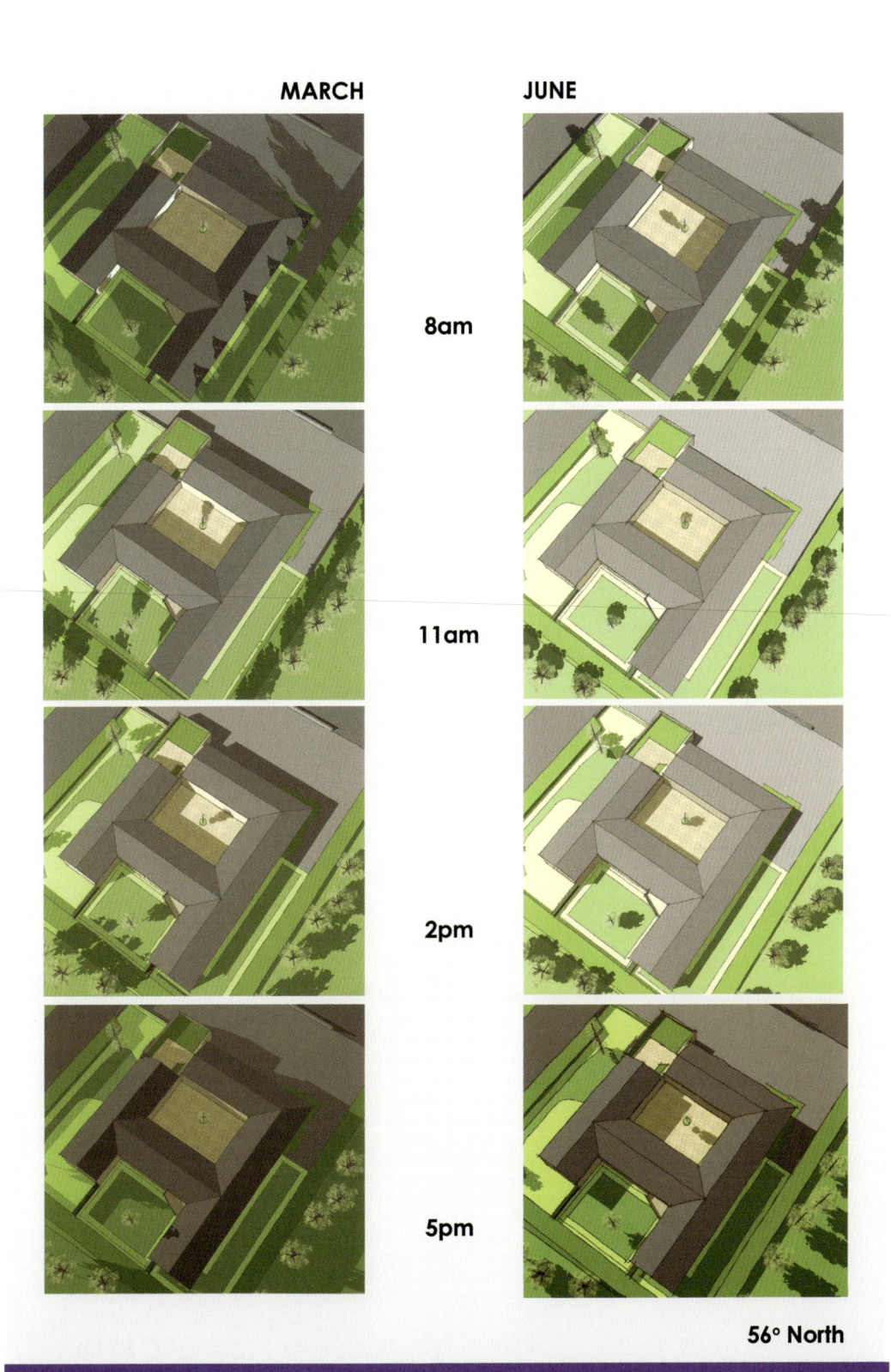

8am

11am

2pm

5pm

56° North

Fig. 62 Sun access throughout the day in the northern hemisphere

Appendix - graphs and plans

SEPTEMBER | DECEMBER

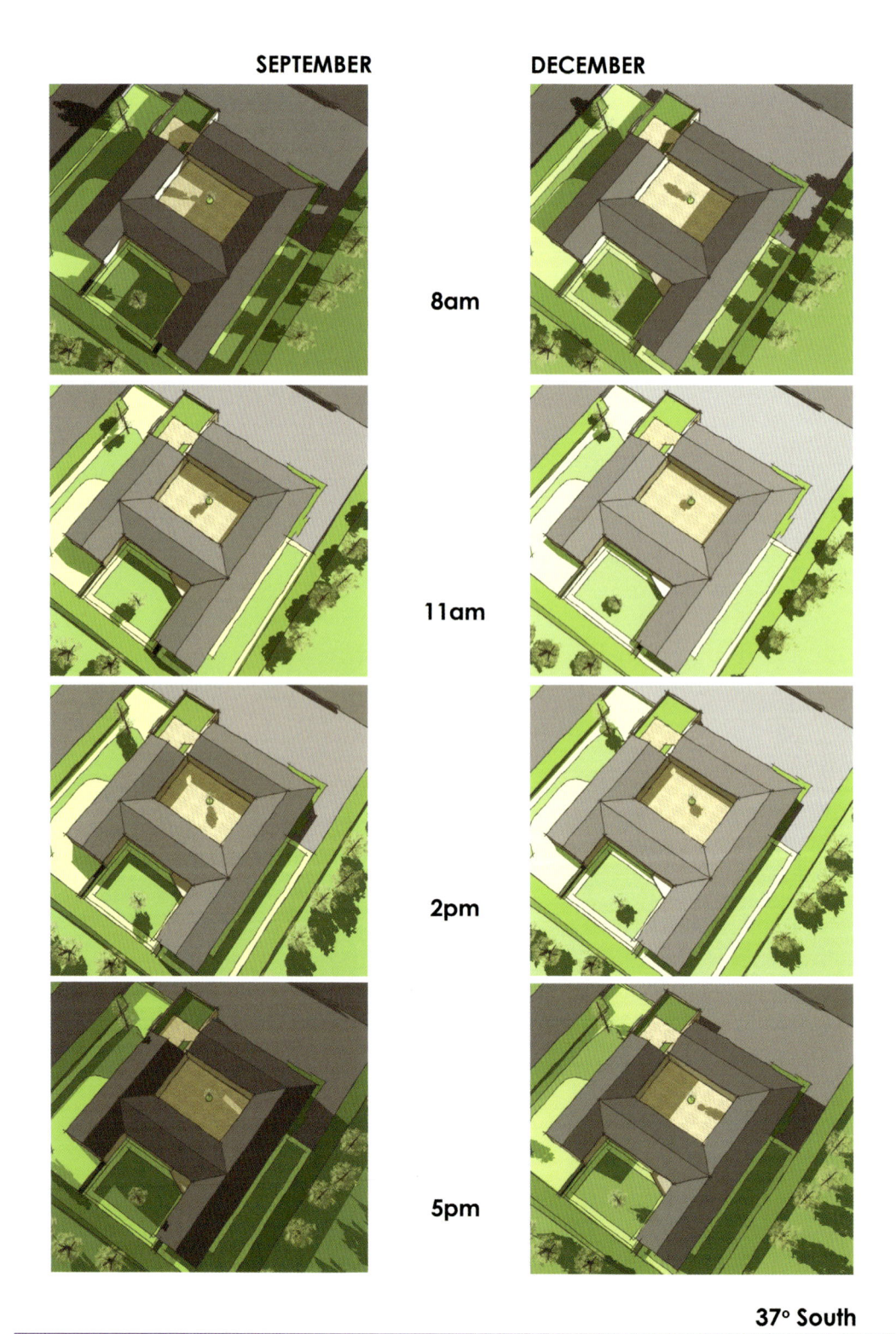

8am

11am

2pm

5pm

37° South

Fig. 63 Sun access throughout the day in the southern hemisphere

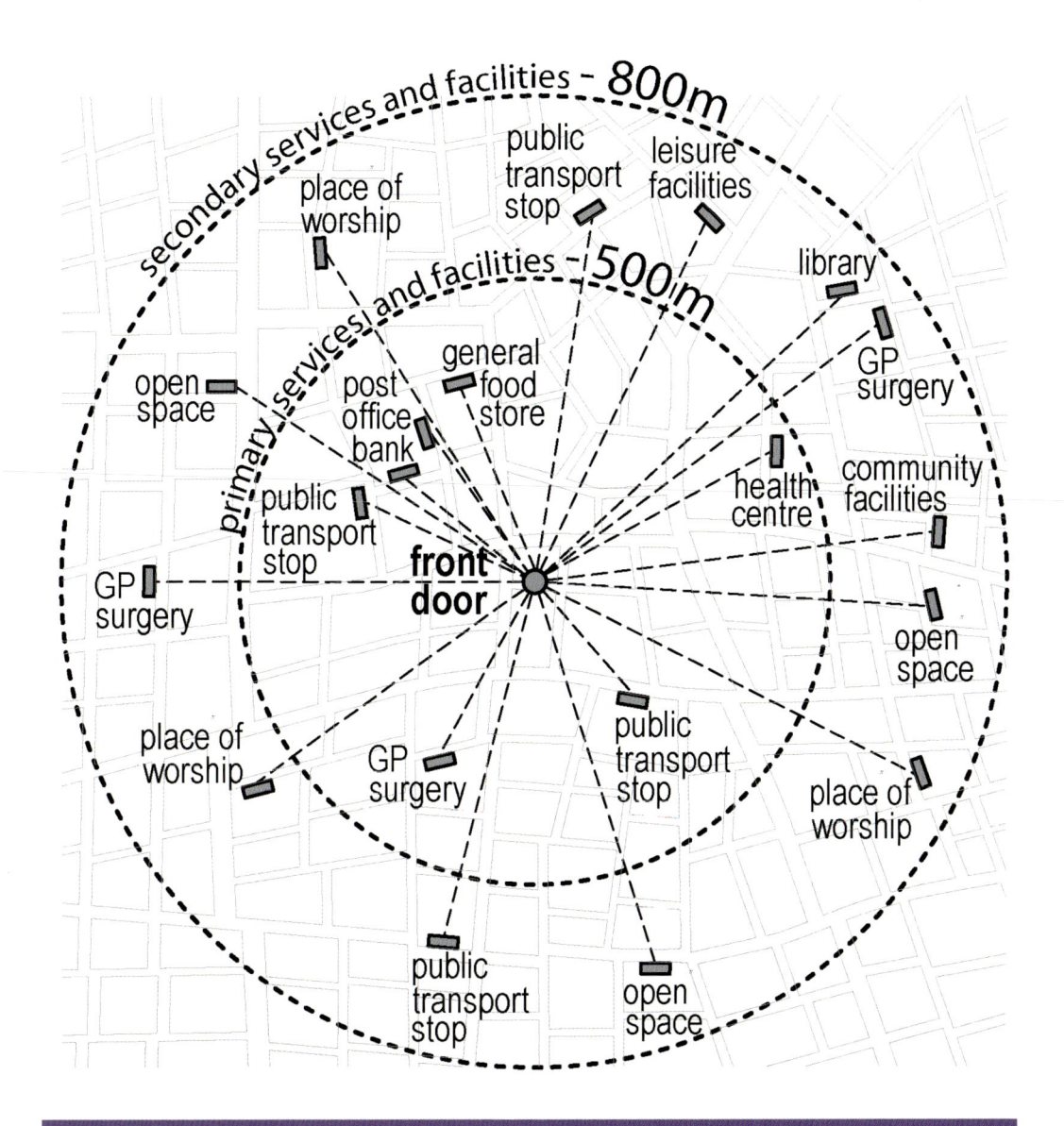

Fig. 88 Primary services and facilities should be within 500 metres of older people's housing and secondary services within 800 metres

Appendix - graphs and plans

217

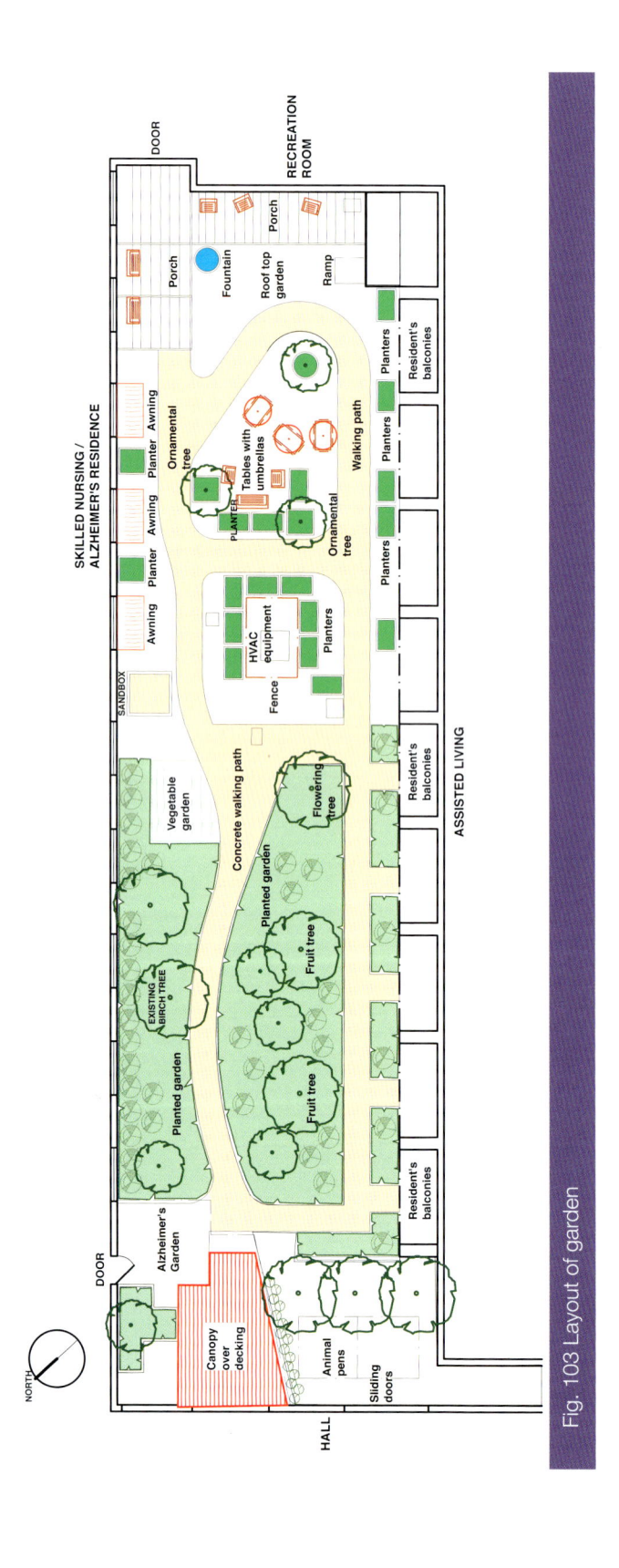

Fig. 103 Layout of garden

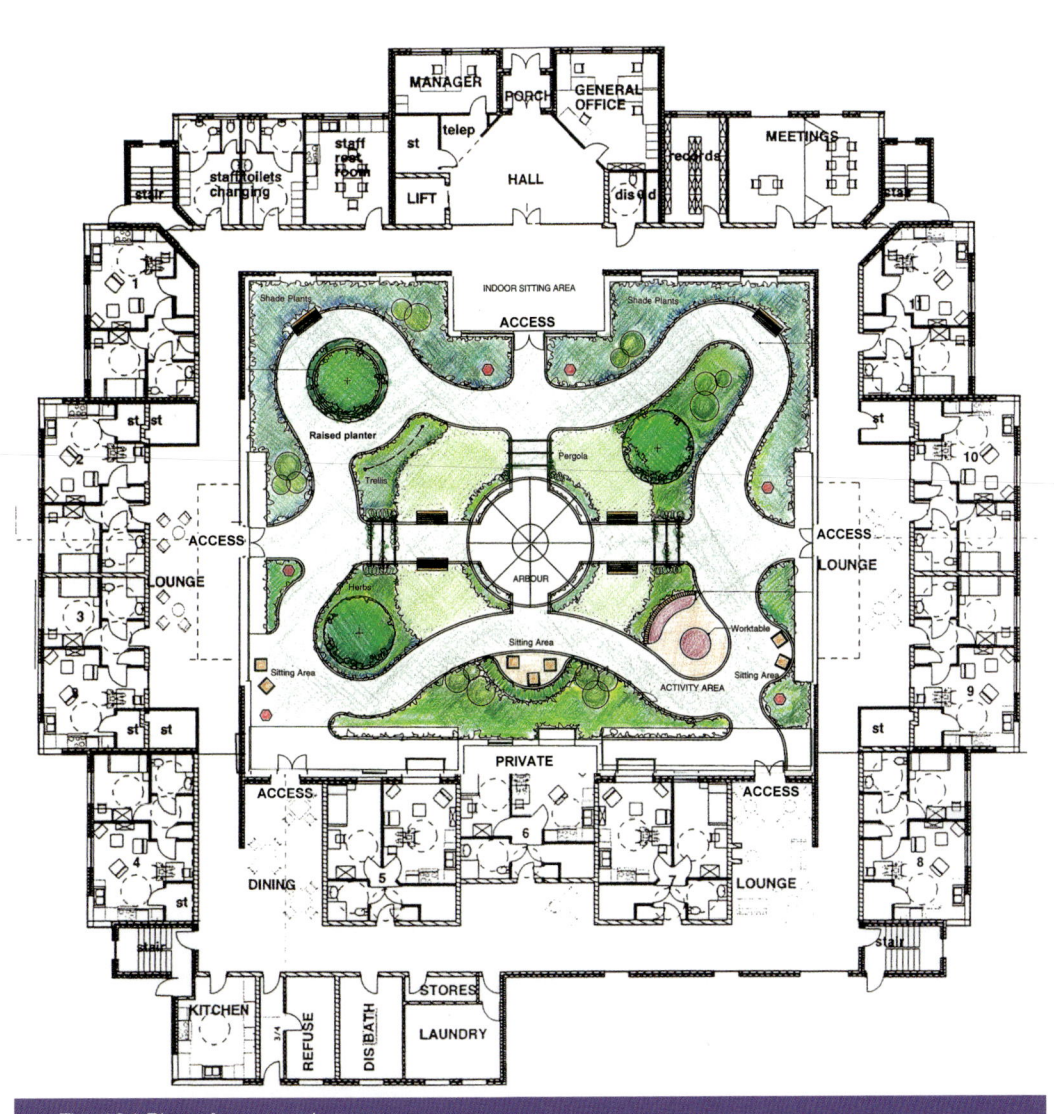

Fig. 134 Plan of courtyard

Appendix - graphs and plans

219

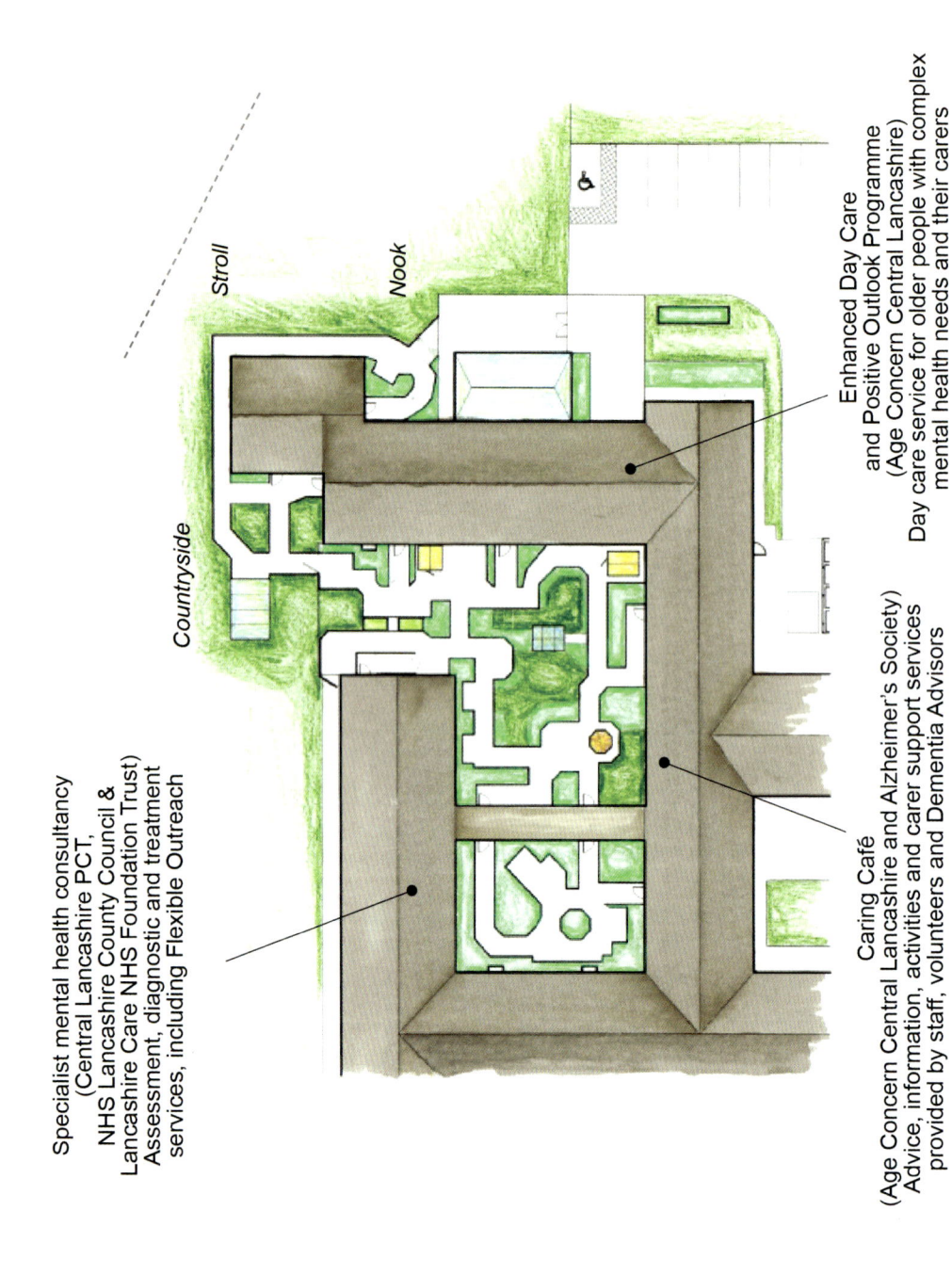

Specialist mental health consultancy
(Central Lancashire PCT,
NHS Lancashire County Council &
Lancashire Care NHS Foundation Trust)
Assessment, diagnostic and treatment
services, including Flexible Outreach

Stroll

Nook

Countryside

Enhanced Day Care
and Positive Outlook Programme
(Age Concern Central Lancashire)
Day care service for older people with complex
mental health needs and their carers

Caring Café
(Age Concern Central Lancashire and Alzheimer's Society)
Advice, information, activities and carer support services
provided by staff, volunteers and Dementia Advisors

Fig. 149 Building and courtyards

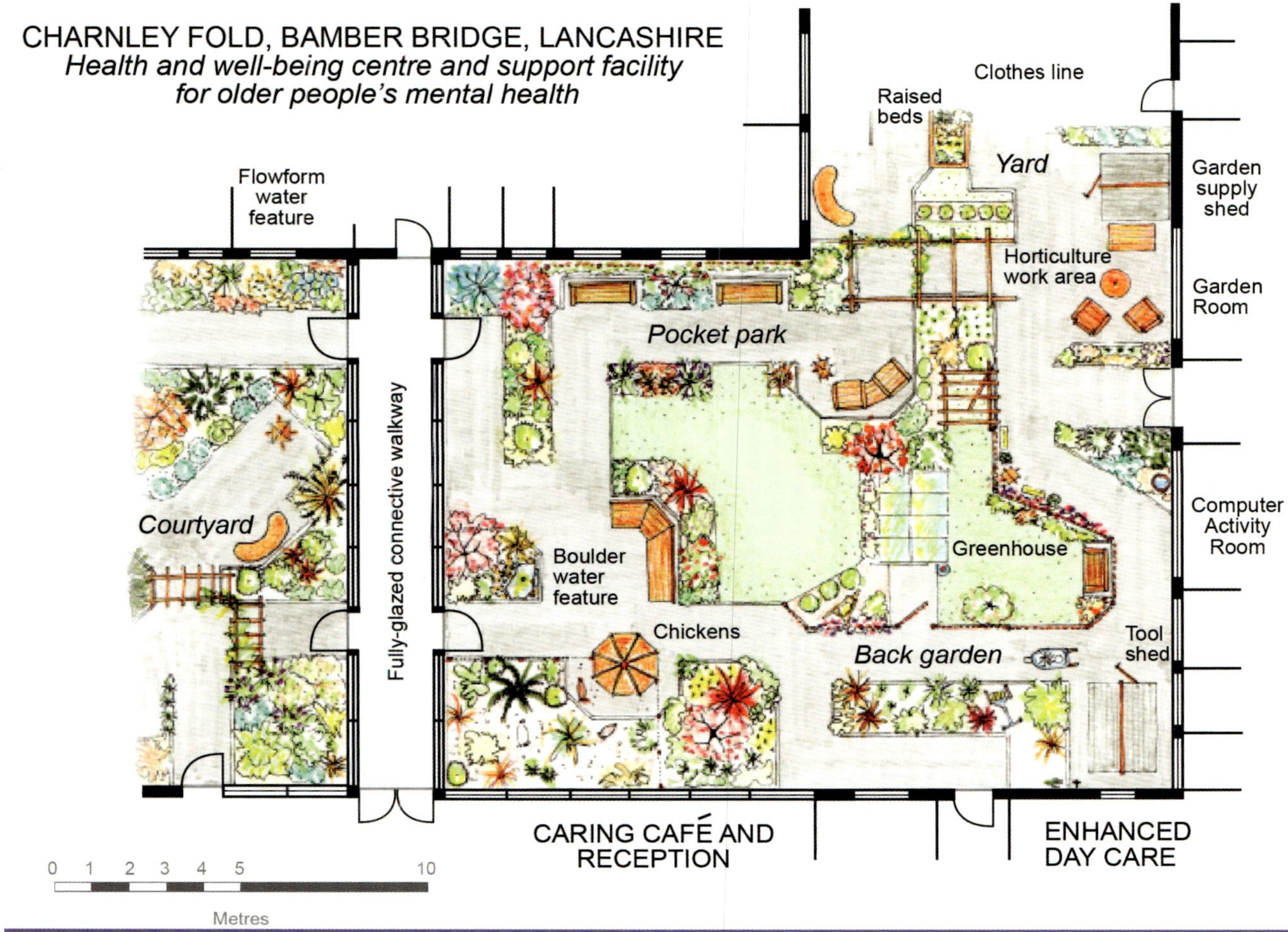

CHARNLEY FOLD, BAMBER BRIDGE, LANCASHIRE
Health and well-being centre and support facility for older people's mental health

Fig. 151 Garden layout

Appendix - graphs and plans

221

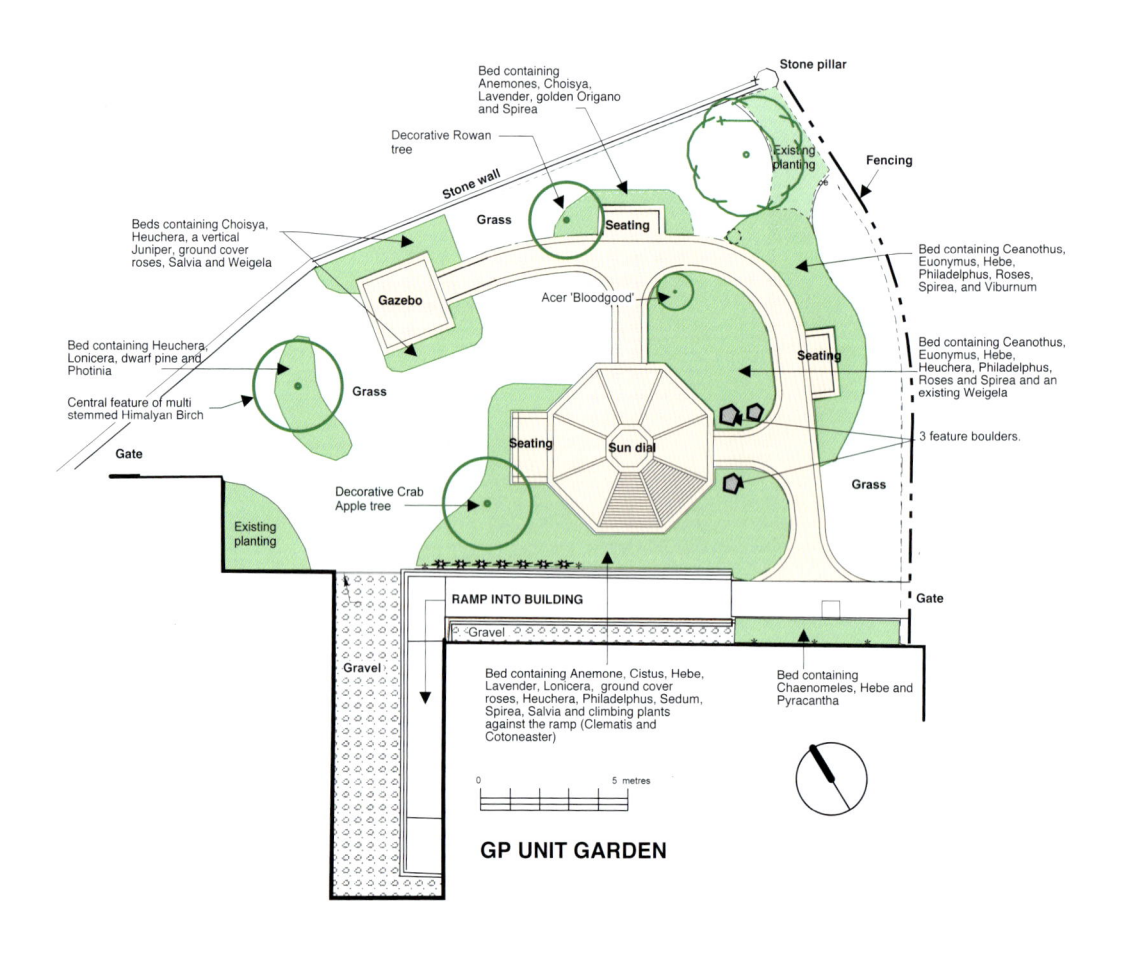

Fig. 167 Plan of GP unit garden

Fig. 171 Plan of Strathmore unit garden

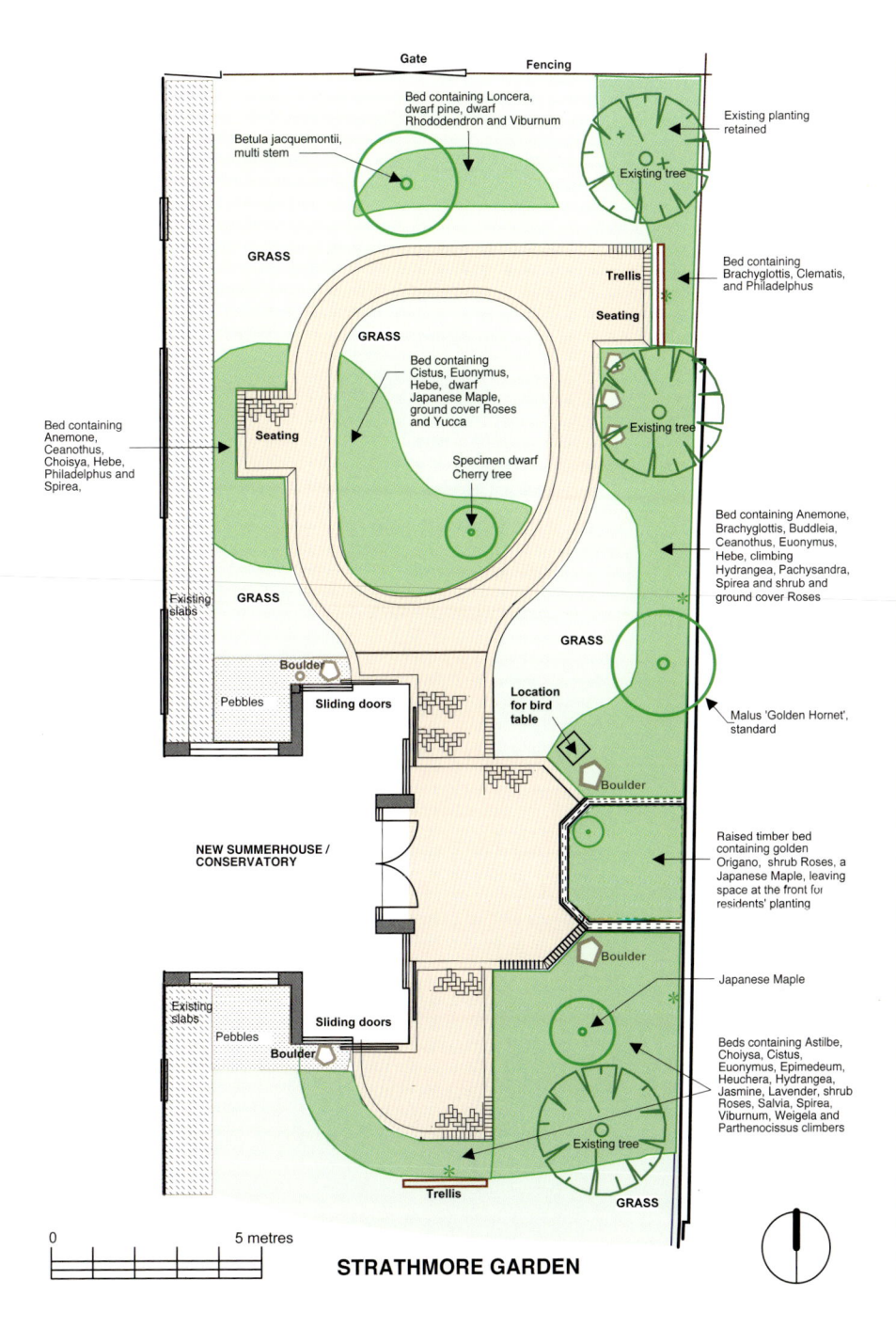

STRATHMORE GARDEN

Appendix - graphs and plans

223

Image credits

Section	Figure	Image Credit
Chapter 1	1	none
Chapter 2	2	Lothian Health Services Archive, Edinburgh University Library (Record Ref: LHB8a/9)
	3	Annie Pollock
	4	Anne Ragnhild Moseby
	5	Legacy Health
	6 & 7	Anne Ragnhild Moseby
	8	Adapted from Namazi and Johnson
	9	Richard Pollock
	10	Annie Pollock
Case study 1	11-14	Clare Cooper Marcus
Chapter 3	15	Mary Marshall
	16	Legacy Health
Case study 2	17 - 22	Yuji Okubo
Chapter 4	23	Martin Saunders Photography
	24 - 26	HammondCare
Case study 3	27 - 32	Hesse Rural Health Service
Chapter 5	33 - 44	Kirsty Bennett
Case study 4	45 & page 87	Ellen-Elisabeth Grefsrød, amended by Annie Pollock
	45 - 48	Ellen-Elisabeth Grefsrød
Chapter 6	49	Burnett Pollock Associates
	50	Annie Pollock
	51 - 54	Burnett Pollock Associates
	55 & 56	Annie Pollock
	57	Burnett Pollock Associates
	58	Pozzoni LLP
	59 - 64	Burnett Pollock Associates
	65	Richard Pollock
	66 - 67	Burnett Pollock Associates
	68	Annie Pollock

Section	Figure	Image Credit
	69	www.edinphoto.org.uk
	70 - 77	Burnett Pollock Associates
	78	Legacy Health
	79 & 80	Clifford McClenaghan, amended by Annie Pollock
Chapter 7	81 - 101	Daniel Kozak
Case study 5	102 - 106	Jack Carman
Chapter 8	107	Clare Cooper Marcus
	108	Annie Pollock
	109	Hesse Rural Health Service
	110 & 111	Annie Pollock
	112	Richard Pollock
	113	Staveley Deputy Manager
	114	Clare Cooper Marcus
	115	Staveley Deputy Manager
	116	Annie Pollock
	117	Hesse Rural Health Service
	118	Annie Pollock
	119	Hesse Rural Health Service
	120	Pozzoni LLP
	121 & 122	Clare Cooper Marcus
	123	Richard Pollock
	124	Clare Cooper Marcus
	125 & 126	Annie Pollock
	127	Ellen-Elisabeth Grefsrød
	128	Pozzoni LLP
	129	Liz Fuggle
	130	Garuth Chalfont
	131	Richard Pollock

Section	Figure	Image Credit
	132	Annie Pollock
	133	Liz Fuggle
Case study 6	134	Clifford McClenaghan and Sally Visik
	135 - 138	Annie Pollock
Chapter 9	139	Pozzoni LLP
	140 - 144	Legacy Health
	145 & 146	Annie Pollock
	147 & 148	Legacy Health
Case Study 7	149 - 155	Garuth Chalfont
Chapter 10	156 - 161	HammondCare
Chapter 11	162	HammondCare
	163 - 164	Garuth Chalfont
	165	HammondCare
	166	Legacy Health
Case Study 8	167 - 172 & page 200	Annie Pollock
Conclusions	173	Pozzoni LLP
	174	'Garden-Use Model' prepared by Charlotte F. Grant and Jean D Wineman (permission granted for use, and adapted by Annie Pollock)

All other images are copyright of HammondCare ©

Important. Research and knowledge in the field of dementia care is constantly changing. As new information emerges, changes in how we support people with dementia become necessary. The authors and publishers have, as far as possible, taken care to ensure that the information given in this text is accurate and up to date at the time of publication. However, readers are strongly advised to confirm the information complies with current legislation and standards or practice. The views expressed within any chapter or case study of this publication remain the views of the individual contributing authors and are not necessarily the views of The Dementia Centre or DSDC, unless otherwise specified.

The Dementia Centre, HammondCare is committed to promoting excellence in dementia care. Older and younger people living with dementia need services to be designed and delivered based on evidence and practice based knowledge on what works. We achieve this through providing research, training and education, publications and information, consultancy and conferences.

The DSDC, The University of Stirling is an international leader in the dementia field, with offices in London, Belfast and Stirling and partnerships throughout the world. Its aim is to improve services for people with dementia and their carers.

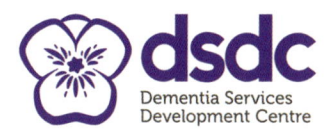

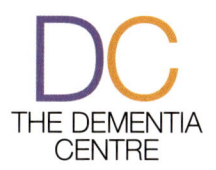

Feedback. The authors and publishers welcome feedback on this book. You can get in touch by emailing hammondpress@hammond.com.au, or by writing c/o The Dementia Centre P.O. Box 5084, Greenwich, NSW 2065 Australia.

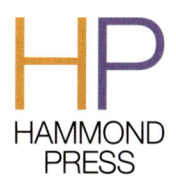

Published by HammondPress and DSDC 2012. The information contained in this document is and remains the joint property of The Dementia Centre, HammondCare and the DSDC, University of Stirling. This content must not be reproduced or transmitted to any third party without the express written permission of The Dementia Centre, HammondCare and the the DSDC, University of Stirling.

ISBN: 978-0-9871892-2-6